Nursing Home Administration

Fouth Edition

James E. Allen

PhD, MSPH, NHA

SPRINGER PUBLISHING COMPANY

Copyright © 2003 Springer Publishing Company, Inc.

Springer Publishing Company, Inc.
536 Broadway
New York, NY 10012-3955

Acquisitions Editor: Sheri W. Sussman
Production Editor: Pamela Lankas
Cover design by Joanne Honigman

03 04 05 06 07 / 5 4 3 2 1

Library of Congress Cataloging-in-Publication Data

Allen, James. (James Elmore), 1935–
    Nursing home administration / James E. Allen.—4th ed.
        p. cm.
    Includes bibliographical references and index.
    ISBN 0-8261-5393-3
    1. Nursing homes-Administration. I. Title.
    [DNLM: 1. Nursing Homes-organization & administration. WX 150 A427n]
RA999.A45A451 2003b
362.1'6'068-dc21

                                                                2002030427

Printed in the United States of America by Maple-Vail Manufacturing Group.

What's New in *Nursing Home Administration*, 4th Edition

This 4th edition of *Nursing Home Administration* covers the NAB (National Association of Boards of Examiners for Long Term Care Administrators) Domains of Practice effective 2002-2007. These are the five domains tested in the national examination required for all persons being licensed as nursing home administrators. NAB develops and tests the following five Domains of Practice:

Part One of this text covers the NAB domain *Leadership and Management,* which comprises 23% (35 test questions) of the national examination for nursing home administrators.

Part Two covers the NAB domain *Human Resources,* which is 15% (23 test questions) of the national examination.

Part Three of this text covers the NAB domain *Finance,* which is 14% (21 test questions) of the national examination.

Part Four covers the NAB domain *Physical Environment and Atmosphere,* which is 13% (19 test questions) of the national examination.

Part Five covers the NAB domain *Resident Care and Quality of Life,* which is 35% (52 test questions) of the 150-question national examination.

Information on the use of computer networks and client–server architecture in the nursing facility.

Updated information on the theories of aging.

Information on the major organizations in the long-term care field with Web site addresses.

Additional information on the use of restraints.

Extensive data from the national federal database on deficiency patterns in nursing facilities during the years 1993–1999. This is the first time national data have been compiled and made available.

First-time information on the number of special-care beds in certified nursing facilities in the United States.

New data on total nursing hours per resident day for U.S. nursing facilities.

Detailed state-by-state information on distribution of U.S. nursing facilities by ownership type, 1993–1999.

New information on percentage of chain-owned and hospital-owned nursing facilities in the United States.

New information on percentage of nursing home residents and facility occupancy rates in the United States, 1993–1999.

New information on percentage of nursing home residents with dementia and other psychological diagnoses in the United States 1993–1999.

New data on percentage of U.S. nursing facility residents who are bedfast or chairbound and percentage with pressure sores, 1993–1999.

New bladder incontinence data, 1993–1999.

New data on percentage of residents in U.S. nursing facilities receiving psychoactive medication and percentage with contractures and physical restraints.

The ideas that shape this work grow out of the concept of nursing home administrator as hero.

To these individuals this book is dedicated.

Contents

PART ONE Management, Governance, Leadership

PART TWO Human Resources

Foreword

Over the past 12 months, the National Association of Boards of Examiners for Nursing Home Administrators has conducted a job analysis to update the role delineation of the nursing home administrator according to the responsibilities involved in nursing home administration. This study is conducted every 5 years to assure that the job analysis accurately represents contemporary practice in nursing home administration. The role delineation is the basis for the national licensing exam that is used to test entry-level competence of Nursing Home Administration.

Having had the privilege to participate in the job-analysis update, it is clear that nursing home administration is truly in an era of change. Rapid change is being driven by many forces that will require today's administrator to anticipate and be prepared to respond quickly to the challenges and opportunities presented.

The long-term-care industry must respond to market demands and market realities that are driven by resident needs and desires, the changes in the health-care delivery system, and the emphasis on cost containment. Regulatory reforms require increased accountability, protection of resident's rights, and a shifting of the responsibility for the cost of long-term care from federal to state and local governments.

Nursing home administration is a multifaceted environment that requires a broad range of knowledge and skill, acceptance of tremendous responsibility, ethics beyond reproach, vision and leadership, and most important, compassion for the residents and their families.

It should come as no surprise that the new role delineation of the nursing home administrator puts the greatest emphasis on resident care. Residents expect to receive quality care in a positive environment, with the right of choice and respect for their dignity. Only competent nursing home administrators will be able to meet the challenge.

There is a lot of discussion and debate today about how competency can be measured, particularly continued competency. The level of competency required for entry in the profession is much easier to measure than continued competency. Nursing home administration today and 5 years from now will require a different set of skills and knowledge. Nursing home administrators will be required to adapt to the changes and to continually evaluate and refine their individual competency as relevant to their responsibility.

Outcomes may be one of the best measures of competency. Successful outcomes are an indicator of competency and a mark of leadership. Successful outcomes result from a process of evaluation; setting realistic goals and objectives; developing a plan; determining the necessary resources, implementation, monitoring, and periodic evaluation, with a change in course when necessary.

Leadership is essential to success. Leaders must create a clear vision, exercise sound management practices, establish clear policy and direction, and establish an environment that includes a human-resources team that shares in a vision supported by clearly defined goals and objectives.

Although nursing home administration is becoming more challenging and more complex, it has never offered greater opportunity. The number of older individuals who require care will continue to grow, as Americans are living longer due to improved health care. In addition, the industry will expand by offering a broader range of long-term care services that include independent living, assisted living, skilled nursing, and subacute care, all within a single community.

You can make a difference in nursing home administration by preparing yourself well for this era of change. That preparation will offer many opportunities for administrators to continue to enhance the quality of care provided to the nursing home resident.

RANDY LINDNER, CAE
Executive Director, National Association of
   Boards of Examiners for
   Long-Term Care Administrators (NAB)
Senior Vice President and General Manager,
   Bostrom Corporation

Acknowledgments

For more than a decade, I have interacted with countless long-term care personnel, from nursing assistants to corporate leaders, in an effort to absorb as much as possible about the industry in all its complexity.

During the past 5 years I have been privileged to participate in the daily life of a local nursing facility where my name tag reads "James Allen PIT" (professor in training). It is impossible for one person to know all that is required to successfully operate a nursing facility. This PIT will remain in training for the rest of his professional career, seeking to understand how to achieve excellence in the administration of the nursing home.

Introduction

Along with the other components of the American health-care system, the nursing home has entered an extended period of change. Second in size only to hospitals, it has already become a $100 billion-a-year industry.

The administrator of a nursing home has one of the most demanding and exciting positions in the health care field, with the quality of life of more than a million Americans depending on her or his leadership skills.

This text provides an introduction to the practice of nursing home administration. The book is divided into five parts: management, personnel, finance, the industry's environment, and resident/patient care. Each section offers a working vocabulary and detailed description of activities associated with it. Each term is defined as it is introduced.

The sections are self-contained and may be studied in any sequence.

The book contains the knowledge that is essential in preparing for licensure or employment as a nursing home administrator.

The nursing home administrator and the director of nursing, are uniquely responsible for the quality of care and quality of life of residents/patients and staff in their facility.

This text, together with additional publications by the author, cover the current domains of practice on which the national nursing home administrator examination is based.

The Nursing Home Administrator's Challenge

LEADERSHIP BY VISION

For many centuries, a village was known far and wide for its porcelain. Especially sought after were its urns: Tall as a person, graceful in form, they were admired for their delicate beauty. But what was the potter to do when, on occasion, a carefully made piece would break? A master potter solved the problem by pouring gold between the shards and thus restoring the urn.

What seemed a broken vessel, useless for any purpose, became with a gold filigree, a unique work of art.

—from ancient Chinese legend (adapted from R. J. Kriegel)

The nursing home administrator's task is that of the creative master potter of legend, restoring as if with gold filigree the joy of living to what appeared to be the shattered life of a resident/patient.

LEADERSHIP BY WALKING AROUND

Typically, it depends on who the administrator and director of nursing are. If they're doing their job, and forceful enough, then you have a good, well-managed facility. But if they're weak individuals, or not paying attention, then care doesn't get up to the rate one would expect.

—Carol Scott, a contemporary experienced observer of the nursing home industry.

List of Figures

List of Tables

PART ONE

Management, Governance, Leadership

1.1 Management Functions

The skilled administrator of a nursing facility is a person capable of organizing the resources and finances available to best meet the needs of the residents. In successfully accomplishing this, the administrator makes innumerable decisions.

Management is decision-making (Barnard, 1969; Dale, 1938; Hitt, Ireland, & Hoskisson, 2001). What the administrator does for the nursing facility is make decisions about what ought to happen in the facility (Johns & Saks, 2001).

Although there is by now an extensive literature describing the field of management theory, authors have returned again and again to a basic set of activities as the best explanation of what managers do (Dale, 1969; Drucker, 1954; Hitt et al., 2001).

Luther Gulick, an early 20th century author, defined the manager's tasks as

Planning
Organizing
Staffing
Directing
Coordinating
Reporting
Budgeting (Gulick & Lyndall, 1937; Hitt et al., 2001)

Several decades later Ernest Dale, in his book *Management Theory and Practice,* differed only slightly in his description. He agreed on the importance of the first four tasks, but consolidated the last four under three rubrics: controlling, innovating, and representing (Dale, 1969).

We will discuss concepts of current management *approaches* such as Total Quality Management (TQM) (Johns & Saks, 2001), quality circles, Continuous Quality Improvement (CQI); and *authors* such as Juran, Peters, and Deming in detail later in this section. Very briefly, at the core, this is what an administrator does:

Forecasts—Projects trends and needs that the facility management must meet in the future.

Plans—Decides what needs to be done and makes a set of plans to accomplish it.

Budgets—Projects costs and establishes categories with dollar amounts for each.

Organizes—Once a plan has been made, decides how to structure a suitable organization to implement the plan, put it into action. This will include the number of people needed for the staff and the materials with which to build or to work.

Staffs—Attempts to find the right person for each well-defined job.

Directs—Provides direction (preliminary training and ongoing supervision) through communication to each employee who thereby learns what is expected of him or her.

Evaluates—Judges the extent to which the organization is accomplishing its goals.

Controls Quality—Takes steps to assure that the goals are accomplished and that each job is done as planned.

Innovates—Leads the staff to develop new ideas that enable the facility to enhance its attractiveness to the community served.

Markets—Assures that the facility successfully attracts and admits the persons it seeks to serve.

The nursing-facility administrator is responsible for assuring that all of these activities are accomplished by the facility. Assuring that forecasting, planning, organizing, staffing, directing, evaluating, controlling, innovating, and marketing is successfully accomplished is providing leadership to the facility (Argenti, 1994).

One approach to leadership that is of particular value in the nursing facility setting is "leading by walking around" (LBWA). LBWA reassures the administrator that facility resources and finances are successfully being used to best meet the needs of the residents. This is one part of the quality assurance process (discussed later in this section).

Another description of the manager's function is that "management is getting things done through other people" (Hitt et al., 2001; Levey & Loomba, 1973). A staff member who becomes a manager may or may not continue to give direct care but also assumes new duties that are entirely managerial in character (Dale, 1969). The new manager is no longer directly responsible for doing specific work, for instance patient care, but ensures that such care is provided. For example, when a nurse who has been giving direct care to patients becomes the director of nurses, this new job entails the supervision of other employees to provide the nursing care needed by the patients/residents.

According to another group of management theorists (Christensen, Berg, & Salter, 1980; Hitt et al., 2001), the general manager (such as a nursing home administrator) performs five functions:

- planning for future operations
- designing and administering decision-making structures (organizing)
- developing human resources and capabilities (staffing, directing)
- supervising current operations (controlling)
- representing and holding an organization responsible to its various constituencies (Christensen et al., 1980, p. xvi)

The administrator's job is to ensure that the appropriate employees do the tasks of the organization at an acceptable quality level (Dale, 1969; Hitt et al., 2001). Many volumes have been written about managing because it is one of the more complex tasks in modern society. In the eighth edition of their text *Policy Formulation and Administration* three professors at the Harvard Graduate School of Business Administration (Christensen et al., 1980) state that what administrators do is ask three questions: Where are we now? Where do we want to go? How do we get there?

A DETAILED LOOK AT WHAT MANAGERS/ ADMINISTRATORS DO

We have described in very general terms what administrators do. But what is actually involved in forecasting, planning, organizing, staffing, directing, evaluating, controlling, innovating, and marketing? Consider the following the basic functions of the manager:

Forecasting (projecting trends into the future): The administrator forecasts the economic, social, and political environment of the organization and the resources that will be available to it.

Planning (deciding what is to be done): The administrator decides what is to be accomplished, sets short- and long-term objectives, then decides on the means to be used for achieving them.

Budgeting (deciding acceptable costs): All facilities must operate on plans that have been translated into budgets that are realistic yet functional.

Organizing (deciding the scheme of the organization and the staffing it will require): The administrator decides on the structure the organization will take, the skills that will be needed, and the staff positions and their particular duties and responsibilities. This includes coordinating the work assignments, that is, the interrelationships among the departments and their workers (Johns & Saks, 2001).

Staffing (the human resources function): The administrator attempts to find the right person for each defined job.

Directing (providing daily supervision, employing good communication and people skills): The administrator provides day-to-day supervision of subordinates, makes sure that subordinates know what results are expected, and helps the staff to improve their own skills. In short, the administrator explains what is to be done and the employees do it to the best of their abilities.

Evaluating (comparing actual to expected results): The administrator determines how well the jobs have been done and what progress is being made to achieve the organization's goals as stated in its policies and plans of action.

Controlling quality (taking necessary corrective actions): The administrator revises policies, procedures, and plans of action and takes necessary personnel actions to achieve more nearly the facility goals.

Innovating (the effective administrator is always an innovator): The administrator develops new ideas independently, combines old ideas to form new ones, searches for useful ideas from other fields and adapts them, and acts as a catalyst to stimulate others to be as creative.

Marketing (identifying and attracting the persons to be served): The administrator assures that the facility identifies the group(s) of persons to be served and successfully attracts and serves the residents/patients it seeks.

These are the basic functions of administrators/managers. The reader may wish to use other words and concepts to describe these functions, or even improve on the model. Certainly administrators do much more than has been described above (Hitt et al., 2001; Pressman & Wildavsky, 1974).

However, if forecasting, planning, organizing, staffing, directing, evaluating, controlling, innovating, and marketing are not successfully accomplished, the minimum leadership responsibilities of a nursing home administrator have not been fulfilled.

The skilled long-term-care administrator is capable of providing leadership that accomplishes each of these tasks in a manner that meets both facility financial needs and resident/patient care needs.

In his book *A Passion for Excellence,* Tom Peters advocates a simple four-part scheme of management's role: care of customers, constant innovation, turned-on people, and leadership (Peters & Austin, 1985). He observes that in both the for-profit and not-for-profit sectors, superior performance over the long haul depends on two things: taking exceptional care of clients (residents/patients in the facility) via service and superior quality (of care); and constant innovation.

Peters observes that although financial control is vital, one does not sell financial control, but rather a quality service or product (excellent care for residents/patients). A facility seldom sustains superior performance merely by having all the beds full; the superior facility sustains itself through innovation in ways to serve residents/patients and promote market development. Efficient management of the budget is vital in an organization such as a university, he states, yet a great university (or nursing facility) is never characterized by the remark, "It has a good budget" (Peters & Austin, p. 4). Just as the superb university is so only by virtue of its success in serving its ultimate customer—the student— the superb nursing home is so only by virtue of its success in serving *its* ultimate customers—the residents/patients and their families and significant others.

Peters advocates a management model based on what he calls "a blinding flash of the obvious" (1985, p. 3): Giving every employee the space to innovate, at least a little. Answering the phones and resident call-buttons with common courtesy. Doing things that work (giving quality care). Listening to residents and families and asking for their ideas, then acting on them. Soliciting staff input, then, as appropriate, implementing it. Wandering around with residents/patients, staff, suppliers, visitors. Obvious common sense? Yes. But it must not be so obvious or more would practice it. All of these are people skills, based on an ability to facilitate communication among staff and residents/patients. All too often, common sense is very scarce.

To achieve Peters' "blinding flash of the obvious" in the nursing facility environment, the administrator normally must cultivate good people-skills (communicate successfully with both residents/patients and staff) to achieve excellence in service to the facility residents/patients and their significant others. People skills will be discussed in more depth later in this section.

1.1.1 Levels of Management

Two additional concepts are worth noting at this point: upper, middle, and lower levels of management and line-staff relationships. The administrator of a large nursing home might assign some of these responsibilities to others. The administrator need not personally perform each of the management tasks, but rather must assure that these tasks are successfully carried out. To accomplish this, management is often divided into three tiers: upper, middle, and lower (Hitt et al., 2001; Katz & Kahn, 1967).

UPPER-LEVEL MANAGEMENT

The upper-level manager is responsible for the overall functioning of the facility, normally interacting directly with the board of directors or owners. This person is responsible for formulating policies that will be applied to the entire facility. The nursing home administrator is an excellent example of upper-level management (Hitt et al., 2001; Mintzberg, 1979).

MIDDLE-LEVEL MANAGEMENT

Middle-level managers report to upper-level managers and at the same time interact significantly with lower-level managers. A good example in the nursing home is the director of nursing who reports to the facility administrator and in turn has managers (e.g., nurse supervisors and charge nurses) reporting to her (Hitt et al., 2001; Mintzberg, 1979).

As the name implies, this staff member interfaces with upper- and lower-level managers. The middle-level manager normally does not make policies affecting the entire facility, as does the facility administrator. However, the middle-level manager does make decisions of policy for managers responsible to her. The middle-level manager must have good communication skills to deal successfully with both the administrator of the facility and the lower-level workers.

The emergence of nursing home chains has implications for the type of management role that local nursing home administrators are being assigned. Some chains allow local facility administrators wide latitude in decision making, in which case the local administrator functions primarily as an upper-level manager. In other chains, decision making is more centralized in the corporate offices, in which case some dimensions of the local administrator's role more nearly resemble that of the middle-level manager.

LOWER-LEVEL MANAGEMENT

As a rule, lower-level managers have direct supervisory responsibilities for the staff who do the actual work, for example, the nurse's aide who physically takes care of the resident in his or her room. The nurse supervisor or charge nurse is a good example of lower-level management in a nursing home facility (Mintzberg, 1979). At this level, managers deal directly with those at the middle level, but not with administrators at the upper level. That is, they are expected to conduct their business through the channel of their middle-level managers.

If the charge nurse wants a change in a policy, he will discuss the matter with the nursing supervisor, who in turn will bring it to the attention of upper-level managers, should this be desirable. The middle-level manager might also make a policy decision without consulting upper-level management, for example, to change the bathing schedule to accommodate an additional workload due to increased occupancy.

Management decisions in nursing home facilities are noticeably more complicated than the simple establishment of lower, middle and upper levels of management. The presence of several professions—physicians, nurses, physical therapists, dietitians, and others—causes decision making in nursing home facilities to be a complex and often delicate task. This is explored later in this section.

1.1.2 Line–Staff Relationships

Line-staff relationships constitute a second important concept in understanding management functions (Dale, 1969; Hitt et al., 2001). A person who is empowered by the administrator to make decisions for the organization is said to have line authority. A person is said to have a staff role if she is advisory to the manager and does not have authority to make decisions for the organization (Robey, 1982).

A LINE POSITION

The administrator must assign to other employees some of the decision-making authority to accomplish the work of the organization. Such employees are line managers. They are empowered to make decisions on behalf of the administrator. The director of nurses is a line position. Therefore, decisions by the director of nursing have the same force as if the administrator made them. The administrator still remains responsible for all decisions made on his behalf by persons to whom decision-making authority has been delegated. Implications of this process for the administrator are explored later under the topic of risk management.

A STAFF POSITION

A staff position, on the other hand, is an advisory role. None of the administrator's authority to make decisions on behalf of the facility is delegated to persons in a staff position. An accountant in the business office is an example of a staff position. Paid consultants, such as a local pharmacist or a registered dietitian, hold staff positions. They are expected to advise the administrator or appropriate others in the facility on what to do, but they have been given no authority by the administrator to make decisions on behalf of the facility.

Smaller nursing home facilities typically do not employ as their food services director a person eligible for registration by the American Dietetic Association. Consequently, to meet federal regulations, they hire such a person as a consultant on a periodic basis. Although the consulting dietitian may be the better trained person, if the nursing home administrator allows this consultant to give direct orders to the food service director, lines of authority in the facility may become confused, and staff morale will suffer. Matters, however, are slightly more complicated. Only a person eligible for registration by the American Dietetic Association may designate diets as prescribed by physicians, and in this case the consultant is making decisions for the facility that an unqualified food service director is not permitted to make.

Or, again, in a very large facility the administrator might hire a specially trained geriatric nurse practitioner to advise the administrator or the director of nursing on nursing functions in the facility. This nurse would normally have no authority to ask or order anyone to do anything in the facility.

It is the director of nursing to whom power and authority to make nursing decisions has been delegated and who therefore makes decisions on behalf of the administrator in the nursing area. The director of nurses can hire and fire, assign work, and give whatever orders are needed to make the facility's nursing activities function because line authority to do so has been delegated to that employee.

If, for example, the administrator permitted the geriatric nurse practitioner, to whom a staff role had been assigned, to tell the director of nurses what to do or to give orders to nurses on the halls, the authority of the director of nurses would be undermined. The director of nurses and nursing staff would be understandably confused about the role of the director of nurses: Does the director of nurses represent the authority of the administrator or is the staff advisory nurse practitioner actually the manager of the director of nurses?

Again, life in the nursing facility is seldom this seemingly uncomplicated. A large number of nursing facilities in the United States are operated by chains with corporate staff who often visit or are assigned to assist a facility for a short period of time. Technically, these corporate representatives may be there only to advise, but facility staff are hardly free to ignore such "advice." Some chains expect their corporate staff to function more nearly as consultants to the local facilities they visit; other chains want them to function as if they exercised line authority in their area of expertise while in one of that chain's facilities. Or, again, when the facility is functioning smoothly the corporate representative might be comfortable with a "take it or leave it" approach to advice given, but in times of crisis that same representative might come in and exercise direct line authority in the day-to-day operation of that facility.

We turn now to a more detailed discussion of some of the activities and skills involved in the management functions. We will begin to explore further some of the complexities of these functions.

1.2 Forecasting

Managerial success belongs to those who prepare successfully for the future. In the nursing home industry, the early 2000s belong to administrators who can anticipate and successfully prepare for rapid change.

TREND ANALYSIS

After nearly two decades of more gradual evolvement, the pace of change in the long-term care field increased visibly with reforms to Medicare and Medicaid, which were contained in the 1987 Omnibus Budget Reconciliation Act and subsequent amendments. The long-term care industry has entered a period in which rapid and far reaching changes can be expected. Some of the causes for this accelerated rate are explored later in parts 1 and 4 of this text.

Forecasting involves trend identification and analysis. Clues to the future are present in trends that the alert administrator can observe. The skill needed in forecasting is the ability to predict accurately the future implications for the nursing facility of new trends to which the current environment may offer clues. For example, several states have moved to be reimbursed for public-paying patients based on the acuteness of their illness. The federal government is actively employing this reimbursement method after the Balanced Budget Act of 1997. Alert administrators in states using other reimbursement approaches can estimate the likelihood that this method may be adopted in their states and make contingency plans to adapt if this occurs.

One apparent certainty is that conventional perceptions of the nursing facility's roles will be challenged in the American health care system. In the past, developments occurred incrementally, at a slow pace. During the 1970s and 1980s, administrators had the luxury of making long-range projections during a period of relative stability in the health care industry under unlimited Medicare and Medicaid reimbursements from the federal and state governments. In today's world, the rate of transformation in the health care field is exponential, shifting so rapidly that it is ever more difficult to predict the shape of the nursing home industry, even from year to year, as Congress and the states modify, sometimes radically, the reimbursement rules.

THE CHANGING CORE

Consider the following. Every 10 years, one fourth of all current knowledge and accepted practices in the health care and other industries will be obsolete. The life span of new technologies is down to 18 months and still decreasing (Kreigel, 1991). Estimates are that people under 25 can expect to change careers every decade and jobs every 4 years, either by choice or because the industry in which they work will disappear and be replaced by others yet unimagined. The core business of the nursing home of the early 2000s may be entirely different from one in the second decade of the 21st century (Kriegel, 1991).

As Kriegel has observed, nursing home administration in the second millennium is a new and unpredictable world, an arena in which we have not played before. The rules will be different and the game itself is changing— the nursing home we went to work for 5 years earlier may have changed entirely. Everything is moving faster in the health field, and new technologies are replacing current technologies more quickly. What the nursing home administrator needs to know to act effectively is changing. Relying on the "tried and truly," observes Kriegel, is dangerous because what was tried yesterday is no longer viable today (p. xvi). Nursing homes that continue to rely on conventional formulas for success will not only miss opportunities for new markets but will also find themselves in the backwash of the health care industry as it metamorphoses into constantly new permutations.

The truth is that for the first time in human history the capacity exists to provide more expensive and effective health care than any nation, including the United States, may be able to afford. The roles possible for hospitals, nursing homes, assisted-living facilities, home health agencies, managed care organizations, and other providers are endless and will remain theirs for the taking over the next few decades as society struggles to absorb health care costs and technologies.

CHANGE ITSELF

As one chief executive officer observed, mankind's cumulative knowledge doubled between 1985 and 1995—and will double again every 5 years (Kriegel, 1991). In the health sciences field this may occur even more rapidly. The U.S. Congress's Office of Technology has warned that the rate of development is too fast for proper monitoring of the effects and will threaten the foundations of even the most secure American businesses (Kriegel, 1991). The staff in nursing facilities are experiencing culture shock: In the 1980s those nurses were considered to be working at a lower technological level than hospital nurses. Today their nurses are busy learning high-tech skills just to be able to treat the sub-acute care residents/patients being admitted to nursing facilities. Almost as soon as rules are established, they become obsolete. By the time we noticed that a nursing home could be started with as little as $12,000 cash from the owner (when combined with federal government incentive loans that are no longer available), a new facility costs $4.5 million.

Survival in the nursing home industry will depend on the ability to forecast the future and to learn entirely new ways of thinking, behaving, motivating, and communicating in the nursing facility. Survival will depend on ability and willingness to change, something that owners and staff do with great reluctance.

1.3 Planning

1.3.1 Why Plan?

AN INTEGRATED DECISION SYSTEM

The purpose of planning is to provide an integrated decision system that, based on the changes forecast by the administrator, establishes the framework for all facility activities (Dale, 1969; Levey and Loomba, 1973; Rogers, 1980). Plans, in essence, are statements of the organizational goals of the facility.

A MEANS OF COPING WITH UNCERTAINTY

Plans are a means of coping with the uncertainty of the future (Hitt et al., 2001; Katz and Kahn, 1967; Levey & Loomba, 1973). All organizations must deal with the outside world in order to survive. Inevitably, events beyond the control of the nursing home will shape the range of options available to the facility and set the context within which it will be obliged to function.

A plan is a prediction of what the facility's decision makers believe they must do to cope with the future. A carefully developed plan makes it possible to compare what actually happens to what was expected to happen. The plan may then be altered to achieve the set goals when external conditions change.

STRATEGIC PLANNING

To survive and prosper, the nursing facility must engage in strategic planning (Noe et al., 2000). "Strategy" comes from the Greek word *strategos,* referring to a general's (the administrator's) grand design behind a campaign or battle. Strategic management is conceiving and implementing the pattern or plan that integrates the facilities' major goals, policies and action sequences into a cohesive whole (Noe et al., 2000). It is the process of analyzing the facility's competitive position, developing the strategic goals, devising a plan of action, and allocating the resources that will best achieve those goals (Noe et al., 2000).

Break-It Thinking

It is important to have a plan, but sometimes it is even more important to abandon it. As Kreigel (1991) has observed, change today is happening at such a fast pace that today's innovations are tomorrow's outworn models. He observes that if it ain't broke today, it will be tomorrow. He cites an architect who finds the pace so fast that he feels like a gunfighter dodging bullets, and an electronics manager who does little besides come up for air and catch his breath in the momentary lull before the next storm (Kriegel, 1991). The nursing facility administrator in this millennium is faced with so many new regulations from the federal and state governments and with the financial pressures merely to survive that it seems difficult to do more than just dodge these bullets. We will explore ways to make an ally of change in part 1.6.3.

1.3.2 Steps in Planning

PHASE ONE: DECIDE WHAT OUGHT TO BE DONE

Few people have the opportunity to plan for an organization from the very outset. Typically in the nursing home field, an individual is hired as the administrator of an ongoing facility. For the purposes of illustration, however, let us follow the planning process that might occur in the creation of a new nursing home.

Suppose that one is asked by the regional vice-president of a mid-sized, publicly traded, for-profit chain of nursing homes to evaluate a medium-sized community (about 50,000 residents) for the purpose of recommending or advising against the building of a nursing facility there. Assume that sufficient funds are available if the decision is favorable. The assumption is further made that if a home is built, the person doing this assessment would serve as its initial administrator.

This individual must appraise the present competitive, economic, and political environment in that community. We will not attempt to provide a complete checklist for arriving at an assessment of a community, but among the major planning considerations might be the following factors.

Governmental Permission

Numerous governmental bodies must grant permission to build a facility. Zoning requirements, building codes, and local fire codes must be met. If certificate of need or similar governmental permission exists to build a new nursing facility legislation, the likelihood of obtaining this is an early consideration. Will approval of all required federal, state, and local government permits be forthcoming (Boling et al.; Hitt et al., 2001; Miller, 1982)? What is the political climate in the town? Is the proposed nursing facility likely to be welcomed, or if not, would permits probably be delayed, disapproved, or interpreted so strictly that costs rise unacceptably?

Competition

What is the level of unmet need for nursing facility beds in the community and its environs? How many competitors are there? What are their present and projected bed capacities? Is there enough unmet bed need to expect that a new nursing home would fill up sufficiently quickly and maintain the desired level of occupancy over an extended period of at least 5, preferably 10, years? What expansion plans do present facilities have? Are other competing nursing homes apt to be built over the next 3 to 5 years? In many communities assisted living facilities are being built beyond the capacity to absorb. What is known about local hospitals? Are they likely to enlarge, shrink, or stay the same? Are hospitals themselves in the process of opening long-term care or expecting to do so? What is known about local home health care agencies? Is it probable that they will aggressively siphon off patients who might currently be candidates for nursing home placement? Is there an active hospice agency? Will they be competition or is a cooperative effort possible, placing selected hospice patients in the proposed nursing facility?

Economic Considerations

Are the expected patients/residents apt to have the present and future income to keep the occupancy level high and with the desired mix of patients/residents? Based on the company's projected daily charges for care, would the facility be competitive with charges by its competitors? Will the community and its surrounding area maintain or improve its

economic condition over the next several years? What are the public and
third party reimbursement trends in this community and state? Can your
company build a facility and charge competitive prices based on present
and anticipated trends in reimbursement for nursing home care?

What are the trends among third-party payers in this community? Are
health maintenance organizations, preferred provider organizations, and
similar third-party reimbursement groups such as health insurance companies hiring case managers to place persons in nursing facilities and
controlling their length of stay and type of care? Are these case managers placing patients at favorable negotiated rates based on acuity levels
of care needs in this community? Is it possible to negotiate bed-hold
contracts with other providers such as hospitals or health maintenance
organizations that would guarantee payment for a specified number of
the facility's beds whether occupied or not? To what extent are Veterans
Administration patient contracts available in this community?

Market Considerations

The evaluator must visualize the desired roles of the proposed nursing
facility in this environment. The considerations mentioned amount to
conducting a *needs assessment* for the proposed nursing home. The perceived unmet needs will influence the role planned for the proposed
facility. Unmet need, however, is not the sole criterion. The company
may seek to create new markets for nursing facility care that does not
currently exist in that community. Increasingly the nursing facility census is made up of a profile of several types of residents/patients. The
long-term resident is only one of several types of patients/residents for
which a facility might be planned. Nursing facility care is now more
frequently characterized by niche marketing, in which facilities offer
identifiable specialized types of care for subacute conditions, ventilator
care, Alzheimer's disease, wound care, and numerous others. These will
be explored at greater length, especially in part 6.

PHASE TWO: SET SHORT- AND LONG-RANGE OBJECTIVES

Let us assume that a decision to build a new 100-bed facility has been
made. The next step is to develop broad goals, objectives, and plans that
will direct the efforts. A broad goal might be to build in keeping with the
architecture of the community in a location convenient to the local hospital.

From a set of broad goal statements such as these, more specific
objectives and plans can be developed. A short-range objective (Hitt et

al., 2001; Kotter, 1982) might be set to have a 100 bed facility in operation within 18 months, and, as a long-range objective, a new wing of 60 additional beds within 10 years.

PHASE THREE: DECIDE ON THE MEANS TO ACHIEVE THE OBJECTIVE

The next logical step is to translate broad planning goals into particular, functional efforts. It is at this stage that allowable cost levels are determined, plans for the building drawn, and the building site purchased.

The planning process has moved from the general to the specific: from broad goals to architectural plans that direct every person connected with the project. In this way, broad goals are translated into specific behaviors for everyone who takes part in realizing these goals.

PLANNING FOR NEXT YEAR

We have used planning for a new facility as the example because this demonstrates the entire planning process. Most planning is shorter range (for the following year). As a practical matter, this planning is usually accomplished when the budget for the next fiscal year is to be developed. An extensive example of the steps of planning for the next fiscal year through the budgeting process is given in part 3.

Once plans have crystallized, the next step is to put them into effect, to make them operational. This is the process of giving plans an organizational form. The form depends on the administrators' perceptions of that structure in particular and behavior of organizations in general.

PLAN TO CHANGE YOUR PLANS

No matter how carefully we plan, circumstances can change at any moment. The three main sources of patients/residents today may be entirely different tomorrow. Perhaps this is why administering a nursing facility will remain a challenging job: Nothing is stagnant in the health care field.

Consider Kriegel's (1991) experiences in teaching people how to prepare mentally for difficult rock climbing. Looking up the mountain from the bottom, one mentally constructs a plan to reach the top. Once the climb begins, however, the view becomes different. Other more promising routes to the top begin to appear. So the climbers would change the route. Mountain climbers come to expect that no matter how well they plan from the bottom of the mountain, they can count on running into the unexpected on the ascent. To those who enjoy finding new ways and improving current modes of doing things in the nursing facility, this is an exciting prospect, an opportunity for creativity. Nursing home administrators who learn to deal with the unexpected, even to thrive on it, will endure in the profession. As management guru Peter Drucker has observed, "No other area offers richer opportunities for successful innovation than [the] unexpected" (Kriegel, 1991, p. 221).

Successful nursing home administrators will assume that once they begin to implement any plan they will meet new people, receive new information, learn of new developments, and see possibilities that they could not have known at the outset. The unexpected cannot be controlled. In the nursing home industry of today, uncertainty and surprise from both the public and private sectors are normal. What *can* be controlled is one's attitude toward the unanticipated. If one accepts that change is integral to living, one can look forward to it and be ready to take advantage of the new opportunities it offers. Accepting the inevitability of change is an attitude that will serve the administrator well.

1.4 Organizing

Organizing is a method of ensuring that the work necessary to achieve a goal is broken down into segments, each of which can be handled by one person (Dale, 1969; Hitt et al., 2001). There must be no duplication of work. Efforts are then directed toward accomplishing the goal by dividing up the work so that each job can be done by one person and by providing a means for coordinating the jobs done by different people, which is the task of the managers.

Descriptions are written for each job. As a rule, an organizational manual containing all job descriptions and several charts is prepared. A job list for each position usually includes the following:

- the objectives (results to be accomplished)
- the duties and authorities of the position
- its relationship to other positions in the organization

It is argued in William Gulick's text that job analysis consists of answering the following questions (Gulick & Lyndall, 1937, p. 103):

- What does the worker do? (worker functions)
- How does the worker do it? (methods and techniques)
- What aids are necessary? (machines, tools, equipment)
- What is accomplished? (products, services produced)
- What knowledge, skills, abilities are involved? (qualifications)

Organizing is the first step in the implementation of a plan. It is the process of translating plans into combinations of money, materials, and people.

All administrators organize their facilities according to some theory of organization. Their understanding of organization is reflected in their day-to-day and year-to-year direction. For some administrators this is a very thoughtful process; for others it is quite superficial. Nevertheless, all of them apply their concept of organization through their behavior in daily decision making.

SYSTEMS

Organizations are systems of interactions among the three available inputs: people, materials, and money (Hitt et al., 2001; Johns & Saks, 2001; Robey, 1982).

A great deal has been written in recent decades about systems theory. This literature appeared after World War II and has paralleled the development of computer applications to management tasks (Boling et al., 1983; Katz & Kahn, 1967; Levey & Loomba, 1973). The systems concept is primarily a way of thinking about the task of managing any organization. It offers the manager a framework for visualizing the internal and external environment of the organization (Katz & Kahn, 1967).

A *system* has been defined as an organized or complex whole, an assembling or combining of things or parts forming a complex or single whole (Johns & Saks, 2001). Stated more simply, the idea of systems helps us to figure out how things are put together. How, for example, do all of the departments in the nursing home relate to one another, to the community, and to the rest of the world that affects them (Johns & Saks, 2001)?

Systems theory is a tool for making sense out of our world by helping to make clearer the interrelationships within and outside the organization. The administrator uses systems theory to determine what is going on inside the facility and between the facility and the larger outside community.

1.4.1 The Organization As a System

Systems descriptions vary from completely nonmathematical to highly sophisticated mathematical models that demand specially trained personnel and computers (George, 1972; Hitt et al., 2001; Mintzberg, 1979). The model we present does not require quantification, although numerical weights could be given each of its elements (DeGroot, 1979; Hitt et al., 2001; Johns & Saks, 2001; Zmud, 1983).

OVERVIEW

In Figure 1-1, we illustrate a systems model that may be useful to the nursing home administrator in daily management of the facility. This model consists of the following elements: inputs, processor, outputs, control, plans of action, feedback, and environment. (For an equally simplified model, see Miller, 1982, pp. 4015–4018; see also Robey, 1982; pp. 134–135).

Organizations like nursing homes use inputs to get work done, which results in outputs. The outputs are evaluated by the residents, their significant others, and the public, which then reacts, and the facility receives feedback. The outputs are also evaluated by the administrators and compared to what was sought. If the results, or outputs, do not conform to organizational policy and action plans, the administrator takes control actions to bring the outputs into line with those planned. All of these activities occur within the constraints placed on the organization by the external environment.

INPUTS

The inputs to any organization can be described as three elements: money, people, and materials. Inputs are elements the facility administrators can change and use to advantage.

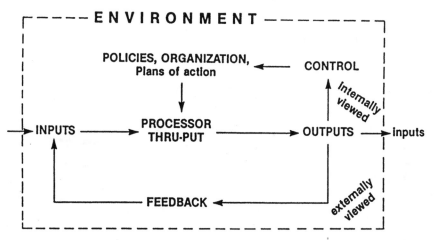

FIGURE 1-1. Simplifieid systems model.

How Can Inputs Be Increased?

A primary concern of the system's administrator is how inputs can be renewed and increased. To accomplish this, organizations take in resources (Hitt et al., 2001; Katz & Kahn, 1967). Just as the human body must have oxygen from the air and food from the environment, the nursing facility must constantly draw renewed supplies of energy from other institutions, from people, and from the material environment.

As patients/residents are rehabilitated and return home, or die, more patients/residents must be admitted into the facility if it is to continue to function. As food is consumed in the dining rooms, more food supplies must be brought in, so that the work of the facility (caring for patients/residents) may continue. As employees leave for other jobs, new staff must be recruited. As the month's cash income is spent paying the facility bills, more revenue from patients/residents must be brought in.

PROCESSOR

The *processor* is the work the organization accomplishes. Organizations transform the energy (inputs) available to them, just as the human body converts starch and sugar into heat and action. The nursing facility cares for patients/residents. Work is completed. Inputs are reorganized (e.g., food supplies are blended into recipes for the next meal). This is sometimes called the throughput. It is the actual work that the organization performs (Hitt et al., 2001; Katz & Kahn, 1967).

The nursing facility takes its inputs (staff, money, and materials) and reorganizes them into active caring for patients/residents. In essence, what nursing facilities do is take money resources from patients/residents and other sources and use those funds to hire staff and provide materials needed (buildings, beds, food, syringes, tissues) to give resident care.

OUTPUT

The results of the work (caring for patients/residents) that nursing facilities do is the *output,* the product of the work accomplished by the organization. The organization exports some product (service) to the environment.

Nursing home produce services to residents/patients. This service may take many forms, as we have noted elsewhere, such as day care as the output for an adult day program, mobility as the output of a physical therapy program, self-feeding as the output of a restorative feeding program, meals served to senior citizens in the community, and so forth. Nursing facilities can and do provide an increasing variety of outputs.

The usefulness of thinking about the administrative tasks within a systems framework will become more evident as we describe the complex ramifications of the work of nursing homes (resident care) that is produced for the community. Later is this section we will examine a number of additional insights provided by viewing organizations as systems.

CONTROL OF QUALITY

For the purposes of exploring the systems diagram in Figure 1-1, control will be described only briefly here at greater length. Control is a most important tool available to administrators in the process of keeping the organization on course. *Control* is the corrective action taken after evaluation of outputs by the organizational decision makers. The intended output may not be achieved.

In the nursing home, the administrator exercises control of quality by comparing the actual care that is given to patients/residents (actual output) with the care called for in the organizational policies and plans of action. This, in our view, is at the very heart of what administrators do. Just as important, every nursing home administrator has the responsibility of comparing the ultimate financial results with the expected financial results. We deal with this in depth in part 3.

Put simply, control of quality is the process of asking if the work accomplished (actual output) by the facility is up to expected standards and, if not, taking corrective actions to remedy the problem (Dale, 1969; Hitt et al., 2001). Here we are discussing the actual standards the organization has established for itself through its policies and plans of action.

There are several standards of care that exist for nursing homes. Among them are the federal requirements for care and standards imposed by each state for a license to operate (Robey, 1982).

POLICIES AND PLANS OF ACTION

Policies and plans are discussed in greater depth elsewhere in this text. For the purpose of illustrating the system configuration we use, let us simply refer to *policies* and plans of action as the guidelines the administrator uses to compare the output (e.g., actual patient care or financial results achieved) with the expected (i.e., the policies and plans of action developed and put into operation by the facility). As the arrows in Figure 1-1 indicate, the administrator uses the organization's *policies* (broad statements of goals and procedures) and *plans of action,* which are the more specific procedures designed to govern the implementation of the policies.

Numerous organizations are geared to set policies and impose plans of action for nursing homes in the United States (Boling et al., 1983; Miller and Barry, 1979; Rogers, 1980). In part, this has been a response to the financing of nursing home care by Medicare and Medicaid.

Congress imposed detailed operating regulations, called requirements (see part 4), on facilities that are prepared to accept Medicare patients (Miller, 1982). Individual states, at the request of Congress, have also issued very specific sets of policies and detailed requirements for facilities that wish to serve Medicaid patients (Rogers, 1980). A number of states leave little room for exercising discretion, while other have dealt with a more permissive hand (Boling et al., 1983).

Nevertheless, there are many areas in which nursing facilities must develop and implement their own policies and plans for action. One such area is food services. Every facility develops policies by which it hopes to control the quality of food served its patients/residents.

To summarize, administrators compare the results obtained with the results expected and then take steps to reorganize the inputs or reorganize the processor (the work itself) to more nearly achieve the desired standards.

FEEDBACK

Feedback is a form of control, but feedback is used here to refer to the external responses to the output (resident care provided, etc.) by the nursing facility.

Nursing facility outputs have many dimensions, such as roles played in long-term care in the community and in providing short-term, and increasingly, sub-acute care to patients who have been hospitalized, before they return home.

Feedback from residents and their families represents a key source of evaluative help to the administrator and staff. Federal survey data indicate that in the years 1993 to 1999, 92% of U.S. nursing facilities had resident councils and 45% had family groups as an additional form of feedback (Harrington, Carrillo, Thollaug, Summers, & Wellin, 2000).

Regulatory Feedback

Inevitably, members of the community and other individuals such as state inspectors and complaint investigators evaluate the results of nursing home efforts to provide quality care to patients/residents. In the 1960s congressional feedback to the nursing home industry resulted in considerable reshaping of the inputs in the industry when lawmakers established the requirements then called the conditions of participation. More recently, the 1987 Omnibus Budget Reconciliation Act, which contained Medicare and Medicaid reforms, imposed even more stringent requirements.

Laws passed by Congress and subsequent regulations prescribe how nursing homes must configure inputs (e.g., the minimum number of staff hours per patient day, square feet or floor space per patient and like issues). As a consequence, the potential freedom to determine operating policies is reduced. It is frequently asserted that the nursing home industry is the second most heavily regulated industry, nuclear power plants being the first. We devote part 4 to these concerns.

External Feedback

Typically, external feedback to an industry is not manifested in such powerful and influential terms as stringent federal and state regulations. The feedback is normally expressed through reactions in the community about quality of work (outputs) being produced. This appears in

- word-of-mouth evaluations
- newspaper articles and radio and TV commentary
- the reputation enjoyed by the facility's staff that leads potential employees to consider it a desirable or undesirable place to work
- the number of potential residents applying for admission to the facility

The reader can add to the list. All of these elements constitute what is referred to in Figure 1-1 as the environment.

ENVIRONMENT

The *environment* consists of all relevant external forces that affect the nursing home facility.

Defining the Environment

Defining the relevant environment of one's organization is perhaps the most complex and least obvious aspect of viewing organizations as systems. The environment consists of opportunities and constraints. One way to conceptualize this is to ask two questions:

1. Does it relate meaningfully to my objectives? If, so it is an opportunity.
2. Can I do anything about it? If not, it is a constraint.

If the answer to the first question is yes and to the second question no, it is a constraint in the relevant environment. If the answer to both questions is yes, it is an opportunity for the facility.

From the systems perspective the entire world is interconnected in one large network. The challenge is to identify the aspects of the external world that now or eventually may affect the facility in its attempt to achieve objectives, such as serving patients and making a profit. This is the first step in the management process: forecasting.

The environment is both a set of constraints within which the facility must operate and a set of opportunities which the facility administration may seize. (Hitt et al., 2001; Pfeffer & Salanick, 1978).

Some easily recognizable constraints in a nursing facility's environment might be

- federal, state, and local regulations
- the number of other facilities operating in the area
- the availability of qualified applicants for positions to be filled in the home
- the availability of foods at affordable prices
- state Medicaid practices and reimbursement policies
- availability and costs of money
- inflation or deflation rates

Some recognizable opportunities might be

- increasing availability of managed care contracts for individual patients at negotiated rates
- the opportunity to offer "higher-tech" services
- the opportunity to identify and serve niches in care needs
- the increasing number of frail elderly who will need nursing care
- pressures for increased number of beds due to the aging of the baby-boom population explosion that followed World War II (1945–1963)

1.4.2 Identifying Systems

The outputs of one system normally become the inputs for the next system (Levey & Loomba, 1973; Hitt et al., 2001), for example, the set of relationships that normally exists among hospitals, nursing homes, home health agencies, and hospice providers.

Hospital patients who no longer need acute care and who need facility-based nursing care (the outputs of the hospital) become the inputs of the nursing facility—new patient admissions. The rehabilitated nursing home resident who no longer needs facility-based nursing care but requires follow-up home care (the nursing home output) becomes the input of the home health agency or perhaps the hospice agency.

We have been using the nursing home as an entity to illustrate the systems concept. We could have selected another level of function within the facility, for instance, the department of nursing.

WHO DEFINES THE SYSTEM?

The selection of what is to be viewed as the system is left entirely to the discretion of the person who describes or analyzes it. This may be one of the more subtle concepts in systems theory. The fact is the user decides what to designate as a system for his or her own purposes. For example, the chief executive officer of a large nursing home chain is accustomed to thinking of the several hundred homes as the system. The individual nursing home administrator may conceive of the departments operating in the facility as the system. The maintenance department manager may consider the department as the system.

One of the virtues of the systems concept is that it is almost infinitely adaptable to the needs of the individual user. Anybody can define any set of interrelationships as the system for purposes of description or analysis. All of us use systems analysis in our everyday thinking about the interrelationships of things around us. The systems theory and model described here is an analytic tool that the administrator can use to solve organizational problems as they arise.

1.4.3 Additional Characteristics of Systems

Social science researchers have identified several characteristics of systems that the reader may find useful as analytical tools.

The output of each system furnishes the stimulus for repeating the cycle (Katz & Kahn). In the case of nursing care facilities, the successfully cared for resident (the desired outcome of the nursing home's efforts) furnishes the source of more inputs: Other persons apply for admission to the facility to replace the resident who has left (Argenti, 1994). The new resident brings renewed energy in the form of a renewed source of continuing income to the facility and thereby furnishes a renewal of the capacity of the facility to continue to pay employees and provide services.

Administrators can view the nursing facility as a dynamic system whose essence is the cycle of activities (providing care to residents/patients, making sufficient income) for which they are is responsible.

ORGANIZATIONAL GROWTH

A nursing home and similar social organizations can grow indefinitely. Scientists speak of the *entropic process,* a universal law of nature that states all organisms move toward death (Hitt et al., 2001; Katz & Kahn, 1967). All of us, for example, realize that one day we will die because one or more of our vital systems comes to a halt. In sharp contrast, a nursing facility or chain not only does not have to die, but can keep on growing, with no time constraints, as long as it receives more energy from the environment than it consumes. In this way organizations can be said to acquire negative entropy (Robey, 1982).

Organizations tend to try to grow, not in every case, of course, but in general. Organizational theorists have called this the tendency to maximize the ratio of imported to expended energy. One social scientist (Miller, 1982) has observed that the rate of growth of an organization, within certain ranges, is dramatic if it exists in a medium that makes available unrestricted amounts of additional inputs. The significance for administrators is that organizations, unlike people, are not subject to disintegration as long as they can keep adding to their resources, and that organizations, like people, tend to try to grow. Between 1965 and 1983 American hospitals added vastly to their expensive equipment and procedures because Congress had made virtually unlimited resources available through reimbursement for whatever the hospitals chose to charge under Medicare. Growth may be qualitative (better care) or quantitative (a larger patient census or more facilities being added to the chain).

MAXIMIZING BASIC CHARACTER

Another important aspect of organizations is that as they grow, organizations attempt to accommodate the world around them to meet their own needs (Hitt et al., 2001; Katz & Kahn, 1967). For example, in planning for an extended care system, the nursing home associations place themselves at the heart of the system. The American Hospital Association, on the other hand, envisions the American health care system with hospitals at its core. The insurance companies are similarly convinced of their own strategic importance at the very center of such a system.

MAINTENANCE FUNCTIONS: ATHEROSCLEROSIS, CONGESTIVE HEART FAILURE

Once in place, organizations become creatures of habit and develop a tendency to resist change. There may be a strong effort to keep the current pattern of relationships with others from changing at all, which is sometimes called organizational hardening of the arteries. Organizations that have become set in their ways will try to maintain the status quo through several devices:

1. Any internal or external situation that threatens to force a change in the organization is countered by employees seeking to retain their old patterns and modes of operation (Johns & Saks, 2001). For example, the nursing home faced with a "disruptive employee" agitating for change will dismiss the employee, will resist change (Bradley & Calvin, 1956; Hitt et al., 2001).

2. When confronted with external changes that might affect the organization, administrators, will try to ignore them. For instance, if their patient census declines while it increases in nearby homes, the tendency will be to find excuses rather than to examine if the others are offering better services.

3. Resisting change, many organizations will attempt to cope with external forces that might require them to change by acquiring control of them. For example, if a nursing home chain is losing patients to a competing freestanding group of facilities, the chain might attempt to acquire those other facilities rather than remedy its own situation (Katz & Kahn, 1967; Hitt et al., 2001).

Nursing facilities and nursing facility chains can fall from a leadership question to trailing the pack. How can this happen? A Massachusetts Institute of Technology study on productivity attributes this possibility to "a deep reservoir of outmoded attitudes and policies" at most organizations (Kriegel, 1991).

Rapid and unanticipated changes are a permanent fixture of the managerial landscape of today. This textbook is about learning to appreciate that change brings opportunities.

BUT WE'VE ALWAYS DONE IT THAT WAY

Once firmly in place, systems, policies, procedures, plans, organizational approaches and assumptions become the standard operations of the facility, its sacred cows. They are sacrosanct because it has "always" been done this way. They are created by the training received in nursing, medical, or physical therapy school. In this way creativity is stifled and competitive strength weakened. Today, anything that remains unchallenged or untouched for very long can become the sacred cow of tomorrow. Sacred cows are difficult to round up for a variety of reasons. They may be untouchable because the state inspectors want it that way, or because they are the administrator's special concern or relate to one department's closely guarded turf.

One corporate executive officer identified the following dearly cherished beliefs:

- *Eliminate budgets* . . . use the computer to give you an up-to-the moment report.
- *Using plans* . . . is like firing a cannonball at a castle—only today's markets are moving targets.
- *Pushing functions down the pyramid* . . . let the department head run the department
- *Sell the purchasing department* . . . let departments buy and be accountable for the supplies they need.
- *Let human resources departments go* . . . let each manager hire, then be responsible for the employee.
- *Let everybody touch the customer* . . . welcome the family and others into the facility.
- *Reject any quality control department* . . . make everybody responsible for quality—you can't inspect quality into something.
- *Discard the time clock* . . . if the employees can't be trusted to work their shift, don't hire them.
- *Eliminate levels* . . . it's hard to build a team among unequals (Kriegel, 1991).

You cannot move fast if you are following a herd of sacred cows. Paper trails represent people trying to keep tabs on other people. All this when the real purpose of systems as we have described them is to empower, not control, people and to liberate staff to experiment with new ways to meet resident/patient needs, not to tie them down. The nursing home industry is full of sacred cows; federal, state, and local officials see to that.

Finally, two other characteristics of organizations should be mentioned.

ORGANIZATIONS GROW INCREASINGLY COMPLEX

New organizations tend to be simple at inception, then become more and more complex as they grow. The human personality is similar. As infants we have few perceptions. As we grow, we begin to build more complex and complicated perceptions of the world around us. The personality we develop is a system with no physical boundaries. A social organization such as a nursing home is also a system with no physical boundaries (Allport, 1962; Hitt et al., 2001; Johns & Saks, 2001; Katz & Kahn, 1967).

Just as the human personality becomes progressively more sophisticated, social organizations move toward the multiplication and elaboration of roles with greater specialization of functions. For example, the mom-and-pop nursing homes of a few decades ago are giving way to increasingly larger and more sophisticated facilities, offering medically complex services.

The organization of American medicine provides another illustration. In 1870, 80% of all American physicians were general practitioners. Today, with the explosion of medical technology, 80% are specialists, and only 20% are general practitioners. As was bound to happen, today one must have 3 years of training to become a general practitioner, who now is called a family practice specialist.

The process of nursing homes grouping into increasingly larger and competing chains (i.e., multiplication and elaboration of roles) has led to increasing the number of possible management jobs available to persons interested in such a career. Middle- and upper-level positions are now available in corporate nursing-home management offices.

ORGANIZATIONS ARE DIFFICULT TO PREDICT

There need not be a single strategy for an organization to achieve an objective. We have argued that organizations are dynamic systems of social interactions. Because the situation is volatile, there is low predictability (von Bertalanffy, 1967; Hitt et al., 2001).

An organization can reach its goals from different starting points and by a variety of routes. If, for example, a small, financially weak nursing-home-chain management staff wanted to take over a financially stronger and larger chain, there are many possible alternatives. They could try to compete more successfully, thus weakening the larger chain, making it more susceptible to takeover. They could attempt to raise enough venture capital to buy out the larger group (Hitt et al., 2001). They could arrange to be taken over by an unrelated corporation with considerable liquid assets, thereby enabling them to buy out the currently stronger and larger chain. More of these and similar concepts will be explored in part 3.

The list of the ten largest nursing home chains has changed rapidly over the past several years. Predictability is equally low in a number of fields, for instance, hospitals, the assisted living industry, the home health care industry, and health maintenance organizations, to name a few.

SUMMARY

In the process of looking at the function called organizing, we have suggested that thinking of organizations as systems is a useful approach to the task of understanding how a nursing facility operates. The systems model is a useful way to visualize the inputs (money, materials, and people) that are available to administrators. The way in which administrators configure and use money, materials, and people will depend on their beliefs about how organizations function.

1.5 Staffing

Staffing is hiring the right persons for the jobs in the organization. It is one of the most difficult tasks the administrator and her/his department managers face because it is seldom possible to predict from an interview and recommendations how a person will work out on the job. The number of variables is almost infinite, and many of them are difficult to recognize beforehand.

Staffing patterns of nursing homes are more prescribed than for most other health care institutions. This is the result of the federal requirements and state regulation, which carefully delineate qualifications for each type of staff position and require minimum staffing in nearly every area of the facility.

One thing is quite clear: The success of the nursing home depends directly on adequate staffing. Nursing care is looking after people. The interactions between residents and staff determine the quality of life in the nursing home. Physical facilities are important, but once they are in place at a minimally adequate level, patient satisfaction with the facility varies directly with satisfaction with the staff performance.

The administrator may choose to delegate coordination of the hiring process to a personnel director or assign it to the individual department managers (normally) with the advice and consent of the administrator. For this reason, we mention the staffing function at this point. The reader is referred to part 2 for a detailed discussion of staffing tasks.

1.6 Directing

Directing is the process of communicating to employees what is to be done by each of them and helping them to accomplish it. An earlier step, organizing, included breaking down the work necessary to achieve the organizational goals into work assignments that can be handled by one person. Directing is an aspect of the organizational activity in which the actual work is done.

Several important management concepts will be included under this heading:

- policy making
- decision making
- leadership
- power and authority
- communication skills
- organizational norms and values
- additional related concepts

Directing involves reference to each of these key concepts to arrive at the goal of a successful program.

1.6.1 Policy Making

The ultimate goal of the administrator is to design a program in which every member of the organization makes the same decisions given the same set of circumstances. To this end, the administrator attempts to persuade the entire staff to carry out their responsibilities exactly as the administrator would like them to.

PURPOSE AND FUNCTION

It is impossible for the administrator to be everywhere at once, 24 hours a day, throughout the facility. It is possible, however, for the administrator to make policies that direct the activities of the employees everywhere in the facility, 24 hours a day. The purpose and function of these policies is to communicate to each employee as exactly as possible what the management expects in any situation on the job.

It is, of course, neither possible nor desirable to establish policies for every conceivable situation. However, a person can provide guidelines or policies that become the framework within which the employee decides what to do in each situation requiring action on behalf of the nursing home facility. In his book *Principles of Management* (1969) G. R. Terry has defined policy as a verbal, written, or implied overall guide that sets up boundaries supplying the general limits and direction in which managerial action will take place.

Policies are used to help keep decisions within the areas intended by the planners, because they provide for some consistency in what employees decide in particular situations, usually under repetitive conditions. Policies reveal the facility administrator's intentions with respect to the behavior of employees, patients/residents, and the public in the future. Policies are decided before the need for employee knowledge arises. A simple illustration might be useful.

It is not possible for management to know when, where, or even whether a fire will break out in the facility. By developing a complete set of procedures for personnel to follow in case of fire, the administrator is able to communicate before the occasion arises precisely what each employee in the facility must do if a fire should occur.

DEFINING POLICIES AND PROCEDURES

The reader may have noticed the use of the word *procedures* in the previous section, rather than *policies*. Writers in the field of management use *policies, procedures,* and *plans of action* as terms to indicate movement from generalized statements of intention (*policies*) to specific spelling out of the method, step by step (*procedures*), for carrying out those policies or plans of action.

It may be useful to think of the following set of concepts, which moves from the general to the specific in setting forth of behaviors the manager wishes the employees to exercise.

EXAMPLE OF POLICIES AND PROCEDURES

Fire Preparedness

General goals or objectives may be stated for the facility. In the area of fire preparedness it might be "to have our facility employees completely prepared to take appropriate action in case of fire." The administrator might then draw up a general policy statement indicating that the head of the housekeeping department would develop a step-by-step plan of action for every department to follow in case of fire. This plan is a *set of procedures,* a highly detailed plan of specific actions that each employee would be expected to follow in case of fire.

Notice that at each level the degrees of freedom within which decisions could be made were reduced. The head of housekeeping could develop a variety of configurations for employee responsibilities, but by the time the individual employee became involved, the degrees of freedom had nearly vanished. The responsibility in case of fire had moved from the general goal or policy of fire preparedness to a detailed set of instructions or procedures to be followed to the letter. "The moment you hear the fire alarm, proceed immediately to station J on the blue wing and report to the nurse in charge" is an example of a procedure.

Food Preparation

The board of directors might set a policy goal of offering an outstanding selection of first-quality food to the residents of the facility. It becomes the responsibility of each progressively lower level of management to actually implement this policy. The food service director must take this communicated policy or goal and develop a series of policies for decision making by the kitchen staff that result in the actual service of an outstanding selection of first-quality food to the residents.

General policies are developed at each level of management. Normally, the amount of specificity increases at each lower level. The food service manager may, for example, announce a policy to the food service supervisor responsible for salads that there be a sufficient variety with specified proportions of crisp fresh lettuce every evening. The supervisor may then write out a step-by-step set of procedures for the kitchen worker who prepares salads.

The set of steps the salad worker is to follow at 4:00 P.M. each day, beginning, perhaps, with removing the lettuce from the refrigerator, is an example of a *set of procedures.* The broad policy of excellence in food service promulgated by the administrator has now been translated into a set of procedures or individual steps for the salad worker in the kitchen to follow every day at 4:00 P.M. to assure the crispness of the lettuce that will be served each evening. It sounds simple, but ask the residents/ patients; too few nursing facilities succeed in serving a sufficient variety of salads with crisp lettuce. Providing interesting salads 365 days a year is but one of hundreds of complex tasks that must be successfully accomplished each 24 hours.

Insertion of a Peripheral Device

A policy statement regarding peripheral devices might read as follows. It is the policy of this facility to permit nurses to insert peripheral devices only after 20 hours of specialized training and certification by the director or nursing that the nurse has qualified.

A procedure statement regarding insertion of a peripheral device and administration of continuous solution might read as follows.

1. Verify physician's orders. Check for allergies.
2. Compare label on solution with order.
3. Wash hands.
4. Assemble equipment and supplies.
5. Inspect solution and container.
6. Close flow clamp on tubing.
7. Attach administration set to fluid container. Hang on IV pole.
8. Prime intravenous therapy tubing by squeezing drip chamber to fill ½ full; open flow clamp until tubing is primed; close flow clamp.
9. Explain procedure to patient, position patient.
10. Apply tourniquet to extremity (optional).
11. Select catheter insertion site, cleanse site with antimicrobial swab; start at center of the site, use a circular motion moving outward.
12. Repeat with antimicrobial swab. Allow to completely dry on skin at least 30 seconds.
13. Don gloves.
14. Place thumb below intended venipuncture site; gently draw skin toward you.
15. For wing-tipped needle, hold needle by the wings, with bevel up, at 45° angle to skin surface; penetrate the skin surface, lower the angle of the needle almost parallel with the skin, pierce the vein.

Observe for blood return; release the tourniquet if one has been applied. Secure wings with tape.

16. Attach IV tubing or extension set, if used for intermittent infusion. Start solution at a slow rate.
17. Observe for signs of infiltration at venipuncture site. Anchor wings of needle with tape.
18. Cover venipuncture site with transparent dressing. Make a small loop with infusion tubing and secure with tape.
19. Check and regulate flow rate according to physician's orders.
20. Place label on dressing, indicating the following: date and time, type, length, and gauge, initials of nurse.
21. Discard used equipment appropriately.

Documentation

Record procedure in the resident's medical record.* Include the following:

- type, length, and gauge of device
- date and time of insertion
- site of insertion
- resident's response
- number of attempts
- type of dressing applied
- solution and rate of administration
- nurse's initials/signature.

SUMMARY

Policies serve as general statements or understanding that guide or channel subordinates' thinking as they make decisions. Policies limit the area within which a decision is to be made and seek to assure that it will be consistent with the overall objectives. Policies tend to decide issues beforehand by establishing the framework and scope of the actions.

The decisions made at each level of management establish the framework for decision making at each successively lower level of management, generally with progressively less discretion to do so. However, each level of management does participate in the policy making process, and policies are made at every level of management. Policy is made by

---

*Adapted from *Nursing Policy and Procedure Manual for Intravenous Therapy,* Medisave Pharmacy/ HealthCare Network, Medisave Pharmacies, inc., Baton Route, LA, 1994, pp. 1–21 plus documentation.

persons at upper, middle and lower levels of management within the nursing home facility. Defining policy making is complicated by this fact.

When do policies become procedures? Sometimes these are separated by a fine line that is hard to distinguish. Generally, a policy is a statement that contains some degree of freedom, some further need for interpretation. Procedures are step-by-step instructions on how a specific task is to be carried out.

1.6.2 Making a Decision

Although decision making can be synonymous with managing, it is difficult to define. G. L. S. Shackle (1957) describes *deciding* as the focal creative psychic event in which knowledge, thought, feeling, and imagination are fused into action (see also Dale, 1969, chap. 23; and Hitt et al., 2001, pp. 26–27, 36–37). Both Dale and Shackle point out the impossibility of a useful formula for decision making. Inevitably, we are left with an imprecise definition of the process. Even so, administrators do make numerous decisions every day.

Making the "right" decision in a given situation is often difficult. It is the nursing facility administrator's job to ensure that all employees make the right decisions for the organization as often as possible (Kotter, 1982).

We define a successful manager as a person who is able, on balance, to make enough right decisions for the organization and *no* disastrously wrong ones.

1.6.3 Leading

Organizations that thrive over an extended period of time depend on *effective leaders,* persons who combine foresight with an ability to guide the organization to take advantage successfully of the opportunities the future offers.

THE GREAT LEADERSHIP THEORY OF HISTORY

A satisfactory description of *leading* is as elusive as one that defines *deciding*. There are, however, those who propose the "great leadership theory of history," suggesting that history is made or measurably influenced by individuals who become leaders. Whatever one might think of their accomplishments, people like Alexander the Great, Genghis Khan, Confucius, Joan of Arc, George Washington, Abraham Lincoln, Margaret Sanger, and Winston Churchill have assumed leadership roles that affected the course of history.

Leadership in the business world seems to be no less crucial to the success of organizations. Between the years 1915 and 1973, Thomas Watson, Sr., and Thomas Watson, Jr., provided leadership to IBM, which came to dominate the computer world during their tenure because father and son combined foresight (successfully predicting the future) with an ability to guide the organization to take advantage successfully of the opportunities offered by the future. It was not until being discharged from a job he had held for 14 years that the senior Tom Watson joined a company that manufactured scales, meat slicers, time clocks, and punch cards for data sorting. He envisioned these punch cards revolutionizing the future, he borrowed money to buy the company, and renamed it. At the time, in 1924, the younger Tom Watson commented, "What a big name for a pip-squeak company that makes meat grinders." (Kriegel, 1991). International Business Machines Corporation had just been born.

In the world of automobile manufacturing there is a general agreement that Lee Iacocca's abilities moved the Chrysler Corporation from near bankruptcy to a position of leadership in the industry. William McWhorter was given responsibility for 103 hospitals that Hospital Corporation of America believed to be irreversibly unprofitable in 1987. Through his personal leadership these hospitals became both profitable and a major leader in the hospital industry.

The leadership provided to the nursing facility by the administrator, director of nurses, and other department managers is no less critical to the success or failure to thrive of each nursing facility.

THE ADMINISTRATOR AND THE DIRECTOR OF NURSING THEORY

There is scant research literature to prove the assertion that leadership by the administrator, director of nurses, and the department heads is key to the success of any nursing facility. Yet even in the absence of such data, there apparently exists a broad consensus among observers of the industry, especially federal and state inspectors, that quality care in a nursing facility does depend on its administrators being able to exercise good leadership skills. Federal inspectors normally try to inspect a nursing facility within 6 months after a change in the administrator or director of nurses, believing that leadership (or lack of it) from these administrators directly affects the quality of care in a facility. When IBM's leadership changed after 60 years, the giant lost its leadership position. The company had ridden the wave of change for 60 years with the Watsons at the helm and usually was ranked #1 in *Fortune* magazine's annual survey of America's most admired corporations. Lou Gertsner, IBM president in the mid-1990s, stated several times that he did not have to have a vision to lead the corporation. By 1995, out of the 500 ranked companies, IBM had dropped from #1 to 281st. Leadership counts. The Watsons inspired IBM to six decades of greatness with a vision. Vision, it seems, also counts (*"America's Most Admired Corporations,"* 1995; Hamel & Prahalad, 1994). Gertsner later developed and implemented a vision of IBM's becoming the service leader in the computer industry and at the beginning of the millennium IBM was regaining its place as the industry leader.

Through forecasting, planning, organizing, staffing, directing, evaluating, controlling quality, innovating, and marketing decisions the administrator is providing leadership to the nursing facility.

LEADERSHIP BY WANDERING AROUND

There are various styles of leadership (for example, democratic, authoritarian, or laissez-faire). One effective style that was mentioned earlier is leading by walking around (LBWA). When walking around and observing such things as staff interaction with residents and families, volunteers and other employees, one can personally evaluate the quality of care being rendered. This is also an opportunity to see if the residents are having any problems and to physically inspect the building and equipment (K. Weddle, RN, personal communication, 1992).

Leadership by wandering or walking around provides opportunity for the staff to speak with the administrator informally. It allows time to observe what is going on and to let the staff know the administrator is interested in them, the residents, and the facility. Leading by walking around is not new to the nursing facility setting. Since the first federal regulations were introduced in 1974, the director of nurses has been required by the government to make 'daily rounds' to see all patients" (§483.28 of the federal requirements). Additionally, in many nursing facilities, each shift is expected to make rounds, reporting on each patient's/resident's condition over the preceding 8 hours. This is how nursing keeps informed of and anticipates each patient's needs for the coming shift.

Through leading by walking around, the administrator receives a daily update on the real world of the facility—in the rooms, hallways, departments, loading dock, and restrooms. This positions the administrator to uncover problems before they become major irritants. Administrators who do not take the initiative to keep informed about facility affairs on a daily basis often become involved in a style of management known as fire fighting. Once small issues become hot issues, a lot of time must be spent extinguishing the flames.

In making daily rounds, the administrator can engage in naive listening, gaining raw impressions of what is happening in the facility, sensing how things are going. Think there's not enough time to get the paperwork done, meet all the other administrator requirements, and still walk daily around the facility sensing its pulse? Sam Walton, the founder of Wal-Mart Corporation, visited every one of his stores at least once a year when he had only 18 stores. By the early 1990s he owned more than 800 stores and he was still visiting all of them at least once a year, riding cross-country with Wal-Mart truck drivers, eating donuts at three in the morning. He thought the checkout clerk the most important employee, and until his death in 1992, every clerk knew that Mr. Sam might be the next customer waiting in the line, observing how the customer ahead of him was being treated.

The future doesn't just happen: Leaders like Tom Watson, Sam Walton, and the local nursing home administrator dream it, shape it, sculpt it.

WALKING, YET MAINTAINING THE CHAIN OF COMMAND

Wandering around the facility talking with residents, visitors and staff appears to violate the traditional concept of chain of command. The administrator is there to hear it firsthand and to communicate firsthand. Ed Carson, the former chairman of an airline who led by walking around, took copious notes on scraps of paper, but never told people down the line what to do or change. He never corrected on the spot what he disliked, but he did promise to get back to the resident, visitor, or employee in a few days. He then discussed each situation with the department head and together they charted a course of action to resolve any problem. And after a few days he would check with the resident, visitor, or employee to see if appropriate action had been taken. He was practicing what he called "visible management" (Peters, 1987; Johns & Saks, 2001).

The basic benefits of leading by walking around are listening (finding out what's happening on the firing line), teaching (communicating the facility's values), and facilitating. Through LBWA the administrator can facilitate the work of employees by asking naive questions, finding out what is frustrating the staff, then running interference and knocking down small hurdles for them. Only the facility that pays excessive attention to details can achieve excellence in resident care. Quality of care means that staff is paying attention to the details that lead to excellent care as they emulate their administrator.

CHOOSING TO LEAD

Riding the Wave of Change

Deciding on one's approach to leading is one of the more important decisions managers ever make. Kriegel compares leading an organization to surfing the waves (Kriegel, 1991). The time to change is when you don't have to, he asserts, when you are on the crest of a wave, not when you are in the trough. In the world of health care administration, surf's up! Waves of change are coming from government, third-party payers, and the patients/residents and their families.

The best surfers (nursing home administrators) are not necessarily the best swimmers (best management theoreticians). The best surfers are those with the following mind-set.

Passion Rules. Catching and riding a wave is fairly simple, but there are many who give lip service to the art. They have the correct equipment and stylish outfits, the right jargon, but spend most of their time on the beach talking about surfing. The best surfers spend their time in the water, rough or calm, looking for the next wave. They are totally committed to surfing—body, mind, and spirit.

No dare, no flair. Good surfers constantly push their limits, continuously trying new moves, going for bigger and bigger waves. They know that no two waves are ever the same, so they ride each one a little differently. Keeping ahead of the wave involves risk taking, constantly challenging yourself and those around you.

Expect to wipe out. For every successful ride there will likely be two or three wipeouts. Sand is part of every surfer's diet. A changing ocean with its dynamic wave patterns and shapes is a source not of fear but of challenge that provides the thrill of surfing. Successful surfers know that if they do not wipe out several times a day they are playing it too safe to keep improving.

Don't turn your back on the ocean. Surfers know they are dealing with an environment beyond their control. They understand that uncertainty and unpredictability are part of the game. They respect the ocean and its power, never taking it for granted. They never turn their backs on the ocean.

Keep looking "outside" The outside waves are those on the horizon. It is important to pay attention to the wave closest to you and also to what is coming. First, there may be a bigger and better wave on the horizon. Second, the wave on the horizon may crash over you as you come up for air after riding the wave closest to you.

Move before it moves you. Surfing involves forecasting and planning for the future. You have to begin moving yourself while that big wave is still on the horizon or it will surge by, leaving you in its trough.

Never surf alone. It is not smart to tackle the complexities of life alone. One needs a backup when emergencies arise. By pooling knowledge and insights, surfers can learn about more exotic spots and trade tips and techniques that work. It is also a lot more fun to have a friend along to "talk story" with as you navigate the complexities of the nursing facility operations. Having someone to share your hopes, dreams, and frustrations leads to more creativity, joy, and effectiveness.

As Kriegel has suggested (1991), the future is coming at us like enormous waves, in set after set, and they are getting bigger. The surf is up in the hospital industry, the assisted living industry, the life care communities, the home health care industry, and the managed care industry. The future belongs to those who decide to ride, to those who welcome the unexpected.

As president of General Electric, John F. Welch became widely regarded as the master of corporate change by shedding 200,000 employees while tripling GE's market value between 1981 and 1993. He believes that every business must be fast and adaptable in order to survive. When people at GE ask if the change is over and can they stop now, he responds that change has just begun, that it is never ending. Change, he asserts, is a continuing process, not an event. He says the administrator's job is listening to, searching for, and spreading ideas—the process of exposing people to good ideas and role models (Welch, 1993). As observed by Dennis Kodner, the days of "business as usual" in the long-term care industry are over (Kodner, 1993). Success in today's world will depend on understanding where the industry is heading, having a vision of the future and developing the capacity to implement change as an ongoing aspect of managing a facility (Kodner, 1993). Connie J. Evashwick thinks that facilities that resist change and continue to function in isolation may survive, but will not thrive in the twenty-first century (Evashnick, 1993).

FIRE IN THE HEART

To be a successful nursing home administrator over a sustained period of years requires that one be excited about the profession. Top performers in all fields have one quality in common: passion. Their drive and enthusiasm for nursing home administration is what distinguishes them. As numerous executive recruiters have observed, "The thing that makes the difference between a good manager and an inspiring, dynamic leader goes beyond competence. It's passion. That is the single quality that is going to lift a person head and shoulders above the rest (Kriegel, 1991).

Passion brings complete commitment to one's work: physical, emotional, and mental. It sustains the successful administrator through the outrages of regulations and an abusive public image of the field. Passion is contagious. An administrator who is enthusiastic about the work can inspire excitement in the nurses and nursing assistants. Knowledge of the field, competence, and experience make a good manager, but a greater commitment gives one the necessary edge to provide the leadership necessary in today's nursing facility.

Of course, passion is not a scientifically measurable component of nursing home administration, but then management is not yet exactly a science. What the nursing home administrator needs is a fire in the heart for continuously improving the quality of the daily life of each resident.

A Continuum of Leadership Styles

In *Leadership and Organization,* Tannenbaum, Wechsler, and Massarik (1961, p. 311), discuss a continuum of leadership styles. This allows us to characterize seven possible positions along the continuum, from manager-centered to employee-centered leadership. Several dimensions are portrayed in Figure 1-2. Under manager-centered leadership, the manager retains a high degree of control and uses authority extensively, less so under employee-centered leadership.

Manager-Centered Leadership

Position 1. The manager simply makes the decision, then announces it (autocratic style).

Position 2. The manager attempts to convince the employees of the value of the decision made.

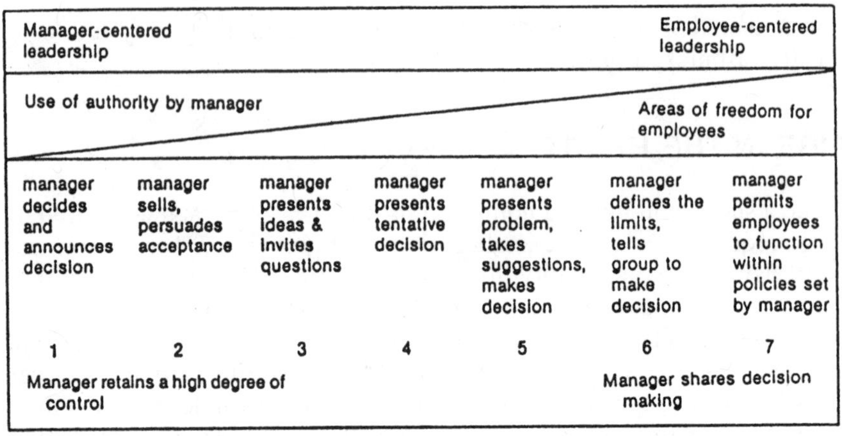

Manager-centered leadership						Employee-centered leadership
Use of authority by manager						Areas of freedom for employees
manager decides and announces decision	manager sells, persuades acceptance	manager presents ideas & invites questions	manager presents tentative decision	manager presents problem, takes suggestions, makes decision	manager defines the limits, tells group to make decision	manager permits employees to function within policies set by manager
1	2	3	4	5	6	7
Manager retains a high degree of control				Manager shares decision making		

FIGURE 1-2. Range of decision-making strategies open to the manager.

Position 3. The manager presents ideas and invites questions, in effect engaging the employees actively in the decision-making process.

Employee-Centered Leadership

Position 4. The manager presents a tentative decision, subject to change; the employees are further involved in the decision-making process itself.

Position 5. The manager presents the problem requiring solution, invites suggestions, then makes the decision.

Position 6. The manager permits the subordinates to make the decision and function within the limits defined by the manager (laissez-faire leadership style) (Johns & Saks, 2001).

DECIDING HOW TO LEAD

At the least, the following three levels of considerations should be taken into account by the administrator who is selecting the leadership style for a particular situation.

First level: Forces in the administrator

- his/her own values

- his/her confidence in the department heads
- his/her own feelings of security or insecurity

Second level: Forces in the employees

The facility administrator can permit greater freedom to department managers who

- have a need for independence (e.g., the director of nurses)
- are ready to assume responsibility for decision making (are professionally licensed)
- are interested in the problem and consider it important (take resident care seriously)
- understand and agree with the mission statement/goals of the facility
- have the necessary knowledge and experience (the R.N. who comes with 2 years' intensive care experience
- are prepared and expect to make decisions (e.g., a trained, licensed physical therapist)

Third level: Forces in the organization

- expectations of the organization's management (position taken by corporation or the board)
- ability of subordinates to function as a group (eight competent department heads who have worked together for 3 years versus five new and three continuing department heads)
- the problem itself (excessive medication errors or in-house acquired decubitus ulcers rates cannot be permitted)
- time constraints (e.g., plans of correction for deficiencies all have correction dates)

LEADERSHIP SKILL REQUIREMENTS

We have already discussed three levels of management: upper, middle, and lower level, each with its own particular skill requirements. Figure 1-3 adapted from Katz and Kahn, shows three different levels of leadership skills.

The Upper-Level Manager

The nursing facility's upper-level administrator is primarily responsible for creating and changing the organization's structure. The chief administrator must understand not only how the organization accommodates to

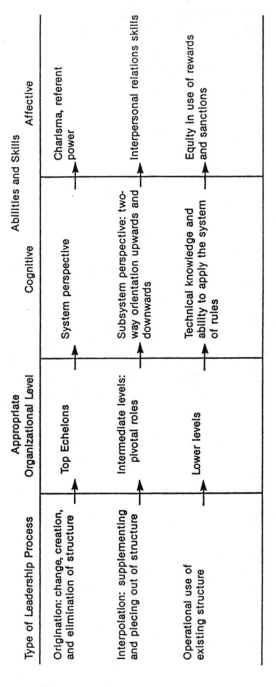

FIGURE 1-3. Three levels of skill requirements for managers. Adapted from Katz & Kahn (1967).

the external environment, but also how all of the subsystems function within the nursing facility itself.

The Middle-Level Manager

The heads of dietary, housekeeping, or other departments are responsible for development of more specific policies that interpret administration policy implications for their departments. The middle-level manager is responsible for implementing the policies of the administration by devising ways to put them into action within the facility. This level of management translates the broader institutional policies by developing more specific ones to control employee behavior. The administrator, for example, may set a goal of preventing acquired decubitus ulcers. The middle-level manager must understand how the subsystems of the organization fit together to achieve the overall goals and has the difficult task of representing to upper-level management the needs of those supervised. To function effectively, middle-level managers must realize that they are the conduit through which action travels in both directions.

The Lower-Level Manager

The lower-level manager (e.g., the charge nurse who supervises a specific group of nurses/nursing assistants) has the responsibility of applying the policies provided by the director of nursing to the hour-by-hour care given. Lower-level managers guide employees according to established policies of the facility. To accomplish this, the rules must be thoroughly understood and applied evenhandedly to all employees under their direction. One particularly important key to effective leadership at the lower level is that employees have a sense of their manager's advocacy. It is not enough simply to be their advocate, however; the manager must be their effective spokesperson.

Procedures can be written by any level of management; in most cases, procedures are written by both middle-level and lower-level managers.

As Figure 1-3 suggests, different skills are needed at the three distinct levels of management.

CHARACTERISTICS OF THE EFFECTIVE LEADER

Katz and Kahn (1967) have characterized an effective leader as a person who

- mediates and tempers the organizational requirements to the needs of persons in a manner that is organizationally enhancing (the facility assists employees having family crises through unplanned time off and other support)

- promotes group loyalty and personal ties (working for the facility becomes a personally satisfying experience)
- demonstrates care for individuals (knows each employee by name and something about that employee's interests)
- relies on referent power (respect from employees and patients/residents) rather than the power of legitimacy and sanctions alone (discussed in 1.6.4)

Tannenbaum et al. (1961) concluded that successful leaders are those who are keenly aware of relevant forces in the situation, who understand themselves and the individuals with whom they are dealing, but also are able to behave appropriately vis-à-vis the situation, making decisions where needed and sharing the decision-making where appropriate.

Tannenbaum considers the successful leader neither strong nor permissive, but rather endowed with a strong instinct (a gut feeling) for determining appropriate personal behavior, and capable of acting accordingly.

Day-to-Day Leadership Requirements

In the daily administration of the typical long-term care facility the administrator will face a variety of situations that call for different kinds of leadership. Recognize appropriate leadership behavior for any specific situation is a valuable insight; the capacity to behave in different leadership styles is an accomplishment of a high order indeed. Much of the flexibility the administrator can exercise in distinctive leadership styles depends on how comfortable she is in wielding power and authority in the management of the facility.

Charismatic Leadership

Although charismatic leadership cannot be consciously chosen by the administrator, it is worth mentioning here (Johns & Saks, 2001). This quality has been described by Max Weber as a magical aura with which people sometimes endow their leaders. It appears when a group has an emotional need for a person who they feel will make the right decision for them. Charismatic leaders are typically unexamined. Their followers do not scrutinize their acts as they would those of their immediate supervisors. Charisma is not an objective assessment and normally requires a psychological distance between the followers and the leader. When charisma is assigned to a leader, the power and authority of the organization is enhanced.

1.6.4 Power and Authority

Power is the ability to control the behavior of others. A person has power when he is able to make other people do what he wants. One writer says this is the ability to motivate someone to do something they would otherwise not do (Argenti, 1994). The administrator of a nursing facility has the power to order employees to act to implement the goals of the facility as expressed in the policies and plans.

Webster's *New World Dictionary* (1968) gives 14 definitions for the word power. An additional half-dozen synonyms indicate that power denotes the inherent ability or the admitted right to rule, govern, determine, control, regulate, restrain, and curb. Power is a complex concept in our culture.

The administrator has the power (from the board or the ownership) to tell employees what to do and to expect them to do it. It is well known that although an organization theoretically provides equal legitimating power to all administrators at the same level, the administrators do not in fact remain equal.

For example, a board of directors that controls five nursing facilities, in theory delegates equal authority to the administrators to act on its behalf in the five facilities. Some of these five administrators might have firm control over employee behavior, while others might be having difficulty convincing employees to do what they request. Why would that be?

RECIPROCITY

Power is a reciprocal relationship. The board of directors or the owners can confer power on the administrator, but the employees and patients/residents must accept that power as permissible if it is to be meaningful. This does not imply disrespect or chaos. The concept of authority or power is more complicated than the mere announcement that power has been given to the administrator by the board or the owners.

French and Raven (1960), Robey (1982), and other writers have identified at least five types of power: legitimate, reward, punishment (coercive), referent, and expert. In light of this, it is important for administrators to be familiar with these types of power and their applications.

Legitimate Power

This describes authority given to a particular position and is associated with the person's position in the organization (Argenti, 1994; Johns &

Saks, 2001). Organizations expect each person to yield to the appropriate authority of others. The administrator has more legitimate power than the director of nurses and so on. When employees or residents/patients respond to legitimate power, their actions are motivated by the level or position of the manager, not to any personality, knowledge, or other characteristics of that person.

Reward Power

The fact that reward is a second type of power is testimony to the mundane reality that employees do not always respond correctly. Administrators are given reward power to induce or persuade employees or patients/residents to do what the administrator asks. If not, certain desired approval(s) may be withheld (Robey, 1982). For example, if the administrator has authority to give a 15% year-end cash bonus to the three supervisors who have best achieved the facility's goals (translation: those who most often responded acceptably to the administrator's instructions), then that administrator has reward power.

Punishment Power

Sometimes known as coercive power, this type of power exists when the employee believes that a manager has the ability (and inclination) to punish unacceptable behaviors. The ultimate punishment power is firing the employee or requiring the resident to leave the facility, but there are many intermediate, less drastic means. Employees who do not observe the manager's rules for functioning in the facility may receive a written warning, a copy of which is placed in the human resources file. Use of punishment power is normally a last resort, after other uses of power have failed. Extensive use of punishment power leads to distrust and fear (Argenti, 1994; Johns & Saks, 2001), which are clearly not conducive to quality resident care.

Referent Power

The power to influence is often based on liking or identifying with another person. When the employees like the administrator and identify with her, they are more apt to do what she wishes. Referent power exists to the degree that employees and residents/patients identify with the administrator. This is both simple and powerful. Employees who do not admire an administrator or do not identify with her are more difficult to control, that is to make them do their work as the organization wishes (Johns & Saks, 2001).

Expert Power

Power can derive from recognition by the employees and residents/patients that the administrator is very skillful, has had considerable training, and is quite knowledgeable in the field of nursing home administration. For the nurse, this acknowledgment comes from the registered-nurse license, and for the physician the license to practice medicine (Johns & Saks, 2001).

POWER FROM OUTSIDE THE ORGANIZATION

It is important to note that expert and referent power, to the extent they are present in the facility, are additions to the power of organizationally given rewards and punishments because expert and referent power cannot be conferred by the organization (Katz & Kahn, 1967). There is literally an increase in the amount of power or control that can be exerted over the personnel and patients/residents, and it is a persistent factor in increased organizational performance.

Expert and referent power can be substituted for power based on punishment. This can mean fewer negative or unintended organizational consequences. It is desirable to promote referent power in addition to, or instead of, power based on rewards and punishment or organizational dictates. Remember, the goal of the administrator is to motivate the members of the organization to achieve the organization's goals.

Expert and referent power are available to all members of the staff. Referent power, in particular, depends on personal and group characteristics and is available to *peers* in the organization. Peer influence is often more readily accepted than influence from superiors. If, for example, one of the nurses is particularly skillful in creating a cheerful atmosphere in the facility, his leadership through referent power gives the nursing facility greater control over the quality of life achieved.

THE ADMINISTRATOR'S POWER IS REAL

Administrators do have power over other people's lives. Christensen, Berg, and Salter (1980) have characterized the power of the chief administrator as potentially "irresponsible" (p. 49). This is not necessarily owing to the use of power in any particular decision or even because of the administrators' motives, but because those affected by the decisions (the employees, patients/residents and their significant others, and even the board or owners) very often have little or no real immediate voice in making some decisions (e.g., when to finally tell employees that the cumulative effect of their behaviors renders them unfit to work at that facility). This can be especially true when most of the power is centralized in the office of the administrator. There are limitations, however, to the administrator's power.

THE ADMINISTRATOR'S POWER IS CONSTRAINED

As we discuss elsewhere, nursing facilities have quite complex lines of authority because of the presence of several professional groups within the facility: physicians, nurses, dietitians, physical therapists, and others. All these groups have professional organizations and loyalties that influence their behavior in the nursing facility. They have authority within their own professional spheres.

The facility administrator's authority is constantly constrained or limited by the influence of the medical, nursing, and other professions over the behavior of its physicians, nurses, nutritionists, and other professionals within the facility. Membership in these professional groups means that in the last analysis, the doctors' behavior may be governed more by professional standards that are enforced by the medical profession than by policies or goals of the nursing facility (Williams & Torrens, 1980). Similarly, nurses are governed by the state's nurse practice act and enforcement board, rather than by the policies or goals of the nursing facility when there is a conflict between the two. The same, of course, is true of the other professionals. This does not mean that the administrator has little or insufficient control, but rather that the authority or power to act is always circumscribed or constrained by the presence of controls exerted by professional groups (Gordon & Stryker, 1983).

The task of achieving control over the behavior of professional employees is a complicated one, requiring tact and ingenuity on the part of the administrator.

1.6.5 Communication Skills

Directing is the process of communicating the organizational objectives to the staff, residents/patients, and their significant others. *Communication* is the exchange of information and the transmission of meaning.

Communication is essential for the survival of any social system. The skills of the administrator in communicating what is to be accomplished and the manner in which it is to be carried out have much to do with the success of the administration in achieving the plan for the facility. Unless the plans of action are successfully communicated to the staff, the plans will, at worst, not be implemented at all, or at best, be only partially carried out.

Steps in the communication process are: (a) someone initiates it; (b) it is transmitted from its source to its destination; and (c) it has an impact on the recipient. Unless or until a communication has made its intended impact on the recipient, it has, for all intents and purposes, not taken place.

COMMUNICATION = INFORMATION = POWER

Communication is the transmission of information, and information is power because it provides a sounder basis for making judgments. The informed person is on more solid ground and is therefore more powerful. Withholding information is also a form of power, inasmuch as the person with the information is in a superior position to make decisions. Good communication is sometimes described as active listening, that is, listening with intensity, acceptance, empathy, and a willingness to assume responsibility for understanding the speaker's complete message (Argenti, 1994).

Systems of Communication

Organizations usually have at least two systems of communication: the formal and the informal communication processes.

The *formal communication* process closely resembles the formal organizational structure of the nursing facility (Dale, 1969). The administrator may send memoranda to the department managers, or the department managers may send them to their staff.

The *informal communication* process exists in nearly every organization. The social groups within the facility define the informal communication process (Dale, 1969; Mintzberg, 1979). Nurses chatting in the lounge communicate informally and exchange much important information in the course of casual conversation.

Direction of Flow

Communication is the flow of information in the organization that social scientists describe as flowing upward, downward, and horizontally. As the words themselves suggest, *upward communication* flows from subordinates to the next upper level of administration. *Downward communication* flows from upper-level management to lower-level members of the staff. *Horizontal communication* is information flowing between persons of equal rank or status.

The closer a person gets to the organizational center of control, the more pronounced the emphasis on the exchange of information. Administrators process information and use it in their decision making. Communicating is at the heart of the management process.

Communicating is an art that managers must master. Communications between administrators and personnel are full of subtleties and shades of meaning. Most communication also has numerous levels of meaning and function and is essential to building a relationship. Any act of communication may answer a question at the moment, but it has different meanings for the persons involved. Managers need to be aware that there are many barriers to full, clear communication. Seldom does any single communication have only one level of meaning (Johns & Saks, 2001; Kotter, 1982).

Barriers to Communication

Agenda Carrying. Each person has her own agenda in every communication situation, is preoccupied with her own concerns and life experiences. The individual filters what is communicated by means of her own perceptions.

Selective Hearing. People hear selectively; that is, they tend to hear what they want to hear, thereby filtering out the unpleasant. A nursing supervisor may wish to communicate to an aide dissatisfaction with one aspect of the aide's performance. To soften the effect, the supervisor may first praise the employee for some other work. The employee may hear the praise and effectively screen out the criticism.

Differences in Levels of Knowledge. Those who have only sketchy knowledge about a topic may process information quite differently from those who may be more knowledgeable. That is, the degree of sophistication varies among listeners and the information they process from a single communication may differ significantly.

The Filter Effect. The manager may be told what the employees believe she wants to hear. It is not easy to give bad news to a superior when one already knows such news is not welcome. Ancient Greek literature recounts that frequently the messenger who brought bad news to the king was killed. The implication of this reaction has not been lost on most organizational members.

It seems that no matter how much middle- and upper-level administrators insist they want to hear bad as well as good news, the employees filter the information toward the known bias of the next level(s) of management. When there are several layers of management through which unwelcome news must filter, the upper management may receive little accurate information. (This is another good reason for the administrator to manage by walking around doing naive listening in the hallways.)

Subgroup Allegiance. Each one of the subgroups in the organization (nurses, housekeepers, patients/residents on a hall) demands allegiance from its members. Tangible and intangible rewards are given in each group, so when a communication arrives it is interpreted in light of the goals and needs of each subgroup and usually not from the viewpoint of the organization as a whole (Johns & Saks, 2001).

Jay Jackson, in *The Organization and Its Communication Problems* (1960), concluded the following:

• People communicate far more with members of their own subgroup than with any other persons (e.g., the nurses have difficulty in learning what the nurses' aides are thinking and feeling)
• People prefer to communicate with someone of higher status than themselves (the aides prefer to talk to the nurses).
• People try to avoid having communication with those lower in status than themselves (the nurses prefer to talk to the doctors, not to the aides except when giving instructions to them).
• People will communicate with those who will help them achieve their goals (persons of higher status have power to create either gratifying or depriving experiences.
• People communicate with those who can make them feel more secure and avoid those who make them anxious. (pp. 443–456)

Status Distance. The nursing home staff is comprised of a broad range of professional and nonprofessional groups (Johns & Saks, 2001). At the top of the status ladder is the physician on whose orders the majority of nursing facility activities depend. Numerous health professionals at the middle level are present in the facility: nurses, geriatric nurse practitioners, RNs, LPNs, therapists of several types, (e.g., physical, occupational, and recreational), dietitians, pharmacists, physician assistants, and others. Toward the lower end of the status ladder are the nurses' aides and housekeepers, few of whom have any formal training. It is difficult for lower-level employees to communicate upward. The administrator must be aware of the status sensitivities of these many groups and be capable of successfully fostering the needed communication among all of them.

Language Barrier. Doctors and nurses speak "medicalese." The pharmacists speak yet another language, and physical therapists have their jargon (Johns & Saks, 2001). In short, given the great variety of professional specialists who must by regulation be employed or retained as consultants, the nursing home administrator and the staff who deal with them have an especially difficult task in assuring that resident care is not compromised through miscommunication among these occupations.

Self-protection. People often fail to communicate information that might reflect badly on them, their friends, or the organization (translation: the administrator should assure herself that the accident report portrays what actually occurred).

Information Overload. The abundance of information flowing in the facility (as many as 50 to 100 separate forms) may produce an information overload that results in the compromised ability of staff to distinguish among communications requiring prioritizing and attention. Bad news travels fast. Good news hardly travels at all.

Others. The administrator must bear in mind that all communication is multidimensional and needs appropriate interpretation to be of use. In sending out a memorandum to employees or engaging in any communication, the administrator must take into account that its effect depends at least on the following:

- The feelings and attitudes of the parties toward each other
- expectations
- how well the subordinate's needs are being met by the organization: if the nursing facility is supportive, the employee receiving administrative communications may be less defensive and more problem-oriented, that is, readier to absorb the communication and comply with the organization's request.

1.6.6 Organizational Norms and Values

DEVELOPING LOYALTY TO FACILITY GOALS

Administering an organization such as a nursing home facility is a complicated process. We have discussed some of the problems encountered by administrators as they attempt to lead employees to perform the tasks required. One of the impediments to accomplishing this is that the organization can never count on the individual employee's undivided attention. This is known as the concept of partial inclusion, or the segmental involvement of people in the job role.

LIMITATIONS ON EMPLOYEE PARTICIPATION

The nursing home defines behaviors that command only a portion of a person's 24–hour day. The facility asks only that during each shift employees perform the tasks or roles prescribed for them and that they have agreed to do (Pfeffer & Salanick, 1978). Unavoidably, however, the whole person must be brought into the work situation (Katz & Kahn, 1967). To deal with this, the employee is asked to set aside the non-job-related aspects of life while at work. This is literally a depersonalizing demand, which most employees find difficult to accomplish, so informal organizations within the organization develop in defense of personal identity.

The result is that people behave less as members of the nursing facility and more in terms of some compromise of their many commitments. For example, when asked about the sources of satisfaction from their jobs, employees often rate their interpersonal relationships with their fellow employees as the most important aspect of their work. Association with the patients/residents follows, while the goals and values of the nursing home facility itself tend to be somewhat low on the list of employee motivation. Administrators and supervisors engage in a constant struggle to gain employee loyalty to the goals of the facility.

There is yet another important limitation to employees' full participation. People tend to interpret the facility as a whole from the viewpoint of their particular section of the organization. This is another reason that upper-level administrators who collect information only from their immediate subordinates may never know what is actually going on.

People tend to exaggerate their importance to the organization as a whole. Loyalties develop to the work area rather than to the whole facility, which is a major source of conflict among departments. The nursing department views the organization from its unique perspective, as do the maintenance, food service, and other sections.

To enable staff to accomplish the necessary work, organizations develop and specify roles (job descriptions) that are carefully prescribed forms of behavior associated with the tasks the organization wants performed. *Roles* are standardized patterns of required behavior (Katz & Kahn, 1967). The nurse's aide is told very clearly what his role is during the 8 hours on the job.

Connecting Roles to Norms

To build loyalty, organizations try to identify roles and the persons filling them with the *norms* or values of the organization, the general expectations for all employees.

Professional standards for nurses and nurse's aides are example of such norms, which are behavior patterns that all members of the group are expected to adhere to. Respecting the personal privacy of patients would be an example of such a norm. By standing in a checkout line in all his Wal-Mart stores each year, Sam Walton was constantly teaching and reinforcing an important norm: Assure that checkout is a pleasant experience, thus stimulating the customer to feel favorable toward Wal-Mart.

Norms are justified by *values*, which are more generalized statements about the behavior expected from staff members. Values furnish the rationale for the normative requirements. Treating all patients with respect for their rights as persons is an example of a broad value statement, justifying the more specific norm that nursing personnel ought to respect each resident's personal privacy. For Sam Walton, building customer loyalty and repeat business might be the general value under which he established a pleasant checkout experience as a norm to be enforced.

System norms and values are attempts to connect employees with the system so that they remain within system values while carrying out their role assignments. It could be said that norms and values furnish "cognitive road maps" (ways to think about the organization and its goals) help personnel adjust to the system.

Nursing facilities' norms and goals revolve around providing the highest quality of life possible for residents. Under Tag F241 the federal government defines resident dignity as caring for residents in a manner and in an environment that maintains or enhances dignity and respect in full recognition of his or her individuality. This involves assisting residents to be well groomed and to dress appropriately, promoting independence in dining and allowing private space and property; speaking and listening respectfully, and focusing on the individual's communication. In 1993, 19.1% of facilities received deficiencies for this, declining to 13.2% in 1996, and rising to 16.3% in 1999.

The reader may want to study Table 1-1, which tracks deficiencies for quality of life by state from 1993 through 1999. Dignity, like many of the federal standards, is a complex concept, interpreted differently state to state and over time. Using the same federal definition, some states recorded dramatic decreases in dignity deficiencies, while other states recorded dramatic increases over the same period of time using the same criteria.

Table 1-1. Percentage of Nursing Facilities in the U.S.
Deficiency Group = Quality of Life: Dignity: F241, 1993–1999

State	Percentage of Facilities with Deficiencies						
	1993	1994	1995	1996	1997	1998	1999
AK	8.3	14.3	7.7	0.0	7.1	7.1	21.4
AL	18.0	21.2	14.1	13.9	12.8	9.7	18.2
AR	6.3	11.2	12.7	9.4	12.9	12.7	11.1
AZ	19.5	29.6	26.8	19.7	16.1	13.2	27.6
CA	52.5	52.1	44.1	40.9	38.9	36.7	40.1
CO	17.0	5.1	4.9	7.4	6.3	6.1	7.3
CT	17.7	4.7	4.0	6.1	4.0	4.0	13.4
DC	66.7	33.3	46.2	16.7	9.1	0.0	0.0
DE	2.7	20.9	9.1	24.3	14.3	25.9	8.8
FL	13.6	23.5	19.7	19.8	22.7	24.7	24.0
GA	15.0	16.6	18.4	9.3	7.7	6.9	9.8
HI	32.0	34.6	40.5	25.0	26.2	43.2	41.0
IA	7.8	6.3	4.9	7.0	6.4	4.3	4.2
ID	27.7	12.8	18.8	9.5	11.7	19.0	19.2
IL	25.4	23.4	23.8	18.6	16.0	21.0	21.1
IN	20.7	21.8	18.0	13.0	16.4	18.3	17.9
KS	20.9	19.1	16.4	9.9	9.2	9.0	8.5
KY	8.5	10.8	9.4	5.0	6.2	14.1	19.9
LA	9.8	9.2	14.1	9.7	9.2	9.1	13.1
MA	10.6	5.7	8.7	4.6	2.6	4.0	5.6
MD	6.3	7.0	16.1	7.2	4.2	7.0	5.2
ME	8.8	17.6	14.8	7.2	4.8	12.7	14.9
MI	23.9	18.2	24.3	14.4	18.5	20.8	25.9
MN	19.2	15.0	16.6	14.2	9.5	14.5	13.7
MO	27.0	13.4	13.1	13.2	8.8	10.6	10.8
MS	39.0	27.2	20.6	8.9	5.5	6.0	18.1
MT	14.7	13.5	11.0	6.5	7.4	5.4	5.2
NC	11.8	14.1	15.3	20.8	24.5	29.9	35.6
ND	7.5	18.5	14.5	24.1	26.7	22.7	18A
NE	13.7	10.9	8.0	8.7	4.3	5.2	6.1
NH	3.0	6.0	0.0	1.4	5.3	1.3	7.6
NJ	9.9	12.2	20.8	12.0	8.6	6.9	8.7
NM	13.0	15.6	10.4	8.9	9.5	24.2	20.8
NV	38.7	65.0	41.7	38.5	34.2	26.8	32.5
NY	9.2	9.4	15.9	12.2	10.0	7.0	14.8
OH	23.0	21.7	19.9	12.1	9.3	10.8	14.7
OK	1.2	5.9	6.0	6.3	4.7	7.4	12.0
OR	8.3	8.7	15.3	14.9	16.4	14.8	24.6

Table 1-1. (Continued)

State	Percent of Facilities with Deficiencies						
	1993	1994	1995	1996	1997	1998	1999
PA	22.8	19.9	13.4	7.5	7.0	72	8.4
RI	15.6	9.8	4.9	1.2	2.2	4.5	5.4
SC	8.1	12.7	18.2	24.8	32.0	23.3	34.7
SD	12.0	12.3	11.7	7.0	3.0	7.0	3.5
TN	20.4	20.5	23.3	14.8	5.3	8.3	9.8
TX	12.1	14.8	11.4	4.1	6.8	7.5	8.2
UT	17.0	12.2	27.6	17.7	14.3	29.2	18.9
VA	10.7	12.5	12.6	10.3	6.8	5.6	5.0
VT	7.3	5.6	27.5	5.4	5.4	11.8	4.8
WA	23.6	19.3	24.5	19.5	29.0	26.2	34.7
W1	14.7	7.5	6.3	5.1	6.5	6.4	6.5
WV	21.3	21.9	16.4	9.1	11.5	11.6	14.2
WY	39.3	29.4	42.1	8.1	41.7	32.5	16.7
US	19.1	18.5	17.7	13.7	13.2	14.1	16.3

Nursing Facilities, Staffing, Residents and Facility Deficiencies, 1993–1999
Department of Social & Behavioral Sciences
University of California San Francisco

Justification of the Facility: "Soft" and "Hard"

Another contribution of organizational norms and values is the moral or social justification for the activities of the nursing facility. This is often in the form of a *mission statement,* which defines the purposes and values held by the facility. The mission statement often appears at the front of the human resources handbook and is the first impression the prospective employee has of the purposes of the facility.

When nursing homes are attacked in the newspapers or subjected to public criticism, staff members look to their administrators for reaffirmation of the facility's worth, enabling them to feel good about themselves and their work there.

The administrator demonstrates what is important—the values that actually guide day-to-day staff behavior—by the way she behaves and what she gives attention to. If the administrator constantly moves around the facility assuring that each resident is getting quality care and enjoying a high quality of life, the employees will probably follow suit. Likewise, if the administrator concentrates instead on getting the paperwork done, meeting regulations, and saving money, that is what the staff will give their attention to. To develop pride in the facility and enthusiasm for its works is the goal of *people management.*

When it comes to achieving long-term success with personnel, soft is hard. In other words, quality care and a high quality of life are soft, but the administrator must be uncompromising and implacable in implementing them. Administrators care deeply about and respect their staff and residents/patients. Yet they must enforce a no-excuses environment when it comes to patient care. The successful administrator is at once tough on values and tender in support of staff who try to implement those values.

In the view of federal nursing home surveyors the nation's nursing home administrators were enforcing a no-excuses approach to meeting residents daily living needs (such as grooming and personal and oral hygiene) 92% of the time in 1993, but only 86% of the time in 1999 (Harrington et al., 2000).

Dreams, Vision, Goals

Another way to conceptualize values, norms, and roles is to equate them to dreams, or vision, goals and behaviors (mentioned elsewhere in this text). Employees are more motivated by and able to accept a vision or dream held by the facility. A dream or vision is a motivating abstract or belief. Dr. Martin Luther King, Jr. could not have motivated the unprecedented number of demonstrators from the steps of the Lincoln Memorial by telling the marchers that he had this or that goal or this or that plan of action. Rather, he moved them by saying that he had a dream, a dream of equality for all Americans. In the same way, a vision of constantly improving the daily life experiences of patients/residents and staff in the facility can be motivating. Specific goals, such as having a full activities program, are secondary to the dream. Goals give employees a target to shoot for and provide feedback, but goals must be guided by something larger— a dream or vision that inspires. Dreams, then, can become goals with wings (Kriegel, 1991), and each goal is a step toward that dream.

Most nursing home corporations publish mission statements that resemble more a list of goals more than a vision or dream (for example, "We seek to be the provider of choice for each community in which we have a facility"). This is fine for the corporate level, but not very motivating to the nursing assistants in their day-to-day struggles to provide care. Deming has observed that goal statements from the corporate level seldom motivate. Many local facilities have corporate goal statements in large print on well-designed wall posters, but these may not be their own goals. Corporate-generated goal statements are subject to the NIH phenomenon: Not Invented Here. Each facility must generate its own vision of what it is seeking.

One major nursing home chain does have a corporate vision that can motivate all employees, as long as the highest level of management stands behind it: "Whatever it takes." With that motto the corporation promises to assist every employee in giving the best quality of care possible to their residents/patients by means of corporate commitment to assist each employee, no matter what it takes. As long as each employee believes he will be supported in his own individual efforts to improve the daily lives of residents/patients and staff, each employee can participate in the dream.

WHY ORGANIZATIONS NEED ADMINISTRATIVE LEADERSHIP

Once all the plans have been developed and the staff hired and trained, why doesn't the organization just run smoothly? Although there are a number of dimensions in any answer to this question, we will discuss only the few that seem especially relevant.

All organizational designs are imperfect (Demski, 1980; Hitt et al., 2001). Differences among the organizational chart, the written policies, and the organization's actual functioning are easily seen. It is commonly recognized that after being instructed by the supervisor, the new worker turns to the groups members to learn what the job requirements really are.

Actual behavior, the actual functioning of the organization, is infinitely more complex, inconclusive, and variable than the plan. Organizational sabotage is an illustration of this is. Any worker who wants to sabotage the facility can do so by merely following organizational law to the letter—doing what is formally stipulated, no more and no less.

Like all organizations, nursing facilities need administrative leadership to cope with the constantly changing external environment that requires internal adjustments. When, for example, three new assisted living facilities open in an area and one's own occupancy rate drops from 92% to 72%, organizational leadership is in order.

Organizations also need leadership to accommodate the changes constantly occurring within. Employees retire or find work elsewhere, the needs of staff and residents/patients change, conflicts develop, physical systems break down, and decisions to repair or replace are called for.

As Kriegel has pointed out, change is here to stay. To meet current challenges it is necessary to adapt constantly. U.S. business leader J. B. Fuqua has observed that whether one feels one has reached the top, or is still climbing, one cannot stay still. The old saying "If it ain't broke, don't fix it" needs to be changed: "If you don't fix it all the time, it will break" (Kriegel, 1991).

1.6.7 Related Concepts

We turn now to several additional concepts worth reviewing in any consideration of attempts by administrators to direct the efforts of the organization.

CORPORATE CULTURE

Corporate culture is the overall style or atmosphere of a facility. The corporate culture governs how people relate to each other in the organization: "This is how we do things in this facility." Corporate culture is important to the organization's survival. The corporate culture at IBM, for example, shifted dramatically from its commitment to "respect the individual" once the Watsons retired (Argenti, 1994).

DELEGATION

The concept of *delegation* is to permit decisions to be made at the lowest possible level. Such authority is given to middle- and lower-level managers, allowing them to make decisions for the organization as appropriate. The essential issue is the determination of the nature of the decisions to be made at whatever level (Johns & Saks, 2001; Meal, 1984; Mintzberg, 1979).

Delegating can be both beneficial and disadvantageous. At optimum operation, delegation should channel the decision making to staff members who are best informed and most skilled at making a particular decision or set of decisions. The negative aspect of this practice is that because the managers have only a partial view of the organization, they consciously or unconsciously may make decisions in a manner that maximizes their area within the organization to the possible detriment of the facility as a whole.

Ultimate responsibility cannot be delegated. The chief administrator is held accountable for the acts of all persons working under facility auspices.

UNITY OF COMMAND

The concept of unity of command emphasizes the importance of each person's being accountable to only one supervisor (Hitt et al., 2001;

Simon, 1960). It is functionally difficult for any employee to answer to two managers, so the facility must be organized to assure this relationship (Robey, 1982).

SPAN OF CONTROL

How many immediate subordinates with interrelated work should a manager supervise? This has been a point of contention for decades. The World War I British general Sir Ian Hamilton insisted that six was the maximum span of control (Argenti, 1994; Hitt et al., 2001); others have proposed different numbers. Decisions in the 1970s by a number of state governments illustrate this issue. Several states had expanded operations to the point that perhaps 100 persons were reporting directly to the governor. It was realized that in this circumstance no one, in actual practice, was supervising these 100 persons. To regain control, several states reconstituted their organizational pattern to include a department of human resources to whose supervisor most of the former 100 reported, leaving perhaps a dozen persons reporting directly to the governor. In the final analysis, the administrator must be certain that each employee is effectively supervised (Robey, 1982).

SHORT CHAIN OF COMMAND

This principle asserts that there should be as few levels of management as possible between the chief administrator and the rank and file (Dale, 1969). Certainly, for the communication purposes of upper-level management, this seems a good principle to follow. It minimizes the number of interpreters through whom information for upper-level managers must be sifted (Johns & Saks, 2001).

BALANCE

Advocates of the principle of balance (Dale, 1969) assert that there is a need for continual surveillance to maintain balance among the following:

- size of the various departments
- standardization of procedures and flexibility
- centralization and decentralization
- span of control and short chain of command

MANAGEMENT BY OBJECTIVES (MBO)

The management-by-objectives (MBO) approach emphasizes setting specific, jointly developed goals with a time period for goal achievement and performance feedback (Argenti, 1994). The theory is to create a process of participation beginning with the lowest levels of workers whose recommendations are constantly moved upward until final selection of the goals to be put into place is made by upper management.

Management by objectives was first put into practice (under this rubric) by Lyndon B. Johnson. As president of the United States he wished to gain meaningful control of the largest bureaucracy under his management, now known as the Department of Health and Human Services (DHHS) (Johns & Saks, 2001).

Although MBO, in theory, meaningfully involves lowest level employees and managers in recommending organizational goals, the real effect is to shift power upward (Swiss, 1983). This occurs because it is the upper-level managers who actually make the final choice among (and modify if necessary) recommendations from the lower levels.

MANAGEMENT INFORMATION SYSTEMS (MIS)

The phrase *management information systems* (MIS) originally came into the literature as a description of computer-based information processing for managers in making their decisions (Argenti, 1994; Dearden & McFarlan, 1966). Withington (1966) defined MIS as the study of how the organization communicates and processes information to maximize the effectiveness of management and to further the objectives of the organization.

The point recognized in MIS is that the manager needs a constant rationalized and organized flow of information in order to make appropriate decisions. In Levey & Loomba's view,, (1973), developing an MIS is as simple as

1. determining one's need for information
2. identifying the sources of information
3. deciding on the amount, form, and frequency of information needed
4. choosing the means of information processing
5. implementing the system

MANAGEMENT BY EXCEPTION

Every day the manager receives numerous verbal and written reports, which usually contain routine information about the functioning of the facility. One way managers can effectively use their time is by turning their attention to any exceptions in the plan of action. If the census, the number of meals served, or their costs are within plan, there may be no need for action. Countless detailed tasks are being completed in acceptable fashion by the staff every day. What merits the administrator's attention are the exceptions to the policies and plans of action originally established for the organization.

The budget is one of the more useful tools for spotting exceptions (Gordon & Stryker, 1983). Getting information about the amount of money that has been spent in the last time period is a reasonably exact control measurement. As long as any department is spending within the agreed-upon budget there may be no need for the administrator's attention. But whenever a departmental budget falls short or exceeds the amounts allocated to it, the administrator should give attention to the exception and take whatever steps necessary to bring expenditures within the budgeted limits. For example, nursing's having to hire an indeterminate number of temporary nurses from an agency is a frequent cause of budget overage. However, too little expenditure by nursing, or, say, by the food service, might be as much a cause for alarm as too great an expenditure. In the first case the facility might be short on the required number of nursing personnel hours per day, and in the second instance the quality of food being purchased and prepared might be unsatisfactory.

Management by exception does not mean that the routine and within-specification behaviors of the facility remain unexamined. It is the routine behaviors of the organization that are being examined for deviations from the norm.

PERT/CPM

Program Evaluation and Review Technique (PERT) and Critical Path Method (CPM) are control tools that show the relationship among the activities that make up a project. The renovation of a wing of a facility, for example, may be mapped out with time estimates for completion of each necessary step—the critical path—which aids in allocating resources (Argenti, 1991).

CONCEPTS OF EFFICIENCY AND EFFECTIVENESS

Efficiency is the ability to produce the desired effect with a minimum of effort, expense, or waste. (*Webster's New World Dictionary,* 1968). Efficiency can be measured by the ratio of effective work to the energy expended in producing it. In systems terms this simply means getting the maximum outputs with the minimum inputs (Hitt et al., 2001; Pfeffer & Salanick, 1978).

Effectiveness is the power or ability to bring about the desired results. A nursing home that sets a goal of achieving excellence in resident care and then does so is said to be effective (Pfeffer & Salanick, 1978). It may not, however, be efficiently achieving excellence of patient care. The home may, for example, be employing a large number of nurses and aides to accomplish excellence in resident care. Yet studies in human resources reveal that when more people are placed on a work shift than are needed, the quality of care is not necessarily improved. The staff may simply divide the work up to lighten the load for everyone or may take more frequent breaks and not actually give additional attention to the residents/patients. In this case, the too heavy staff/resident ratio may lead to both inefficiency and ineffectiveness (Robey, 1982).

The solution is to assign the optimum known number of staff needed to provide excellent care to a specified number of patients/residents, and then manage their time so that the amount of work and quality are optimized. In this way, the manager achieves both efficiency (the desired effect with a minimum of effort, expense, or waste) and effectiveness (the desired results). Given enough resources and appropriate consultation, almost any nursing home administrator can achieve effectiveness. What is essential today is to be both effective and efficient.

1.6.8 History of the Concept of Management

Administrators have been managing organizations, large and small, for thousands of years. It is believed that some 5,000 years ago the Sumerian civilization (Iran and Iraq today) developed a script to control business accounts (George, 1972). Clay tablets recording business transactions of that ancient time have been found by archaeologists. We have records of Cheops, an Egyptian king who built the Great Pyramid about 2900 B.C. We know that this monument covered 13 acres and employed 100,000 laborers for 20 years and that nearly 9,000 lower-, middle-, and upper-level managers administered the project (George, 1972). In ancient Greece, music was used to govern motions in the production lines. In the fifth century B.C., Plato reports in *The Republic* a dialogue between Socrates and a Greek general about the extent to which management is a transferable skill. The general, it seems, was incensed that the Athenian Assembly had just appointed as the commander-in-chief of the army the manager of the Athenian chorus, who had shown himself to be an excellent fundraiser and chorus director. Socrates argued that if the man could run the chorus well and raise the necessary revenue, then he could also be a good general (George, 1972). Fifteen upper-level executives of General Motors more recently expressed the same view of their own ability to manage almost anything during a 15-month study of their skills, which was conducted by a Harvard Business School professor (Kotter, 1982). Managers' opinions of their capabilities have not changed much over the last 5,000 years.

SCIENTIFIC MANAGEMENT

By the 1800s the early scientific management movement was underway in England as an outgrowth of the industrial revolution. The managers at Soho Foundry of Boulton, Watt and Co. were concerned with market research and forecasting, planned site location, machine layout study, production standards and planning, standard components, cost controls, cost accounting, employee training, work study and incentives and employee welfare (Argenti, 1994; George, 1972).

During that epoch a management literature began to appear, but there was little recognition of the principles of management we have discussed. Current management philosophy in the West seems to have evolved from four schools of thought, although various writers refine them even further (Levey & Loomba).

HUMAN RELATIONS MANAGEMENT

At the end of the 19th century a group of writers emerged who believed management could be an exact science. They focused on the physical activities involved in production (Drucker, 1954; George, 1972). Frederic Taylor conducted research in a Philadelphia machine shop, demonstrating with time and motion studies that work then done by as many as 450 shovelers at Bethlehem Steel could be accomplished by as few as 150, provided they received instructions to improve their effort. Frank Gilbreth's time and motion studies are well known, and Henry Gantt developed his now widely used Gantt Chart with its task and bonus plan and standard hour concept.

Early in the 20th century, Henri Fayol identified management "universals:" to plan, to organize, to command (tell others), and to coordinate (control). Fayol thus developed one of the earliest formulations of a general theory of management. "Process school" members, such as Fayol and James Mooney, focused on departmentalization, coordination, and organizational form—the issues we have discussed under "organizing in this book." (Johns & Saks, 2001).

During the 1920s and 1930s, a group of theorists led by Elton Mayo described management as consisting primarily of human relations skills. According to them, successful organizations fulfill not only the employees' economic needs but also their social and psychological needs.

Sponsored by the National Research Council, Mayo conducted several experiments at the Hawthorne manufacturing plant to determine the effect of illumination on output (Johns & Saks, 2001). He found that production rose for the experimental group when illumination was increased. But the control group also produced more, although it had no increase in illumination. Illumination was then reduced to the barest minimum in both groups, yet their production continued to rise, the apparent reason being the increased attention they were given by the managers (George). Mayo's experiments convinced him that human factors exercise the most powerful influence on employee behavior because of the workers need to participate in social groups. Work arrangements, he concluded, besides meeting production requirements, must meet the employee's need for social satisfaction on the job. Unfortunately, the "behavioral school" experienced a low predictability rate (Barnard, 1938; Dale, 1969; Johns & Saks, 2001).

COMPUTERS AND MANAGEMENT

Various names are applied to management theory that emerged after World War II (Johns & Saks, 2001; Levey & Loomba, 1973). Its major thrust has been systems theory, which is our approach here, and mathematical quantification is the hallmark of these theories. This is made possible by the development of computers that are capable of processing enormous quantities of intricate data (Johns & Saks, 2001). Some members of the management science schools believe that almost everything can be quantified, which may be so. However, the problem remains that people assign the mathematical weights to each factor quantified, and then others must interpret for themselves the meaning they attach to the quantified results (Demski, 1980).

Whatever one's personal views about quantification, it is clear that computers are affording managers access to information that previously was too laborious, too expensive, or too slow to obtain on a timely basis (Miller & Barry, 1979). Computers are already a major management tool at regional and national offices of nursing home chains. Computerization of the local nursing facility is now nearly mandatory to process the minimum data set, patient care planning, and other types of necessary reporting. Jackson, Peter, Rosenberg, and Peck (1995) observed that computers are the only means to keep up with the regulatory process (p. 13). Others view the computer as a way to expand communication capabilities and perform data analyses that enhance decision making (Hegland, 1995; Johns & Saks, 2001).

Managing is an exceptionally complex, multidimensional task not yet fully understood by the social sciences. Much has been learned, however that can be useful to the nursing home administrator in his efforts to ensure a caring environment while running the nursing facility as a good business operation. Nursing facilities will, of necessity, enter the E-commerce business in seeking admissions and developing marketing strategies (Hitt et al., 2001). The internet is increasingly driving mergers and acquisitions in industry, and nursing homes are not exempt (Hitt et al., 2001).

Computer systems are now virtually mandatory at both the corporate and local facility level. Worker skill in the use of new technologies must be comprehended and supported by the administrator, including computer-aided med passes and government mandated computer-to-computer reporting not only for billing, but for resident care through the minimum data set (MDS) patient record (Maddox & Sussman, 2001; Noe et al., 2000).

The nursing facility front office will need to utilize advanced office technology to keep up with Medicare, Medicaid, and other third-party billing (Johns & Saks, 2001).

SUMMARY

In this section, we have examined a number of concepts: policy making, decision making (Argenti, 1994), styles, power, authority, need for communication skills, norms, and values. We have touched lightly on a number of concepts guiding the administrator in attempts to direct the efforts of the nursing facility and have indicated that the administrator, in providing day-to-day guidance for the staff, ensures that they know what is expected of them.

Having done this, administrators may be tempted to rest on their laurels. This could be a fatal error in judgment. We have demonstrated that organizations are volatile systems that may or may not respond to the administrator's direction. The only way an administrator can be certain that the nursing facility is in fact making appropriate progress toward implementing its policies and plans of action is by comparing the outputs (results of organizational work) with the intended results. This is the process of evaluating and controlling for quality.

1.7 Comparing

CONTROLLING QUALITY

Because all organizational designs are incomplete, the quest for quality is frustratingly elusive, both in industry and in the health care setting. The quest for quality in the nursing facility is especially challenging because of its organizational complexity and, more often than not, very limited resources.

Even so, or maybe because of this circumstance, perhaps the most valuable functions managers perform for the facility are comparing (evaluating) and controlling the quality of facility outputs. *Comparing* is judging the extent to which the actual results of the facility's efforts achieve the outcomes proposed in the plans. *Controlling* is successfully taking the steps necessary to adjust the policies and plans of action to achieve stated goals more satisfactorily.

One problem in controlling quality it that it obliges the manager to take sometimes unpleasant corrective actions to keep the facility on target. This may involve advising staff members that the work result is not suitable, or informing department managers that the actual outputs (level of performance) are unsatisfactory. This is invariably an awkward business and is often avoided by managers who hope the situation will correct itself or that the problem will simply disappear. But matters usually get worse and require attention for solution.

1.7.1 Some Requirements for Effective Control of Quality

We will discuss several of the current methods used for controlling quality such as the Deming method, benchmarking, reengineering, and Continuous Quality Improvement (CQI)/Total Quality Management (TQM) (Johns & Saks, 2001).

There are at least nine conditions that any method for effective control of quality should observe.

1. Goals must be translated into policies and plans of action that are clearly stated, known, and measurable.

2. The appropriate measurements must be identified. If the wrong measurements are used to compare actual to expected outputs, no quality control system, however sophisticated, can truly inform and manage quality.

3. Limits to deviations from the goal/policy/plan of action have to be set. The manager must have predetermined and known outside limits for each output (quality goal) being controlled.

4. Information in useful form must go to staff at appropriate levels. It needs to be timely, easily understood, and unambiguous, so that the employee cannot use lack of clarity as a pretext for nonconformity.

5. Policies of actions to be taken when limits are exceeded (quality not achieved) must be known to the managers responsible for controlling outputs. Clear statements of policies are crucial for influencing staff members to take corrective actions when needed.

6. Corrective actions must be taken. To maximize the probability that managers will take necessary corrective actions, an effective system of rewards and punishments is needed to encourage them to do so. When middle-and lower-level managers sense any softening in the administrator's determination to enforce the quality control policies, there will be a simultaneous softening of the quality control effort.

7. A system must be set up for the constant renewal of control measures to account for any changing organizational goals (as expressed in new or modified plans of action) that are responses to changes in the external or internal environments of the organization. Middle-and lower-level managers may interpret discarded portions of the quality control system as evidence that all of the quality control system is no longer in force. Eternal vigilance is the price of a quality control system that remains effective over an extended period of time.

8. To remain effective, the quality control mechanisms themselves must be functional and valued at each level of management to remain effective. If the staff responsible for enforcing quality controls do not feel the measures are acceptable and productive, excuses will be found not to rely on them.

9. Limitations of the scope and capabilities of the quality control system itself must be kept constantly in mind. They are, as we shall see, never perfect. It is not possible to devise an organizational quality control system that does not need the good judgement of concerned employees to arrive at an interpretation of what the organization "really wants" in any situation (Hitt et al., 2001; Zmud, 1983).

1.7.2 Diagnosing Organizational Quality

In caring for their patients, physicians base treatment protocols on their medical diagnoses, which they interpret from the patient's presenting symptoms. In the same way, administrators are organizational diagnosticians who manage the nursing home facility by using judgments based on their interpretation of presenting organizational symptoms. Physicians diagnose and treat patient illnesses; administrators diagnose and treat organizational illnesses. In the literature, organizational illnesses are often referred to as organizational pathologies. Organizational pathology is the study and diagnosis of what is believed to be a problem adversely affecting the nursing facility (Johns & Saks, 2001).

In part 5 we will explore resident care concepts, including such diagnoses as atherosclerosis (narrowing and hardening of the arteries, allowing less blood to flow), aortic stenosis (stiffening of the main blood vessel supplying the body, reducing the amount of blood reaching the limbs), and congestive heart failure (CHF, a progressive reduction of the heart's ability to pump enough blood), which often lead to peripheral vascular diseases (reduced blood flow to the limbs). Organizations suffer from similar pathologies (disease processes), reducing their effectiveness and ability to function.

Managers have always sought to achieve quality control in their organizations, but this remains one of the more elusive aspects of successful managing. A number of studies have been conducted to discover quality indicators for nursing facilities. One group of researchers followed 300 veterans who were discharged to 11 nursing homes for 6 months and arrived at three indices that significantly indicated nursing-home quality as measured by mortality: (a) number of registered nurse hours; (b) the nursing process itself; and (c) physical features supporting optimal functioning (Braun, 1991; Hitt et al., 2001).

THE W. EDWARDS DEMING APPROACH TO ASSURING QUALITY IN ORGANIZATIONS

Born in 1900, Dr. Deming helped the U.S. Census Bureau prepare for the 1940 census with statistical techniques that used sampling rather than 100% participation surveys. After World War II he was invited to Japan by the Supreme Command for the Allies to assist in preparations for the 1951 Japanese census. In brief, Dr. Deming became a major force in the quality control movement in Japan that is believed by many to have helped vault Japan into its position as a world leader in the production of quality products.

Dr. Deming was not "discovered" in the United States until his appearance on June 24, 1980, in a television documentary entitled "If Japan Can . . . Why Can't We?" (Molloy, 1994; Walton, 1986) This led to his immediate broad popularity in this country. Dr. Deming lectured to enthusiastic American corporate executives, even while wheelchair-bound, until a few weeks before his death at the age of 93. His 14 points and seven deadly organizational diseases, along with their potential application to the nursing home industry, are explored next and are described in Walton (1986, pp. 34–37ff.). At first blush, Deming's points may seem too focused on the manufacturing plant, yet the thrust of his observations have application to nursing facility operation.

Deming's Fourteen Points

1. *Create and publish to all employees a statement of the aims and purposes of the . . . organization. The management must demonstrate constantly their commitment to this statement.* The role of the corporation, Deming argued, rather than to make money, is to stay in business and provide jobs through innovation (Argenti, 1994), research, constant improvement, and maintenance. The nursing home chain's goal, then, is to stay in business (not to "provide skilled care" or, if publicly owned, to pay dividends) and to provide jobs. This is to be accomplished through innovation (discovering current health care needs and foreseeing future health care needs); research (finding out how effective current care is, finding new ways to give better care); constant improvement (of the experience of being a resident/patient in their facilities); and maintenance (keeping everything in working order).

2. *Learn the new philosophy, top management and everybody.* Don't tolerate poor care giving and sullen service to residents; mistakes and negativism in approaching residents and other staff are not acceptable.

3. *Understand the purpose of inspection, for improvement of processes and reduction of cost.* Focus on the resident's daily experience, not on nursing summaries and plans of care. Mass inspection means inspecting the product as it comes off the line or at major stages. Defective products are thrown out or reworked, which means paying employees to give less than quality care and then paying them again to correct poor care (preventing decubiti is easier and less expensive than curing decubiti), and this does not lead to corrective actions. Quality, he argues, comes not from inspections but from improvement of the process, that is, keep the focus on improving the care giving process, not on the quality of the nurses' notes or doctor's orders, but rather on achieving an improved level of care. Keep focused on improving the resident's daily experience.

4. *End the practice of awarding business on the basis of price tag alone.* Buying the lowest priced often means buying low quality. The goal should be to identify a single quality supplier for any one item in a long term relationship, for example, food vendors. The goal should be good, dependable quality of a long period of time, consistently good food supplies, medical supplies, physical therapy, pharmacy supplies, and the like.

5. *Improve constantly and forever the system of production and service.* Management's job is to continually look for ways to reduce waste and improve quality, that is, don't use expensive medicine cups as water cups while doing medication rounds.

6. *Institute training.* Too often nursing assistants, licensed practical nurses, and even the directors of nursing learn their jobs from workers who were never trained properly. Workers are forced to follow poor instruction sets and cannot do their jobs because no one told them how.

7. *Teach and institute leadership.* The nurse supervisor or department head's job is not to tell nursing assistants what to do or punish, but to lead, (i.e., to help employees do a better job), learning by objective methods who needs individual help (for example, sort out the nursing assistants whose work is not in an acceptable range). This will pay real dividends in safer resident care and reduce risks at a facility.

8. *Drive out fear. Create trust. Create a climate for innovation.* Create an atmosphere in which employees feel secure enough to ask questions, take positions, admit errors and learn by them, rather than whitewash get an incident or write an erroneous accident report.

9. *Optimize toward the aims and purposes of the company the efforts of teams, groups, staff areas.* Facility staff often compete or have goals that conflict: nursing versus dietary, nursing versus housekeeping (who cleans up the spill?), dietary versus activities, versus nursing versus housekeeping, and who is responsible for the resident's afternoon tea?

10. *Eliminate exhortations for the workforce.* Deming believed these never helped anybody do a good job; instead, let people put up their own slogans.

11. *Eliminate numerical quotas for production. Instead, learn and institute methods for improvement. Eliminate management by objectives. Instead, learn the capabilities of processes, and how to improve them.* Numbers take account only of numbers, not quality or methods. Quotas usually guarantee inefficiencies and high cost. Most CQI programs set numerical quotas in nearly every departmental area. Employees become focused on attaining these quotas themselves. Achieving the numerical goal becomes the employees' goal and focus, not improving the resident's daily experience. Deming agrees that the goal of quotas is laudable but can become ends in themselves, and the employee will meet the quota at any price, regardless of the damage to the facility (for example, the nurse who is determined to pass medications at or below the prescribed error rate disregarding a small crisis that needs managing during the medication pass).

12. *Remove barriers that rob people of pride of workmanship.* People are eager to do a good job and are distressed when they can't because of misguided supervisors, faulty equipment or defective materials. If there are too few nursing hours per resident day to permit the nursing assistants or the rest of the staff to make Mrs. Jones's experience that day a good one, they may use the proverbial excuse "We're working short today" in answer to numerous resident requests. Whenever possible, avoid using nursing pool personnel who don't know the residents and all too often don't care.

13. *Encourage education and self-improvement for everyone.* Both management and the staff will have to be educated in the new methods, including teamwork and statistical techniques.

14. *Take action to accomplish the transformation.* Deming, like most others who prescribe quality-improvement programs, emphasized a need to involve top management in any quality improvement effort, but emphasized that it takes both managers and the workers to succeed. (Melum & Sinioris, 1992, p. 222).

Seven Deadly Diseases

1. *Lack of constancy of purpose.* Keep the focus on staying in business, including long-range plans, not on making dividends next quarter or paying good dividends this year; that is, the workers need to feel that the corporation is preparing for the future and will stay in the business of giving health care.

2. *Emphasis on short-term profits.* Don't worry about paying a dividend.

3. *Evaluation by performance, merit rating, or annual review of performance.* These, Deming felt, destroy teamwork and nurture rivalry. Performance ratings build fear, leave people despondent, bitter, and beaten, and encourage mobility of management.

4. *Mobility of management.* Job-hoppers don't understand the facility and are not there long enough to follow through on long-term changes needed for quality and productivity (e.g., three directors of nurses in 1 year, three administrators in as many years).

5. *Running a company on visible figures alone.* The most important figures, Deming argued, are unknown and unknowable, such as, resident satisfaction. Point: The achievement of a nursing facility's staff cannot be reduced to numbers alone.

6. *Excessive medical costs.* What more should be said on this issue?

7. *Excessive costs of warranty, fueled by lawyers who work on contingency fee.* Successful malpractice suits against nursing facilities continue to raise the cost of required insurance.

To prescribe Deming's diagnosis for all corporations is like a physician writing the same prescriptions for all his/her patients regardless of the stage of the diseases the patients present. Deming was prescribing corrections to organizational illnesses that he felt existed in the United States. Essentially, he was pointing to excesses—good ideas taken too far, or becoming mindless rules in themselves. What's right and what's wrong with organizations changes over time, and like the swinging of a pendulum, so do Deming's list of deadly organizational diseases. But he has some enduring messages for American industry and the nursing facility, powerful reminders of how difficult it is for the facility to constantly focus on the resident/patient. Other analysts make different diagnoses and have written their own prescriptions to assist organizations in achieving and maintaining quality.

BENCHMARKING

Benchmarking is a management tool by which an organization seeks to improve its business practices by comparing them with the best practices of other organizations (Argenti, 1994; Hitt et al., 2001). The Westinghouse Corporation uses benchmarking as a quality control tool within its total quality improvement process for "identifying best practices, wherever they exist, implementing and communicating those practices throughout Westinghouse to improve competitive performance and preserve our core competencies" (Argenti, 1994).

A Five-Step Description

Benchmarking studies not only the very best practices of other corporations, but also seeks any clearly better practices as sufficient to justify a benchmarking effort. Spendolini (1992) describes benchmarking as consisting of five steps:

1. deciding what to benchmark
2. forming a team
3. identifying benchmark partners
4. collecting and analyzing the benchmarking information
5. implementing the new methodology (Spendolini, 1992).

Benchmarking is a measuring process resulting in comparing performance measures, but it also describes how the superior performance is attained. The practices that lead to exceptional performance are called enablers. Benchmarking, then, results in two types of outputs: (a) measures of comparative performance, and (b) enablers, the theory behind the more successful process being benchmarked.

A Four-Step Description

Another writer describes benchmarking as a four-step process (Argenti, pp. 61–62):

1. Selecting and defining the process to be studied. What should we benchmark? Who should we benchmark?
2. Gather as much information as possible about the process, then communicate with the organization being benchmarked through telephone surveys, written questionnaires, and on-site visits.
3. Analyze the information gained to determine the magnitude of the performance gap, and identify the process enablers that facilitated the performance improvement at the organization chosen as a benchmark.
4. Adapt, improve, and implement the benchmarked process in one's own organization.

For example, most major nursing home chains strive to serve a predominantly private-paying and Medicare eligible clientele. One chain has consistently achieved this to a far greater extent than most. Chains that, despite their goals, have a low census of private-paying and Medicare patients/residents might seek to benchmark the successful chain, that is, study and learn the process by which that one chain achieves the resident mix noticeably more successfully than the rest.

Benchmarking at St. Jude's: Nursing homes might benefit from the benchmarking effort of St. Jude's Hospital in southern California. Concerned that their admissions area might be discouraging patients by its complexity, cold attitudes, long waiting periods, and confusing directions, the hospital managers benchmarked hotels, the true professionals on admissions. Out of this effort came plans for a doorperson, a bellperson to carry bags, a concierge to advise about the hospital itself, and computerized admissions. Larger signs were installed in the lobby, which was freshly painted, and music now greets the incoming patients (Kriegel, 1991).

Deming warned that it is a hazard to copy, that it is necessary to understand the theory of what makes the benchmarked process more successful. He cautioned, "Adapt, don't adopt" (Argenti, 1994). The process enablers that result in high private census in a more successful nursing home chain reflect a specific business environment and corporate culture. It may or may not work when introduced into the chain seeking to raise its own private-paying census.

TOTAL QUALITY MANAGEMENT/CONTINUOUS QUALITY IMPROVEMENT

The earliest quality and quality-control publications that led to the current Total Quality Management (TQM) literature may have been initiated by Walter A. Shewhart at Bell Telephone Laboratories in the 1920s. His work was published as *Economic Control of Quality of Manufactured Product* in 1931 (Hitt et al., 2001; Melum & Sinioris, 1992). In his 1979 book, *Quality is Free: The Art of Making Quality Certain,* P. B. Crosby advocated 14 points somewhat similar to the Deming's (Melum, & Sinioris, 1992). An extensive literature on TQM has emerged and is explored in depth in the 1992 American Hospital Association book *Total Quality Management: the Health Care Pioneers* (see Melum & Sinioris, 1992; see also Molloy, 1994).

Definitional Difficulties

Total Quality Management is difficult to define precisely because it is a philosophy of total organizational involvement in improving all aspects of quality of service. There is no single set of steps that has gained broad acceptance as the TQM methodology. However, the basic concept is similar to Deming's fifth, point which is "improve constantly and forever the system of production and service." This view is that it is too expensive to maintain quality by inspections and more efficient to produce quality in the first place. To achieve this, responsibility for quality is ultimately placed with the workers who actually produce the service or product. This is sometimes called "quality at the source." In this scheme the quality departments are focused on training employees in quality control and implementing the quality control concepts throughout the organization (Noe et al., 2000). Employee empowerment in decision making, the use of teams in the organization, and the use of individual responsibility for services and customer service are characteristics of most TQM efforts (Argenti, 1994; Johns & Saks, 2001; Johns & Saks, 2001).

According to Melum and Sinioris (1992), TQM is a customer-driven approach that applies the scientific method to improve organizations' systems. In their view, the focus on quality is total, including every aspect of an organization—its services and products, its suppliers, business procedures, management systems, and human resources. To them, total quality management is a process of continuous improvement, a process of continuously striving to exceed customer expectations (see also Johnson, 1994). Problems in the organization are viewed as problems with the processes used, not with individuals, processes that can be improved using total quality management approaches.

Six Factors for Success

Six factors are viewed as keys to a successful Total Quality Management program.

1. *Visionary leadership:* This must come from the CEO, middle-and lower-level managers via a quality vision statement with goals. Deploy them throughout the organization to empower employees to implement TQM, to evaluate and recognize TQM progress, to promote commitment to customers, and to serve as role models of TQM behavior. CEO and managers act as coaches, not bosses. Coaching implies mentoring employees, assisting them in developing needed skills to perform their jobs (Argenti, 1994; Johns & Saks, 2001; Noe et al., 2000).

2. *Commitment to customers:* Anticipate, meet and exceed the expectations of internal and external customers, linking reward systems to customer satisfaction.

3. *Trained teams:* The entire workforce must participate in teams, applying TQM in their daily work. Use managers as trainers. Quality is the leading agenda item at all meetings.

4. *Physician involvement.* Involve physicians in TQM training so they function as TQM enablers for the nursing staff.

5. *Processes.* Have a management process in place that plans and organizes the overall managing of the organization. Have an improvement process that solves specific problems, improves specific processes, and maintains these changes over time.

6. *Avoid a separate TQM system.* Make the TQM management the sole management process in the organization.

Experience suggests that it takes 5 to 10 years to fully implement a TQM process. The three steps to accomplish this grassroots transformation are

1. Direct TQM through the quality implementation plan.
2. Educate on quality to empower people.
3. Align management systems to integrate and sustain TQM (Melum & Sinioris, 1992).

The Threefold Process

J. M. Juran, another important figure in the managing-for-quality movement, summarizes the process of managing for quality as threefold (Juran, 1988):

1. *Quality planning:* Decide who the customers are, what their needs are, develop features that respond to their needs, develop processes to respond.

2. *Quality control:* Evaluate the actual outputs, compare output to expected output, act on the difference.

3. *Quality improvement:* Establish the needed infrastructure, identify improvement projects, establish project teams. Train, motivate, empower the teams to diagnose the causes, find remedies, and maintain gains (Melum & Sinioris, 1992).

STRUCTURE, PROCESS, OUTCOME

Structure

When the nursing industry began to assume its present size and shape in the late 1960s, quality measurements were primarily focused on structure, that is, an adequate physical plant, the proper equipment, enough trained staff, enough income. The idea was that Medicare, Medicaid, and state nursing home inspectors should ensure that the structure needed to give good care was in place. Structure, in the systems model we have described above, is the inputs (Hitt et al., 2001). The quality of care, however, remained unsatisfactorily low (Bliesmer, 1993).

Process

Attention of the federal and state inspectors was then expanded to include both structure and process. Inspecting for process meant ensuring that all the organizational arrangements believed to be needed were in place. Process is the portion of our systems model described earlier, appropriately enough, as the processor, that is, the work the organization accomplishes. Structure measures the capacity to give resident/patient care. Process measures the way in which resident care is given. For example, are the Minimum Data Sets (MDS) appropriately filled out? Is a well-developed plan of care in place? Are all the resident assessment protocols triggered by the minimum data set appropriately filled out and being followed?

Outcome

Even after measuring for both structure and process, Congress ruled in 1987, through the Nursing Home Reform Act, that inspectors must focus not only on structure (capacity to give care) and process (the giving of care), but also on the outcomes of the care giving. Outcome, the third part of our systems model above, is the result of the effort made, the measurable impacts on the resident/patient in the case of the nursing facility. Outcome focuses on measuring whether residents are in fact enjoying a high quality of life, full enjoyment of the patients' rights established by Congress in 1987, and high quality nursing and medical care.

Some examples of outcome measurements may be in order. Congress, in the federal requirements, phrased these outcome measures in the following manner.

§483.25 Quality of Care Each resident must receive and the facility must provide the necessary care and services to attain or maintain the highest practicable physical, mental and psychosocial well-being, in accordance with the comprehensive assessment and plan of care.

There follow a number of outcome measures to be enforced, for example, a resident's abilities in activities of daily living do not diminish unless circumstances of the individual's clinical condition demonstrate that diminution was unavoidable. This reasoning is extended to vision and hearing, urinary incontinence, range of motion, mental and psychosocial functioning, nasogastric tubes, accidents, nutrition, hydration, special needs, unnecessary drugs, and medication errors (Maddox & Sussman, 2001). Regarding pressure sores, for example, the outcome requirement is that a resident who enters the facility without pressure (decubitus) sores does not develop pressure sores unless the individual's clinical condition demonstrates that they were unavoidable.

After the 1987 Nursing Home Reform Act, the Centers for Medicare and Medicaid Services (CMS) looked at outcomes. CMS no longer specified structure (a specific infection control committed with designated members), nor process (activities successfully identifying and tracking infections). Rather, CMS looked, initially, only at outcome: Are infections being successfully controlled in the facility? Today, if infections are not being successfully controlled, CMS will look at the facility's processes and structure for controlling infections, but no longer specify what structure or process the facility must use.

Today nursing homes are inspected for and required to successfully achieve acceptable levels of structure, process, and outcome. We turn now to explore a few of the methods for maintaining organizational quality that have been advanced and used by the business and health care world in recent years. The majority of problems that arise in any organization occur because the process is broken.

ESTABLISHING AND JUDGING QUALITY IN THE NURSING FACILITY

Nearly every nursing facility in the United States has its own mission statement with accompanying goals for quality of resident care and resident life.

Often, local facilities write their own mission statements with quality goals carefully spelled out in statements of policy and procedures for the facility.

Whose quality goals matter? In the daily life of the American nursing facility it is the quality goals of CMS (formerly HCFA, Health Care Financing Administration) that ultimately matter. Administrators seldom judge their success or failure by corporate or facility standards. Rather, the administrators' feelings about success or failure are dictated by CMS's quality standards embodied in the Federal Requirements and Guidelines to Surveyors. This has come about because CMS surveys every facility on a nearly annual basis, decides whether the facility is deficiency-free, and if not may impose civil money penalties as high as hundreds of thousands of dollars. CMS requires that its quality judgments (survey results) be displayed prominently for all who visit the facility and it posts survey results on the Web for everyone to see. The practical reality is that CMS's judgments become, for most facilities, both the *de jure* (by law) and *de facto* (by practice) quality standards for nursing facilities in the United States. And if the surveyors are really unhappy they can put the facility on a fast track to decertification (ending Medicare and Medicaid eligibility) and prohibit new admissions until they are satisfied with the facility's plan for correcting the deficiencies. Given the razor-thin operating margins of most facilities, the inability to admit new residents, even for a short time, can induce traumatic economic woe.

For the first time a national data base of the federal government's judgments about the quality of care and quality of life in American nursing facilities is available. These data will be presented at appropriate places in this text.

FEDERAL STANDARDS: MINIMUM OR MAXIMUM?

The literature, and often surveyors themselves, describe the federal requirements as minimum standards. They *were* minimum standards when structure was evaluated by federal surveyors. Now, after more than 20 years of intense federal continuous-quality-improvement efforts, federal standards, if achieved, are maximal and state of the art. If all federal requirements for favorable outcomes are achieved, a remarkably high quality of care is being achieved. It is an ongoing process. Minimum data set 1.0 was followed by MDS 2.0 and MDS 3.0 with continuous quality improvements to come.

QUALITY OF CARE: 1993—1999

In Table 1-2 an overview shows that on most of the federal tags (each tag has an "F number" and spells out a specific federal requirement) the

Table 1-2. Percentage of Nursing Facilities in the U.S. with Deficiencies for Quality of Care: 1993–1999

		Deficiency Group = Quality of Care						
FTAG	Description	1993	1994	1995	1996	1997	1998	1999
F309	Quality of Care	11.3	13.8	12.2	12.8	14.4	17.2	21.0
F310	Activities of Daily Living Maintenance	8.3	5.7	4.1	2.8	2.7	2.5	2.1
F311	Appropriate ADL Treatment	5.6	5.2	5.1	5.0	5.0	5.6	6.4
F312	ADL Services	7.6	7.7	9.0	10.0	10.4	12.0	14.0
F313	Vision and Hearing	0.5	0.4	0.6	0.5	0.5	0.6	0.7
F314	Pressure Sores	18.0	15.0	15.6	15.0	16.1	17.1	18.0
F315	Catheter Prevention	1.1	1.3	1.1	1.2	1.3	1.4	1.3
F316	Incontinence Care	11.8	12.0	12.1	10.4	10.4	10.9	11.5
F317	Range of Motion Maintenance	0.7	0.7	1.0	1.0	0.8	0.7	0.9
F318	Limited Range of Motion Services	8.3	7.1	8.3	8.4	8.7	9.2	9.7
F319	Mental and Psychosocial Services	4.5	5.1	4.6	3.3	2.8	2.4	2.6
F320	Maintenance of Psychosocial Functioning	0.3	0.3	0.3	0.2	0.3	0.1	0.2
F321	Nasogastric Tubes (tube feeding)	0.3	0.2	0.2	0.1	0.1	0.2	0.1
F322	Nasogastric Care	5.2	5.2	4.6	4.1	4.1	4.5	5.3
F323	Accident Environment	19.7	19.7	18.3	16.2	16.6	18.0	18.7
F324	Accident Prevention	6.2	7.2	8.0	9.2	11.9	14.7	17.3
F325	Nutrition	9.4	9.4	8.1	8.1	8.3	8.1	9.9
F326	Therapeutic Diet	5.6	5.0	3.7	2.2	2.3	2.0	2.2
F327	Hydration	3.6	3.5	3.2	3.1	2.5	3.2	5.3
F328	Special Needs	5.2	4.1	3.7	3.6	3.3	3.6	4.4
F329	Unnessary Drugs	16.1	12.7	10.8	11.0	10.6	10.7	11.6
F330	Antipsychotic Drugs	2.4	2.1	1.5	1.3	1.1	1.2	0.8
F331	Drug Reduction	2.6	2.3	1.7	1.2	1.2	1.2	1.0
F332	Medication Errors	8.3	7.4	6.4	5.2	4.9	5.7	7.4
F333	Significant Medication Errors	4.8	4.0	3.3	2.4	2.5	3.1	3.6

Nursing Facilities, Staffing, Residents and Facility Deficiencies, 1993-1999
Department of Social & Behavioral Sciences
University of California San Francisco

quality of care achieved was very high, and in most categories exhibits improvement, for example, reduction of unnecessary drugs from 16% in 1993 to 11% in 1999. It is on the more subjective tags that the degree of compliance was judged by CMS to have declined: F309 quality of care and F324 accident prevention, in particular. On most tags, facilities were in compliance well over 90% of the time.

Table 1-3 demonstrates dramatic improvement in every category except self-determination, which remained the same. Except for the highly subjective F241 (dignity) and F 253 (housekeeping), nursing homes achieved remarkably high in providing quality of life to residents.

Figure 1-4 reveals that a remarkably high 17% of facilities had no deficiencies in 1999 and a similarly remarkably low 5.7 average number of deficiencies per facility. When one considers the approximately 330 federal requirements on which deficiencies are given, 5.7 per facility represents .0172% deficiency among the 330 per facility. The percentage of facilities reporting no deficiencies in the U.S. increased from 11.4% in 1993 to 17.5% in 1999, a 54% increase during the period. The percentage of facilities with no deficiencies varied by state from 1.5% in Washington to 48.5% in New Jersey in 1999.

It may be no surprise that the number of deficiencies per facility began rising in 1998. The federal government implemented a crack-

Table 1-3. Percentage of Nursing Facilities in the U.S. with Deficiencies for Quality of Life: F240–F258

		Deficiency Group = Quality of Life						
FTAG	Description	1993	1994	1995	1996	1997	1998	1999
F240	Quality of Life	1.4	1.5	0.7	0.3	0.2	0.2	0.2
F241	Dignity	19.1	18.5	17.7	13.7	13.2	14.1	16.3
F242	Self-Determinatiori/Participation	2.6	2.6	2.5	2.3	2.2	2.5	2.6
F243	Resident and Family Groups	0.9	0.7	0.9	0.5	0.5	0.5	0.6
F244	Listen to Group	1.4	1.3	0.6	0.3	0.5	0.5	0.3
F245	Participate in Other Activities	0.2	0.1	0.2	0.1	0.1	0.1	0.1
F246	Accomodate Needs	17.1	15.5	14.2	10.1	8.6	9.0	9.4
F247	Notice Before Room Change	0.6	0.6	0.4	0.2	0.2	0.2	0.2
F248	Activities Program	12.0	12.2	12.2	9.5	8.3	8.1	8.6
F249	Activities Director	1.1	1.2	0.9	0.5	0.6	0.5	0.5
F250	Social Services	8.8	9.4	8.6	8.7	7.8	7.5	7.8
F251	Social Work Qualification	0.9	0.6	0.4	0.3	0.2	0.2	0.3
F252	Environment	15.5	14.1	11.5	8.0	6.7	7.2	7.3
F253	Housekeeping	19.5	18.3	16.9	15.1	13.3	14.4	15.3
F254	Clean Linens	3.6	3.4	2.9	2.2	1.7	1.7	1.7
F255	Private Closet	1.0	0.7	0.5	0.1	0.1	0.1	0.1
F256	Adequate Lighting	2.2	1.6	1.1	0.7	0.5	0.5	0.5
F257	Comfortable Temperatures	1.7	1.6	1.1	0.9	0.9	1.1	0.9
F258	Comfortable Sound	2.4	2.6	2.3	2.3	1.8	1.7	1.7

Nursing Facilities, Staffing, Residents and Facility Deficiencies, 1993-1999
Department of Social & Behavioral Sciences
University of California San Francisco

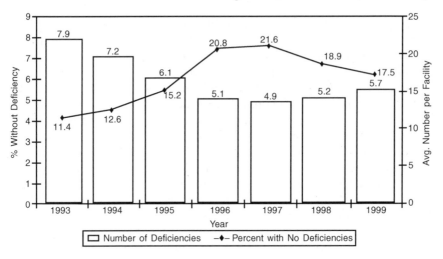

FIGURE 1-4. Average number of deficiencies and percentage without deficiencies.
Nursing Facilities, Staffing, Residents and Facility Deficiencies, 1993–1999, Department of Social & Behavioral Sciences, University of California San Francisco.

down on nursing homes at the behest of the president and consumer organizations at the same time federal funds to facilities were being decreased due to the draconian reductions required by the Balanced Budget Act of 1997.

1.8 Innovating

The effective manager is always an innovator. *Innovating* is the process of bringing new ideas into the way an organization accomplishes its purposes. It is the result of the administrator's studying the changes that are constantly occurring in the organization itself and the environment in which it functions. Innovating is an act of leadership. It is the manager's role to be the sensor of the organization for those external and internal changes that will have an impact on its well-being (Hitt et al., 2001; Johns & Saks, 2001).

The manager is not necessarily the innovator, but does have the task of assuring that innovation occurs within the organization. To achieve this, the manager can develop new ideas, combine old ideas into new ones, borrow and adapt ideas from other fields, or stimulate others to develop innovations (Dale, 1969; Hitt et al., 2001).

To focus on the resident/patient and his or her family and significant others is to be in constant contact with the changing needs of residents. Nearly all staff have contacts with residents and with those close to the residents. If practical innovation is sought from all staff, the staff must become outwardly focused adaptive sensors, listening and adapting to changing needs.

WELCOMING INNOVATIONS

Change is hard work. We have discussed the importance of carefully formulated policies that the administrator can implement through detailed plans of action. Edward Wrapp observed that "good managers don't make policy decisions; rather, they give a sense of direction and are masters at developing opportunities" (Wrapp, 1984, p. 8).

Wrapp addressed the question of why the good manager shies away from very precise statements of objectives for the organization. According to Wrapp, the effective manager finds it impossible to set down specific objectives that will be relevant for any extended period of time. The external environment changes continually, he observes, and the organization's strategies have to be continually revised to take these changes into account. He concludes that the more explicit the statement of strategy, the more difficult it is to persuade the employees to turn to different goals when needs and conditions change (Johns & Saks, 2001).

The Value in Imprecision

Wrapp (1984) believes that goals or objectives are communicated over time through a consistent pattern of operating decisions. We also advise guarding against a degree of specificity in goal and policy statements that would discourage change.

All of the forces that tend to lead to an organizational resistance to change are formidable enemies of the manager who is obliged to introduce changes to keep the facility in tune with the environment (Johns & Saks, 2001). The nursing home facility administrator must keep policies precise enough to guide employee decisions and at the same time continually introduce change into the facility, which is not an easy task (Johns & Saks, 2001).

Innovating

A nursing facility's staff will innovate only if the administrator intentionally introduces changes in the organization that are responses to perceived changes in the environment, and then encourages others to do the same. Innovation is the process of finding new solutions for creating a good quality of life for residents and staff. Not all new solutions will work; the administrator must encourage and praise new solutions that fail as well as the ones that succeed, otherwise staff will stop making suggesting.

Innovation requires being in constant touch with the new—new requirements, new employment trends, new benefits, new resident activities. To be innovative is to respond with flexibility to changes in the environment. Most organizations fight innovation. Hospitals fought the introduction of birthing suites until women arranged to be delivered outside the hospital in home-like suites.

Innovation by Memo

Tom Watson, the executive who led IBM to its position of strength in the computer field, met with great resistance in introducing new technology

(Hitt et al., 2001). In the 1950s, he attempted to move IBM from vacuum tube technology to the new transistor technology. He was aware that the Japanese were already using tiny transistors effectively while IBM continued to use acres of large vacuum tubes to accomplish the same tasks. IBM engineers had spent their lives in vacuum tube technology and weren't about to adopt the new transistor technology. After months of unsuccessful coaxing, wheedling and cajoling, an exasperated Watson wrote a memo in which he stated that after June 1, 1958 no more vacuum tubes would be used in IBM product development ("America's Most Admired Corporations," 1995).

Innovating is not limited to the IBMs of the world. Stodgy old-line corporations are successfully using innovation. In recent years the Kellogg Company has created entire new markets for its cereals by marketing them to adults. Who would have predicted that an obscure company with the unlikely name of Minnesota Mining and Manufacturing (3M) would be one of the most innovative U.S. corporation in the 1980s and the years beyond (e.g., Post-it™)?

Rearranging Nursing Duties

A Washington, D.C., facility, faced with difficulties in finding nurses and pressures on nurses' time to perform administrative functions, tried replacing the charge nurse with an assistant administrator. Initially this person made out the nurse assistant assignments; ensured that supplies and linen were available to the nursing assistants and the nurses; resolved any logistical problems with transportation, dietary, and housekeeping; and coordinated any immediate and long-term maintenance and housekeeping needs for the unit. This new employee made rounds daily, or more often, ensuring that residents' needs were being met and that nurse aides were following nursing directives (walking, turning, and repositioning residents as required). This freed the nurses to concentrate more on resident assessment, medication administration, and care conferences. In this case, everyone wins. The facility enables the more expensive nurse time to be devoted to good nursing care, and the residents' quality of care and level of satisfaction is improved by a unit manager who is practicing leading by walking around (LBWA).

The American health insurance industry grew out of an innovation developed by hospital administrator in Texas. Faced with a drastically reduced cash flow in the Depression because patients had little money, he devised a plan to create a regular cash flow to this hospital, Baylor University Hospital, from the one group that still had a steady income: school teachers who were paid from public taxes. For 50 cents a month, he offered up to 14 days of prepaid hospital care per year. The teachers bought the idea and the United States health insurance system was born.

An AIDS Policy Innovation

Although innovation is an expected part of the job description of the chief executive of a large nursing home chain, it can occur at the local level even in highly centralized chains. AIDS patients are now routinely admitted to most nursing home facilities. During a time when no AIDS patients were being admitted in a certain state, including all facilities owned by a large chain, a local nursing facility administrator decided it was time for a new policy. She announced her determination to admit AIDS patients to her facility, persuaded corporate officials not to interfere, orchestrated a 9-month-long intensive preparation period for her staff, residents/patients, and significant others at the end of which she began routinely admitting AIDS patients with hardly a ripple in the daily life of the facility. Her census was better, the staff were proud, the residents/patients and their significant others were comfortable, and the corporation changed its policies.

Innovators tend to be survivors of change. The future belongs to those organizations that are successful in constantly innovating over time. The early years of the twenty-first century hold promise to innovators in the nursing home industry.

Success today requires that, compared to your competitors, you be more creative, more customer focused, more cost conscious.

1.9 Marketing the Long-Term Care Facility

1.9.1 The Turn to Marketing

Why, one might ask, should the nursing facility administrator be concerned with marketing? High occupancy rates seem guaranteed for the foreseeable future. Many, if not most, nursing facilities have resident waiting lists (Midgett, 1984). In addition, the proportion of Americans who will need nursing facility care is expected to increase yearly at least through the middle of this century. Waiting lists are becoming even longer in some facilities in response to Medicare's prospective payment method (diagnosis-related groups), which places even more and more pressure on hospitals to rapidly discharge acute care patients to nursing homes or, increasingly, home health agencies for periods of subacute and managed care. Even so, a number of factors are coming together that may threaten any seeming guarantee of continued high occupancy rates.

FORCES LEADING TO COMPETITION

Narrowed Profit Margins

The ability of a nursing facility to survive economically is affected by an increasing variety of pressures such as federal and state reimbursement policies, the types of services offered by the facility, and the sources of resident payment. Over the past decade government regulators who pay for care of Medicare and Medicaid residents in nursing facilities have sought ways to narrow the margin of facility profit to achieve mandated government cost savings.

At the same time, facility costs have increased in meeting the additional regulatory requirements under the 1987 Nursing Home Reform Act and subsequent amendments. The Americans with Disabilities Act, the Family and Medical Leave Act, and the more rigorous universal precautions requirements all add costs, often unreimbursed, to providing care. Profitability is threatened by rising human-resource costs, particularly as the level of acuity increases. One geriatrician has observed that over the next 10 years, if present trends continue nursing facilities will be forced to have nearly as many staff as hospitals do.

The patient profile of the typical nursing facility is shifting toward increased levels of acuity and a growing number of sources of payment from providers such as health maintenance organizations, workers' compensation, long-term care insurance, the Veterans Administration, and private insurance companies.

Reduction of Federal Influence in Shaping the Product Mix

Product design in nursing facilities—that is, the mix of services and business activities—was heavily influenced from the 1960s through the 1980s by product and price decisions that were made by the Medicaid and Medicare agencies. The payment policies of the states' Medicaid offices, along with Medicare claims authorities, were predominant influences on prices charged and services offered in the industry (Hitt et al., 2001; Ting, 1984).

In the coming decade most facilities will have multiple payment sources such as insurance companies and the increasing number of affluent older residents. Survival of the average facility will increasingly depend on the administrator's being able to find a niche—to identify and successfully market the offerings of the facility to defined groups of persons who need the emerging types of services now available.

Always Mess with Success

The most cogent reason for marketing the nursing facility is that if *you* don't mess with your success, your competitor will. It is easy to be blinded by one's short-term success. Whenever a facility feels it has achieved premier status as the best caregiver in the community, whenever it starts taking its success for granted, it will lull itself into complacency and slack off.

The computer world is littered with such companies. Between 1984 and 1988, DEC (Digital Equipment Corporation) captured a big chunk of IBM's mid-range computer sales, then rested on its laurels only to be wiped out a year later when its winning (and only) design suddenly became obsolete. IBM did the same thing when Tom Watson, Sr., retired.

No sooner did DEC and IBM began plateauing then they began plunging.

Adequate nursing facilities (public opinion notwithstanding) abound. Simply doing a good job of marketing the facility will not provide the necessary edge to succeed in today's pressure-packed health care marketplace. Good only puts you with the rest of the pack. Good isn't good enough.

1.9.2 The Marketing of Health Care

In 1977, the United States Supreme Court ruled illegal any self-imposed restrictions by health and other professionals against advertising services or prices that result in keeping the public ignorant or inhibiting the free flow of commercial information (Kinnear & Bernhardt, 1986). As a result, over the past two decades the marketing of professional health services has become an increasingly accepted practice. In 1978, it was estimated that hospitals in this country employed only 3 marketing executives. A decade later, more than 2,000 marketing executives were working for United States hospitals (Califano, 1986).

HEALTH CARE PROVIDERS BEGIN TO MARKET

Hospitals have turned to marketing because the occupancy rates across the United States have fallen in each of the past several years.

To increase occupancy rates, hospitals are competing with one another, introducing out-patient surgery and other service centers, nursing facilities, and home health agencies for patients in an attempt to distinguish themselves from their competitors (Inguanzo & Harju, 1985).

According to Kotler and Clarke, competition occurs when two or more organizations seek to serve the same individual or group in an exchange process. An exchange requires (a) at least two parties, (b) that each party offer something the other values, (c) that each party be capable of communicating and delivering what is valued, and (d) that both are free to accept or reject the offer (Johns & Saks, 2001; Kotler & Clarke, 1987).

Competition for patients among public, not-for-profit, and for-profit hospitals is a new experience. Faced with assisted living facilities and home health agencies that increasingly siphon off residents who, until recently, would have entered a nursing facility, administrators of nursing facilities are similarly encountering a need to market their services.

DEFINITION OF MARKETING

The American Marketing Association defines marketing as the process of planning and executing the conception, pricing, promotion, and distribution of ideas, goods, and services to create exchanges that satisfy both individual and organizational objectives (Kinnear & Bernhardt, 1986). The nursing facility is in the business of marketing services. Nearly half of every dollar spent by American consumers is spent on services (Berkowitz, Kerin, & Rudelius, 1986).

Levey and Loomba, in *Health Care Administration: A Managerial Perspective* (1984), argue that health care marketing had its beginnings in a spate of articles first appearing in 1973. They comment that the spread of marketing to hospitals and nursing facilities was inevitable because of forces such as lowered occupancy rates and increasingly marginal net income due to lowered reimbursement rates. Marketing is currently regarded as a central consideration in health services administration. It is the effort to improve the interaction between the organization's goals and the persons whose needs the organization seeks to serve.

Why is it increasingly necessary to pay special attention to the fit between the goals of the nursing facility and the needs of the persons it seeks to serve? To assure that the facility will stay in business, of course (Peters, 1987).

The following steps in marketing are described by Levey and Loomba (1984) as

1. the audit
2. market segmentation
3. choosing a market mix
4. implementing the plan
5. evaluation of results
6. control

This should look familiar. It is a restatement of the management steps described in part 1 of this text. Kotler and Clarke observe that marketing is a "managerial process involving analysis, planning, implementation, and control" (Kotler and Clarke, 1987).

MARKETING AS MANAGERIAL THINKING

Marketing employs the management techniques we have discussed and recommended throughout this book, using a vocabulary developed specifically for the marketing field. Its purpose is to identify and satisfactorily serve the institutional nursing-facility needs in the community.

Marketing provides a useful vocabulary, another way of thinking about how the nursing facility can successfully identify and satisfy an expanding array of health care needs.

Marketing, as a variation on managerial thinking, focuses sharply on the idea that success for the facility depends on bringing about a voluntary exchange of values (services) with the target persons.

END TO THE PRODUCTION ORIENTATION

Fifty years ago, the focus of health care providers was on designing a quality hospital or nursing facility, correctly assuming that if it were built, patients would fill it (Fine, 1984). This is a production orientation, which holds that the facility's task is to deliver care the health professionals know is good for the residents and that the sales task is to stimulate potential residents' interest in what the facility has decided to offer. This is seller's-market thinking.

Angry Mothers

For decades women communicated their displeasure to hospital officials, who were in a seller's market, about the intensely institutional atmosphere and rigid rules surrounding the delivery rooms in the obstetrics departments. There being no competition, the hospitals ignored these complaints. Angry women in New York and then in other cities established birthing centers with homelike atmospheres. A dramatically lower obstetrics occupancy reflected both the end of the baby boom and the dissatisfaction of female customers who ere choosing to deliver in the birthing centers and hospital officials suddenly decided that the warm atmosphere of birthing centers could be provided after all in the nearly empty hospitals. Hospitals now routinely compete with each other and with birthing centers to see who can provide the most pleasing accommodations and flexible birthing rules.

Kotler and Clarke commend the market orientation now taking hold in health care facilities. In this approach the main task of the provider is to discover the needs and desires of potential customers and satisfy them through product design and price, delivering appropriate and competitively viable services (Kotler & Clarke, 1987; Star, 1989). This is market-centeredness, which focuses primarily on customer needs, wants, perceptions, preferences, and satisfaction. Kotler and Clarke advocate a responsive organization, one that makes every effort to understand, serve, and satisfy the preferences and needs of its residents and their sponsors within the constraints of budget and good clinical practice. Satisfaction is defined as a state that a resident feels when a service has fulfilled his or her expectations (Kotler & Clarke, 1987). Health care services are increasingly a buyer's market. Long-term customer satisfaction with the manner in which the facility is being run is one of the major factors in keeping a nursing facility at or near capacity (Peters & Austin, 1985).

SPECIAL CONTEXT OF NURSING FACILITY MARKETING

Local residents want people they know and trust to care for Mom and Dad. The administrator who is visibly active and creates a presence in the community can create an atmosphere of trust through such networking (Evans, et al., 2000).

The nursing facility faces two special challenges: (a) the requirement to maintain a societal marketing orientation, and (b) public ambivalence toward the nursing facility itself. In the societal marketing orientation, the primary task of the nursing facility is to determine the needs, desires, and best interests of residents and to configure the facility to deliver satisfaction that preserves and enhances the residents, their families' and society's well-being.

Both short-term and long-staying residents may wish to be allowed to remain in their beds, to avoid exercise, and to eat only foods they can taste (typically foods high in sugar). But society has determined through the development of nursing facility regulations that residents must be urged to get up each day, to dress and move about the facility to maintain blood flow, to exercise when feasible and practice good oral hygiene, and to eat the balanced diet mandated by federal and state regulations. The nursing facility is thus obligated to encourage residents to engage in behaviors that society has determined are in the residents' interest, which are sometimes contrary to their preference.

A second sense in which nursing facility marketing is a special context is public ambivalence toward the nursing facility. This is a complex, little understood, but frequently expressed problem area. Who among us does not wish to live into healthy and robust old age in our own homes with all our senses and abilities intact? None would welcome the situation of the typical nursing facility resident who may have three or four chronic illnesses that require a physician's care, takes six or more medications daily, has a limited ability to perform the activities of daily living and needs 24-hour-a-day nursing care. There is much more approach/avoidance involved in public feelings toward the care in nursing facilities than toward hospitals where normally the patient expects (hopes) to be healed and returned to active community life. Entering new marketing areas must be done with great forethought. An improperly analyzed niche can become a new cost center rather than the desired profit center.

1.9.3 Developing a Marketing Strategy

NEED FOR A MARKETING STRATEGY

Organizations must continually adapt to changes within and outside the organization. An adaptive organization systematically monitors the external environment and revises its mission, strategies, and objectives to take advantage of emerging opportunities.

A constantly evolving marketing strategy is needed because continuous changes occur in the demographic, technologic, regulatory, economic, political, reimbursement and social environment, which leads to changing demand for nursing facility services. New competition appears, new client demands develop, values change.

Competition for the potential nursing home client is increasing. On the acute care side, hospitals are showing increased interest in converting empty acute-care wings to nursing home–type beds. Some hospitals are even building new nursing homes on their grounds or nearby to create a new revenue stream. From another perspective, home health care agencies are increasingly providing sophisticated nursing care such as intravenous feeding in the patient's home, which was previously performed mostly in hospitals and in only a few nursing facilities. Thus, acute care patients may increasingly go directly home, bypassing the nursing facility. Then there are the assisted living facilities bursting onto the scene that promise to let their residents "age in place" (read: never have to go to a nursing facility).

A *marketing strategy* includes selecting a target market or markets, choosing a competitive position, and developing an effective marketing mix to reach and serve the identified customers (Hitt et al., 2001; Kotler & Clark, 1987).

A *market* is all the people who have an actual or potential interest in using the facility's services. A facility may select among several market coverage strategies. It may concentrate on one market or market segment (called *market concentration*), by choosing, for example, to serve only Medicaid residents or the facility may decide to offer only one service for all markets (called *product concentration*), perhaps by serving only Alzheimer's patients regardless of their funding source. Another option is *market specialization,* that is, serving only one market segment, such as persons who need rehabilitative care and are expected to return home within a specified brief period of time. Or, it may prefer to work in several product markets, serving both Alzheimer's and other brain-damaged persons of all ages (known as *selective specializations*).

CREATING NEW MARKETS, NEW NICHES

Tom Peters distinguishes between market sharing and market creation. Those using the market-share mentality focus on how they can attain a desired share of the present market. Market creators are those who attempt to create a new market (Peters, 1987). Opening a ventilator unit in a nursing home, for example, was a new phenomenon in the late 1980s. Up to that point, ventilator care had mostly been confined to hospitals, and entrepreneurial nursing home administrators created a new long-term care market by opening this kind of unit in their nursing facilities (Hitt et al., 2001). These administrators convinced third-party reimbursement officials to move ventilator patients out of hospitals and into nursing facilities, thus creating a new, larger long-term care market. In the 1990s the market for nursing-home ventilator beds became saturated in several parts of the country. Time to create the next niches. Survival for both individual facilities and nursing facility chains is becoming increasingly tied to specialization in market niches, in which one can gain a reputation for excellence, in order to keep census at the needed levels.

WHICH NICHE?

Table 1-4 shows the number of beds in special care units for Alzheimer's, AIDS, and hospice from 1993 through 1999. The number of dedicated Alzheimer's beds was 76,538 in 1999. This number is still less than 5% of the total certified beds in the United States.

The number of dedicated AIDS beds was 2,002 in 1999, a fraction less than 1% of all beds from 1993–1999. The number of hospice beds was 3,121 in 1999, but this number is also less than 1% of all beds in the United States. This reflects the general trend to provide hospice care either in the home or in hospitals

Table 1-5 shows that there were 18,256 rehabilitation beds in special units in certified nursing facilities in 1999. All three categories represent only about 1% of certified beds in the United States. There were also 4,726 ventilator beds reported in special care units in 1999. There were 568 dialysis unit beds surveyed in 1999.

Examining Tables 1-4 and 1-5 state-by-state reveals large differences in approach among the states. Many require additional and expensive services in units that are designated "special care," thus many facilities accept residents in each of these special categories but do not maintain

Table 1-4. Total Number of Special-Care Beds in Certified Nursing Facilities in the U.S., 1993–1999

State	Alzheimers							AIDS							Hospice						
	1993	1994	1995	1996	1997	1998	1999	1993	1994	1995	1996	1997	1998	1999	1993	1994	1995	1996	1997	1998	1999
AK	0	22	22	0	0	0	22	0	0	0	0	0	0	0	0	0	0	0	0	0	0
AL	281	352	254	305	383	515	464	2	0	0	0	0	0	0	21	23	23	28	45	15	15
AR	12.6	254	265	377	393	556	470	20	18	18	0	0	1	0	11	1	1	18	8	3	2
AZ	1,191	1,362	1.402	1.317	1,336	1,694	1,116	0	185	140	157	31	141	0	115	157	150	67	18	82	19
CA	3,898	4,760	4,001	3,936	3,978	3,893	4.794	102	350	356	460	186	94	400	391	660	694	428	356	554	717
CO	1,606	1,749	1,741	1,594	1,840	2,047	2,135	0	15	15	0	10	5	5	76	175	171	161	72	107	66
CT	1,001	1.179	1,118	1,209	1,573	1,338	1,501	0	114	106	60	187	24	30	11	34	47	48	172	27	22
DC	46	10	10	0	36	64	49	0	0	0	0	0	0	0	9	0	0	0	9	9	9
DE	232	235	138	227	324	189	277	0	0	0	0	0	0	0	0	0	0	0	0	0	0
FL	2,350	2,871	2,388	2,921	3,677	4,234	4,620	214	210	67	208	65	217	80	86	189	87	384	96	102	187
GA	606	907	927	822	785	903	930	0	6	6	0	0	0	0	59	2T7	274	225	6	179	179
HI	90	60	60	50	88	102	51	0	10	10	0	0	0	0	6	10	16	6	88	6	0
IA	784	875	877	1,025	1,107	1,245	1,405	0	12	12	0	0	0	0	76	5	5	39	66	67	63
ID	430	428	428	427	412	492	460	0	0	0	0	0	0	0	16	15	16	14	2	0	2
IL	2,932	3,487	3,694	4,OT8	4,167	5,186	5,852	100	169	159	174	44	44	44	147	169	173	239	90	44	118
IN	2,163	2,688	2,631	2,471	2,765	2,827	3,163	39	49	49	68	58	39	39	31	254	164	163	91	36	14
KS	646	1,387	1,202	1,503	1,456	1,914	1,893	6	6	6	0	0	0	0	2	65	64	61	1	63	4
KY	204	209	137	295	483	260	284	2	12	14	12	14	14	16	11	14	10	98	1	6	24
LA	671	804	960	949	1,234	1,181	1,619	12	98	108	120	36	14	12	0	73	73	72	11	4	15
MA	1,349	1,660	1,506	1,956	2,725	2,724	2,910	15	15	15	0	0	0	0	15	15	48	63	58	0	58
MD	401	608	602	1,016	1,191	743	717	16	155	143	98	125	48	163	20	32	20	1	22	3	120
ME	332	443	405	589	862	843	934	9	9	9	9	9	9	9	13	2	12	3	3	9	8
MI	739	778	649	859	1,263	1,354	1,181	0	0	0	0	0	0	0	51	62	90	25	23	169	59
MN	1,856	2,129	Z329	2,259	2,636	2,706	3,037	25	191	191	18	37	18	18	33	179	185	27	30	30	28
MO	1,804	2,645	2,400	2,793	3,389	3,536	3,462	2	4	4	0	4	16	0	12	43	43	163	30	92	4
MS	0	100	100	181	189	189	137	0	0	0	0	0	0	0	0	0	0	0	2	0	2
MT	292	396	381	408	404	408	607	0	0	0	0	0	32	0	0	1	1	3	0	4	4
NC	798	1,207	1,285	1,295	1,349	1,330	964	10	8	8	8	8	0	0	0	5	5	0	62	124	0
ND	119	142	134	129	67	217	301	0	0	0	0	0	0	0	0	0	0	0	0	0	0
NE	456	709	684	794	822	857	910	0	0	0	0	0	0	0	14	16	5	19	18	19	12

Table 1-4. (Continued)

State	Alzheimers							AIDS							Hospice						
	1993	1994	1995	1996	1997	1998	1999	1993	1994	1995	1996	1997	1998	1999	1993	1994	1995	1996	1997	1998	1999
NH	515	553	526	577	669	712	624	0	0	0	0	0	0	0	0	50	so	50	50	0	51
NJ	541	364	443	686	513	658	280	120	0	60	69	60	60	0	6	6	6	126	12	12	3
NM	207	295	310	269	379	382	542	0	0	0	0	0	0	0	1	2	3	0	0	0	0
NV	252	232	232	248	168	256	311	0	0	0	0	0	0	0	1	4	4	2	0	2	0
NY	1,566	2,113	2,055	3,029	2,421	3,235	3,653	449	611	620	1,082	1,088	811	1,027	321	156	134	41	23	44	46
OH	3,081	3,500	2,591	4,105	4,372	4,810	5,121	21	244	244	103	41	23	16	2	40	189	628	256	265	198
OK	635	729	832	917	1,129	902	1,007	13	29	0	29	0	0	0	4	9	11	11	243	2	142
OR	761	835	664	698	848	893	829	0	0	0	0	0	0	0	5	4	5	80	78	72	77
PA	2,791	3,634	3,372	4,267	5,280	5,353	5,375	25	45	29	4	34	34	16	45	25	64	32	270	230	234
RI	246	468	508	573	420	559	607	0	0	0	0	0	0	0	0	0	0	0	0	0	0
SC	60	175	333	377	745	746	482	0	0	0	0	0	0	0	0	a	8	0	0	0	0
SD	169	215	226	191	216	231	245	0	0	0	0	0	0	0	1	0	1	2	0	1	11
TN	259	300	256	378	340	359	412	0	7	7	16	0	0	0	0	4	4	10	0	0	1
TX	2,210	2,795	2,872	3,056	2,863	2,928	3,044	24	51	51	12	0	25	0	48	35	237	230	42	8	11
UT	431	487	445	499	591	826	614	6	6	6	0	0	0	0	0	0	0	3	8	9	57
VA	1,027	753	724	885	828	739	1,103	40	12	12	29	27	17	5	a	0	0	5	1	10	12
VT	147	154	163	116	137	87	153	0	0	0	0	0	0	0	0	0	0	0	0	4	0
WA	1,643	1,879	1,721	1,804	1,928	2,013	2,095	76	100	30	77	75	75	75	177	198	48	209	241	212	318
WI	2,387	2,195	2,255	2,724	2,847	2,980	3,328	12	52	52	2	2	2	11	236	347	371	300	238	146	208
WV	102	143	53	0	0	10	173	0	0	0	0	0	36	36	0	0	0	0	0	0	0
WY	319	237	299	276	332	303	275	0	0	0	0	0	0	0	1	0	0	1	1	3	1
US	46,752	56,512	53,810	61,460	67,960	72,529	76,538	1,360	2,793	2,547	2,815	2,141	11,799	2,002	2,074	3,364	3,512	4,085	2,843	2,774	3,121

Nursing Facilities, Staffing, Residents and Facility Deficiencies, 1993-1999
Department of Social & Behavioral Sciences
University of California San Francisco

Table 1-5. Total Number of Special-Care Beds in Certified Nursing Facilities in the U.S., 1993–1999

State	Rehabilitation							Ventilator							Dialysis						
	1993	1994	1995	1996	1997	1998	1999	1993	1994	1995	1996	1997	1998	1999	1993	1994	1995	1996	1997	1998	1999
AK	16	16	16	15	0	0	0	0	0	0	0	0	0	0	0	0	0	0	0	0	0
AL	29	309	176	384	301	265	363	43	37	37	17	62	46	87	0	0	0	0	0	0	0
AR	0	178	192	70	82	82	170	1s	6	12	7	18	46	23	0	0	0	0	0	14	0
AZ	75	96	100	188	184	236	194	30	64	38	87	93	165	0	0	64	60	75	0	60	0
CA	2,787	3,461	3,062	3,470	2,409	2,331	2,337	849	1,195	1,155	1,236	976	1,156	1,134	3	77	99	52	14	19	272
CO	319	239	236	203	213	215	365	10	70	73	54	56	13	1	0	7	7	4	22	5	14
CT	774	1,166	1,031	1,236	1,517	1,455	1,064	81	136	136	130	133	43	66	2	20	0	4	4	4	0
DC	78	66	0	0	0	33	0	0	0	0	0	0	14	14	0	0	0	0	0	0	0
DE	148	59	59	69	59	59	0	9	60	56	30	34	8	35	8	0	0	0	0	0	0
FL	641	1,189	1,073	1,101	1,218	1,101	1,940	314	450	497	496	361	465	269	4	0	0	69	17	44	18
GA	110	321	275	197	163	263	265	8	8	8	32	32	39	10	0	0	0	0	0	2	2
HI	0	10	10	0	22	0	0	0	10	10	0	0	0	0	0	10	10	0	0	0	0
IA	34	40	57	133	135	112	148	0	9	9	57	31	0	8	0	0	0	10	4	1	0
ID	34	112	147	89	135	119	126	0	4	8	4	12	4	4	0	0	0	0	0	0	0
IL	1,334	1,937	1,921	1,408	1,588	1,584	1,775	148	353	343	334	402	366	352	14	23	33	2	33	13	12
IN	413	515	424	766	628	567	401	342	175	398	140	126	71	38	0	0	0	19	19	0	1
KS	126	329	215	160	147	125	122	6	5	5	14	8	0	0	0	2	2	0	0	0	0
KY	58	86	91	131	78	109	146	650	230	60	67	97	13	99	0	0	0	0	0	2	0
LA	59	103	139	278	299	249	77	24	83	93	102	114	94	66	22	1	33	0	0	2	6
MA	655	1,017	1,070	962	637	515	437	187	235	121	190	171	118	76	0	0	0	2	0	2	0
MD	76	240	361	454	362	93	247	51	50	41	76	150	99	79	10	512	11	10	34	6	0
ME	34	15	15	143	174	197	244	0	3	3	0	25	0	1	9	9	9	9	9	9	9
MI	190	221	144	237	253	337	398	136	94	101	71	110	100	so	1	0	0	0	1	1	0
MN	269	495	632	748	872	958	1,010	16	57	56	47	47	43	48	0	148	148	0	0	12	12
MO	86	174	184	168	152	185	124	46	34	34	42	47	32	20	1	5	5	so	0	1	0
MS	0	33	43	49	98	187	268	0	0	0	0	0	8	8	0	0	0	0	0	0	0
MT	30	46	46	14	35	26	40	0	0	0	0	0	8	0	0	0	0	0	0	8	0
NC	297	388	328	M	312	137	0	103	146	152	164	154	166	144	10	0	0	0	0	0	0
ND	0	29	29	0	0	0	0	0	0	0	0	0	0	8	0	0	0	0	0	0	0
NE	160	136	136	182	162	176	206	106	55	55	59	63	62	76	6	0	0	0	2	0	0

Table 1-5. (Continued)

State	Rehabilitation							Ventilator							Dialysis						
	1993	1994	1995	1996	1997	1998	1999	1993	1994	1995	1996	1997	1998	1999	1993	1994	1995	1996	1997	1998	1999
NH	142	86	62	118	90	72	100	50	62	62	72	6	0	12	0	50	50	50	50	0	5
NJ	190	142	142	223	350	388	95	109	127	107	106	148	201	131	0	0	0	9	0	0	3
NM	0	29	29	0	0	16	0	0	1	1	1	0	0	0	0	0	0	0	0	0	0
NV	0	0	0	0	47	37	61	0	13	12	1	144	26	46	0	0	0	20	0	0	2
NY	450	258	505	883	914	1,557	1,183	152	152	113	196	403	400	506	4	10	10	0	3	9	4
OH	424	518	367	723	986	884	1,035	287	474	457	706	803	593	512	1	1	3	0	27	0	0
OK	49	114	129	99	247	165	316	19	42	46	25	23	14	9	6	3	3	1	a	8	U
OR	179	139	118	121	97	104	209	4	1	1	10	16	0	1	0	4	4	2	4	0	1
PA	715	923	846	1,060	831	923	795	231	263	237	240	289	510	434	12	1	1	5	3	3	15
RI	138	64	64	114	76	164	227	14	22	0	0	0	25	10	0	0	0	0	2	0	
SC	0	71	148	216	120	151	0	0	0	0	0	8	4	12	0	0	0	0	0	3	0
SD	0	48	48	79	61	50	61	0	24	24	36	36	36	36	0	0	0	0	0	0	0
TN	254	159	109	183	62	175	165	12	73	85	77	3	56	15	0	1	1	9	0	1	0
TX	247	278	299	233	336	145	150	44	161	141	164	159	93	56	10	18	18	4	0	4	0
UT	156	180	214	139	114	100	115	20	6	12	12	0	5	0	6	0	0	10	0	0	0
VA	265	351	363	394	322	222	307	124	131	108	142	134	80	57	0	0	0	0	0	0	0
VT	32	60	120	60	80	112	112	1	0	0	0	0	0	0	0	0	0	0	0	0	0
WA	169	139	133	187	365	198	268	94	107	172	85	66	64	58	10	0	13	6	1	4	126
WI	618	1,030	990	842	822	785	522	56	103	103	95	76	72	53	0	2	2	4	10	10	10
WV	0	32	20	0	0	36	68	2	34	0	0	0	40	40	0	0	0	0	0	36	36
WY	24	0	0	19	29	0	0	0	0	0	0	0	0	0	0	0	0	0	0	0	0
US	12,884	17,647	16,918	18,754	18,184	18,000	18,256	3,806	5,365	5,172	5,423	5,692	5,406	4,726	139	968	522	426	265	283	568

Nursing Facilities, Staffing, Residents and Facility Deficiencies, 1993-1999
Department of Social & Behavioral Sciences
University of California San Francisco

separate units for such residents. Finding and establishing niches must be done carefully—what may be a great marketing tool may be cost-prohibitive in practice. Many administrators have found that the unbelievably high ventilator reimbursements barely cover the increased costs of service.

Developing niches is becoming increasingly important because as we will see in part 4, average occupancy rates dropped from 88% in 1993 to 82% in 1999, a trend that can portend economic disaster for the average facility's financial solvency, which we discuss in part 3.

DEVELOPING A MARKETING STRATEGY FOR THE FACILITY

Step One: The Audit

A first step in developing a marketing strategy is the audit. *Auditing* is the process of identifying, collecting, and analyzing information about the external environment. Marketers typically characterize a market as potential, available, qualified, served, and penetrated. The *potential market* is all the people who express some level of interest in a defined market offer. Discounting those who are interested but unable to pay defines the *available market:* those who have the interest, the funds, and access to the market offering. The *qualified available market* is those who have interest, financial means, access, and quality (for example, who meet the requirement for 24-hour-a-day nursing care). The *served market* is that segment of the qualified available market that the facility makes an effort to attract to the facility. Those who are admitted to or served by the facility constitute the *penetrated market,* the actual consumers of the services offered.

It is necessary to estimate the extent of demand for a service the facility might offer. Total market demand is the total volume of services that would be bought by a defined available number of persons in a specific geographic area in a defined time period in a stated marketing environment under a specific marketing program (Kotler & Clarke, 1987). Market forces measure the number of services that the facility could expect to be purchased under such a specific marketing plan.

In forecasting future demand Kotler and Clarke suggest the facility examine three things: (a) uncontrollable environment factors such as the economy, technological changes, reimbursement formula changes, and broad changes in the health care system such as the emergence of managed care; (b) new competition from other providers (e.g., new facilities, new services, new marketing budget); and (c) intraorganizational factors such as the condition of one's facility, possible new services, and promotional efforts programs (Kotler & Clarke, 1987). Forecasts may be based on what people say they will do, are actually doing, and have actually done in the past.

Step-Two: Market Segmentation

Market segmentation is using the audit information to divide the people who are potentially to be served into identifiable subgroups. Subgroups may be longer- and shorter-term residents who come for rehabilitation then return home, or groupings such as private pay patients and public-pay patients. Further, a nursing home chain might segment the market it seeks by geography: region of the country, urban or rural, density, and climate. Markets can be segmented by demographic characteristics such as age, family size, sex, educational level, occupation, or religion. Psychographic social classes can also be used (life style, personality). Those who are by nature gregarious and who thrive on extensive personal interactions, for example, are good candidates for application to life care communities. In addition, behavior tendencies can be used to segment markets; benefits sought (for example, a life care community benefit set), user status (within age limits and able to pay), and readiness stage (persons over a certain age, retired, and actively seeking a care giver) all identify market segments (Hitt et al., 2001).

Step Three: The Marketing Mix

Determining the market mix consists of deciding what types of residents to approach and in what proportions. Most facilities find it useful to identify specific groups of the people they are seeking to serve. This is more feasible and necessary in urban settings than in rural areas where choices of whom to serve may be more limited by geography and income.

Most facilities will consciously choose a *product mix,* that is, the set of all product lines and items the facility intends to offer. A *product line* in the nursing facility setting is a set of services within the product mix that are closely related due to functional similarity, for example, being made available to the same type of persons, or marketed through the same channels. A facility may choose to serve a combination of heavy-care patients from the local hospital who can expect to return home or die shortly as one group, plus another group of persons who enter as light-care patients and are expected to remain in the facility for the foreseeable future. A *product item* is a distinct unit within a product line that is distinguishable by purpose in some other characteristic. The facility may, for example, within the heavy-care group, especially solicit persons being fed intravenously or needing tracheostomy care.

Step Four: Implementing and Evaluating the Plan

Implementing the marketing plan is the process of managing organizational behaviors and outreach activities to attract residents with the identified characteristics in the proportions desired.

Creating awareness among potential consumers that the services exist, assisting them in deciding, and assuring that they are satisfied with the quality of services provided by the facility is the process of *marketing implementation* (King, 1963). An ongoing evaluation of the effectiveness of the marketing efforts is necessary.

THE MARKETING OF SERVICES

Nursing facilities are primarily in the business of marketing services. A service is an activity or benefit that one person can offer to another that is intangible and does not result in the ownership of anything (Kotler & Clarke, 1987). According to Berkowitz, Kerin, and Rudelius (1986), services have four characteristics that differentiate them from durable goods: intangibility, inconsistency, inseparability, and inventory.

The Characteristics of Services

Intangibility. Services cannot be touched, sat in, or driven like a car: They are intangible. Health care that the resident expects to receive in a nursing facility cannot be experienced directly before entering the facility. Nursing facilities can, however, make services appear more tangible (for example, a TV advertisement portraying attentive care being given to a resident at the facility) (Berkowicz, Kerin, & Rudelius, 1986).

Inconsistency. The marketing of services differs from marketing tangible goods like an automobile because the quality of service can be inconsistent from day to day or even from one shift to the next. Quality that endures over time can be built into a car through consistent assembly-line procedures and quality checks, but the service received at the hands of the nurses or nursing assistants on any given day can vary widely depending on the mood of the employee.

Inseparability. A third characteristic of service marketing is that the consumer does not separate the service from the deliverer of the service or the setting in which service is given. The nursing home may be giving excellent nursing care, but if the bathrooms smell bad and are dirty the patients' and visitors' perceptions of the facility, including their perceptions of quality of nursing care, are affected. The services given and the service provided are inseparably linked in the consumer's mind.

Inventory. Idle production capacity (that is, the presence of an unoccupied bed in a health care facility) is a fourth characteristic of service marketing. The inventory carrying costs of empty nursing home beds is high: Empty beds may cost as much as 70% of the cost of occupied beds due to fixed and variable costs (discussed in part 3).

In *Marketing Long-Term and Senior Care Services,* Midgett (1984) asserts that if a nursing facility carefully apportions the number of subsidized and private-pay patients, it can provide better accommodations and services for both. This is true because in many states the public reimbursement rates are at or below costs, forcing providers to subsidize publicly paying patients by shifting these costs to the bills of private-paying patients. (Sinioris & Butler, 1983).

CONSUMER DECISION MAKING

Marketing texts typically characterize *consumer decision making* as (a) problem recognition, (b) information search, (c) alternative evaluation, (d) purchase decision, (e) post-purchase evaluation (Berkowitz, Kerin and Rudelius, 1986).

Kotler and Clarke (1987) describe it in a similar way (a) need arousal (trigger factors such as a hospital episode), (b) information gathering, (c) decision evaluation, (d) decision execution, (e) post-decision assessment.

The decision for a person to enter a nursing facility is often a complex one shared by several participants. The decision making unit may consist of the following:

- *initiator*—the daughter, for example, who suggests looking into nursing facility care
- *influential friend*—for example, acquaintances already in local nursing facilities or who have convalesced in one
- *decider*—the person who ultimately forces some part of the decision, perhaps the son who decides he cannot provide the new level of care needed
- *buyer*—the person who will pay the bills, if not the resident
- *user*—the person who will be the new resident or nursing home service user (Hitt et al., 2001; Kotler & Clarke, 1987)

Decisions are based on the consumer's perceptions of whether the service provided by the nursing facility will meet their needs (Goldsmith & Leebow, 1986; Kotler, 1986; Peters & Austin, 1985). Research suggests that physicians typically have a major influence on patient decisions (Smith, 1984), and recommendations from local physicians can provide the facility with a sustainable advantage (Ghemawat, 1986). Hospital discharge planners are an important group whose image of the facility and communication with it can also provide a competitive edge (Kotler & Clarke, 1987).

EFFECTIVE MARKETING TOOLS

A personal tour through the building that includes meeting staff and patients is one of the most effective marketing tools available to the facility (Butler, 1986; Skelly, 1986). During the visit or visits the potential clients, usually the children or close friends of the prospective resident, are gathering impressions on which they will make judgments of the facility. Subliminal perceptions often become the key factor. Subliminal perceptions are factors which the decision maker is not consciously aware of, such as the general appearance of the facility, absence of odors, the friendliness of the staff, and appearance of the patients (Robertson, Zielinski, & Ward, 1984).

One writer has argued that image is credibility (Peterson, 1986). Numerous ways are available for creating a positive image for the facility in the community. Developing a community advisory board, hosting neighborhood open-houses, publicizing enthusiastic families and volunteers, and cosponsoring community events such as local arts festivals are but a few of the avenues available to facilities (Anderson, 1986; Kotler & Clarke, 1987; Ruff, 1986; Jerstd & Meier, 1986; Sweeney & Lewis, 1986; U.S. Department of Health and Human Services, 1985).

ADVERTISING

Many facilities have begun to advertise their services. Advertising consists of non-personal forms of communication conducted through paid media with a clear sponsorship program (Kotler & Clarke, 1987). The purpose of advertising is to motivate the target audience to move through the following buyer-readiness states toward actual use of facility services (Kotler & Clarke, 1987):

- cognitive (awareness that the facility is available)
- affective (favorable image of facility when comparing it to alternatives)
- behavioral (conviction; for example, ask physician to "place mother there")

Nursing facilities are increasingly focusing on serving the customer (Hauser, 1984; Rosenberg & Van West, 1984).

REFERENCES: PART ONE

Allport, F. H. (1962). A structuronomic conception of behavior. *Journal of Abnormal and Social Psychology,* 3–30.

Allport, F. H. (1993). *Institutional behavior.* Chapel Hill: University of North Carolina Press.

American Hospital Association. (1990). *Hospital statistics, 1989–1990 edition.* Chicago: Author.

American Hospital Association. (1990). *Trends among U.S. registered hospitals,* 1989–1990 edition. Chicago: Author.

America's most admired corporations. (1995, March 6). *Fortune,* p. 66.

Anderson, C. C. (1986). Local arts festival raises facility to new heights. *Provider, 12,* (4), 50–55.

Argenti, P. A. (1994). *The portable MBS desk reference.* New York: Wiley.

Barnard, C. I. (1938). *The functions of the executive.* Cambridge, MA: Harvard University Press.

Berkowitz, E. N., Kerin, R. A., & Rudelius, W. (1986). *Marketing.* St. Louis, MO: Mosby.

Bliesmer, M. (1993). Research considerations: Nursing home quality perceptions. *Journal of Gerontological Nursing,* 27–34.

Boling, T. E., et al. (1983). *Nursing home management.* Springfield, IL: Charles C. Thomas.

Braun, B. I. (1991). The effect of nursing home quality on patient outcome. *Journal of American Geriatrics Society, 39,* 329–338.

Butler, R. L. (1986). Nursing homes gain consumer confidence. *Provider, 12*(11), 48.

Califano, J. A., Jr. (1986). *America's health care revolution.* New York: Random House.

Christensen, C. R., Berg, N. A., & Salter, M. S. (1980). *Policy formulation and administration* (8th ed.). Homewood, IL: Irwin.

Dale, E. (1969). Management: Theory and practice (2nd ed.). New York: McGraw-Hill.

Dearden, J., & McFarlan, F. W. (1966). *Management information systems: Text and cases.* Homewood, IL: Irwin.

DeGroot, M. H. (1970). *Optimal statistical decisions.* New York: McGraw-Hill.

Demski, J. S. (1980). *Information analysis* (2nd ed.). Reading, MA: Addison-Wesley.

Drucker, P. F. (1954). *Practice of management.* New York: Harper and Row.

Evashwick, C. J. (1993, Fall). Strategic management of a continuum of care. *The Journal of Long-Term Care Administration,* 13–24.

Fine, S. H. (1984, June 16). The health product: A social marketing perspective. *Hospitals,* 66–68.

French, J. R. P., Jr., & Raven, B. H. (1960). The bases of social power. In D. Cartwright & A. Zander (Eds.), *Group dynamics: Research and theory* (2nd ed.). Evanston, IL: Row, Peterson.

George, C. S., Jr. (1972). *The history of management thought* (2nd ed.). Englewood Cliffs, NJ: Prentice-Hall.

Ghemawat, P. (1986). Sustainable advantage. *Harvard Business Review, 64*(5), 53–58.

Goldsmith, M., & Leebov, W. (1986). Strengthening the hospital's marketing position through training. *Health Care Management Review, 11*(2), 83–93.

Gordon, G. K., & Stryker, R. (1983). *Creative long-term care administration.* Springfield, IL: Charles C. Thomas.

Gulick, L., & Lyndall. (Eds.). (1937). *Papers on the science of administration.* New York: Institute of Public Administration.

Harrington, C. H., Carrillo, M. S., Thollaug, S. C., Summers, P. R., and Wellin, V. (2000). *Nursing facilities, staffing, residents, and facility deficiencies, 1993 through 1999.* University of California at San Francisco, Department of Social and Behavioral Sciences.

Hamel, G., & Prahalad, C. K. (1994). *Competing for the future.* Boston: Harvard Business School Press.

Hauser, L. J. (1984, September 1). 10 reasons hospital marketing programs fail. *Hospitals,* pp. 74–77.

Health care initiatives in hospital risk management. (1989, July). United States General Accounting Office (GAO-HRD-89-79.

Health care TV advertising up 40% for first half of 1986. (1986, October 20). *Hospitals, 16.*

Hegland, A. (1995, March). Computer power. *Provider,* 44–54.

Hitt, M. A., Ireland, R. D., & Hoskisson, R. E. (2001). *Strategic management: Competitiveness and globalization* (4th ed). Cincinnati, OH: South-Western College Publishing.

Inguanzo, J. M., & Harju, M. (1985, January 1). Creating a market niche. *Hospitals,* 62–67.

Jackson, F. W., Peter, W., Rosenberg, M., & Peck, R. (1995). Nursing home software: Explore the future. *Nursing Homes, 44*(1), 12–15.

Jackson, J. (1960). The organization and its communication problems. In A. Grimshaw & J. W. Hennessey, Jr. (Eds.), *Organizational behavior: Cases and readings.* New York: McGraw-Hill.

Jerstad, M. A., & Meier, P. (1986). Advisory board a valuable "two-way link" to community. *Provider, 12*(11), 60–63.

Johns, G., & Saks, A. (2001). *Organizational Behavior* (5th ed.). Toronto, Canada: Addison Wesley Longman.

Johnson, L. (1994). TQM: A process for discovering the obvious in your facility. *LTC Administrators, 28*(1), 1, 10.

Juran, J. M. (1988). *Juran's quality control handbook* (4th ed.). New York: McGraw-Hill.

Katz, D., & Kahn, R. L. (1967). *The social psychology of organizations.* New York: Wiley.

King, H. (1963, June). Effective marketing can maintain census. *Contemporary Administrator,* 39–41.

Kinnear, T. C., & Bernhardt, K. L. (1986). *Principles of marketing* (2nd ed.). Glenview, IL: Scott, Foresman.

Kodner, D. L. (1993, Fall). Long-term care 2010: Speculations and implications. *Journal of Long-term care Administration,* 82–86.

Kotler, P. (1986). Megamarketing. *Harvard Business Review, 64*(2), 117–124.

Kotler, P., & Clarke, R. N. (1987). *Marketing for health care organizations.* Englewood Cliffs, NJ: Prentice-Hall.

Kotter, J. P. (1982). *The general managers.* New York: Free Press.

Kriegel, R. J. (1991). *If it ain't broke.* New York: Warner.

Levey, S., & Loomba, N. P. (1973). *Health care administration: A managerial perspective.* Philadelphia: Lippincott.

Levey, S., & Loomba, N. P. (1984). *Health care administration: A managerial perspective* (2nd ed.). New York: Lippincott.

Maddox, G. L. (et al.) & Sussman, S. W. (2001). *The encyclopedia of aging* (3rd ed.). New York: Springer.

Meal, H. C. (1984). Putting production decisions where they belong. *Harvard Business Review, 84*(2), 102–111.

Melum, M. M., & Sinioris, M. K. (1992). *Total quality management: The health care pioneers.* Chicago: American Hospital Publisher.

Midgett, M. (1984). Skilled nursing facility marketing. In W. J. Winston (Ed.), *Marketing long-term care and senior care services* (pp. 77–81). New York: Haworth.

Miller, D. B. (Ed.). (1982). *Long-term care administrator's desk manual.* Greenvale, NY: Panel.

Miller, D. B., & Barry, J. T. (1979). *Nursing home organization and operation.* Boston: CBI.

Miller, J. G. (1955). Toward a general theory for the behavioral sciences. *American Psychologist,* 10.

Mintzberg, H. (1979). *The structure of organizations: A synthesis of the research.* Englewood Cliffs, NJ: Prentice-Hall.

Molloy, G. E. (1994, October). Quality is the administration job #1. *Nursing Homes,* 36–39.

National Citizens' Coalition for Nursing Home Reform. (1989, September-October). *Quality Care Advocate.* Washington, DC: Author.

Noe, R., Hollenbeck, J. R., Gerhart, B., & Wright, P. M. (2000). *Human resource management: Gaining a competitive advantage* (3rd ed.). Boston: McGraw-Hill.

Omnibus Budget Reconciliation Act (OBRA). (1991, September 26). Medicare and Medicaid. *Federal Register, 56*(187), 48825–48922.

Peters, T. (1987). *Thriving on chaos.* New York: Harper & Row.

Peters, T., & Austin, N. (1985). *A passion for excellence: The leadership difference.* New York: Random House.

Peterson, S. (1986). Take note: Image is as image does. *Provider, 12*(11), 36–39.

Pfeffer, J., & Salanick, G. R. (1978). *The external control of organizations.* New York: Harper & Row.

Pressman, J. L., & Wildavsky, A. B. (1974). *Implementation.* Berkeley: University of California Press.

Robertson, T. S., Zielinski, J., & Ward, S. (1984). *Consumer behavior.* Palo Alto, CA: Scott, Foresman.

Robey, D. (1982). *Designing organizations.* Homewood, IL: Irwin.

Rogers, W. W. (1980). *General administration in the nursing home* (3rd ed.). Boston: CBI.

Rosenberg, L. J., & Van West, J. H. (1984, November-December). The collaborative approach to marketing. *Business Horizons, 29*–35.

Ruff, K. A. (1986). Families and friends can help educate. *Provider, 12*(11), 46–47.

Shackle, G. L. S. (1957). *Uncertainty and business decisions: A symposium* (2nd ed.). Liverpool, England: Liverpool University Press.

Showalter, J. (1984). Quality assurance and risk management: A joinder of two important movements. *Journal of Legal Medicine, 5,* 497.

Sinioris, M. E., & Butler, P. (1983, June 1). Basic business strategy: Responding to change requires planning, marketing, and budgeting strategies. *Hospitals, 57.*

Skelly, G. (1986). Is food service a part of your marketing strategy? *Provider, 12*(11), 58–60.

Smith, S. M. (1984). Family selection of long-term care services. In W. J. Winston (Ed.), *Marketing long-term and senior care services* (pp. 101–113). New York: Haworth.

Spendolini, M. J. (1992). *The benchmarking book.* New York: American Management Association.

Star, S. H. (1989). Marketing and its discontents. *Harvard Business Review, 89*(6), 148–154.

Sweeney, M., & Lewis, C. (1986). Neighborhood nursing home program opens the right doors. *Provider, 12*(11), 70–71.

Swiss, J. E. (1983). Establishing a management system: The interaction of power shifts and personality under federal MBO. *Public Administration Review, 43*(3), 238–245.

Tannenbaum, R., Wechsler, I., & Massarik, F. (1961). *Leadership and organization.* New York: McGraw-Hill.

Ting, H. M. (1984, May). New directions in nursing home and home healthcare marketing. Healthcare financial management, pp. 62–72.

U.S. Department of Health and Human Services Administration on Aging. (1985). *On finding, training, and keeping volunteers from dropping out.* (DHHS Publication No. 348). Washington, DC: U.S. Government Printing Office.

U.S. Department of Health and Human Services Administration. (1989). *Health U.S.: 1988.* (DHHS Publication No. PHS 89-1232). Hyattsville, MD: Author.

von Bertalanffy, L. (1967). Der organismus als physikalishes system betrachtet. In D. Katz & R. L. Kahn (Eds.), *The social psychology of organizations.* New York: Wiley.

Walton, M. (1986). *The Deming management method.* New York: Perigee.

Webster's new world dictionary. (Nth ed.) (1968). New York: World.

Welch, J. F. (1993, December 13). A master class in radical change. *Future, 83.*

Withington, F. G. (1966). *The use of computers in business organizations.* Reading, MA: Addison-Wesley.

Wrapp, H. E. (1984). Good managers don't make policy decisions. *Harvard Business Review, 84*(4).

Zmud, R. W. (1983). *Information systems in organization.* Dallas, TX: Scott, Foresman.

PART TWO

Human Resources

2.1 Organizational Patterning of the Nursing Facility and Its Staff

COMPLEXITY OF THE STAFF'S ORGANIZATIONAL TASKS

The goal of Total Quality Management is that human resources in every unit arrive at a level of daily performance reflecting a passion for quality (Hitt et al., 2001; Johns & Saks, 2001). This goal is more easily articulated than accomplished, as the multitude of regulations can seem overwhelming. It is often said, only partly in jest, that the nursing home industry is the second most regulated industry, with nuclear power the first. But even that may no longer be true. The nuclear power industry is being deregulated while legal constraints on the nursing home industry are being tightened.

Remembering the array of requirements to be met by each facility is beyond the capacity of a single person. As regulations continue to proliferate, the average nursing-home administrator must increasingly depend on department heads and their staffs to be the experts in each area.

The decision on how to staff a nursing facility depends on many variables. An overarching consideration is the level of medical complexity of care to be delivered. Changes in case mix will normally result in altered staffing patterns. Admission of several medically complex patients/residents may lead to employment of an additional experienced registered nurse and the retraining of most of the floor nurses (Maddox et al., 2001). Admission of several lighter-care residents may call for additional aides rather than additional registered nurses. In this section we present options in organizational form, and a staffing pattern that a 100–bed facility with an average level of intensity might consider.

ORGANIZATIONAL PATTERN FOR A 100-BED FACILITY

Figure 2-1 shows the organizational pattern and staffing levels for a 100-bed facility as recommended in the federal government regulations in July, 1970. This listing of the essential functional areas is still valid.

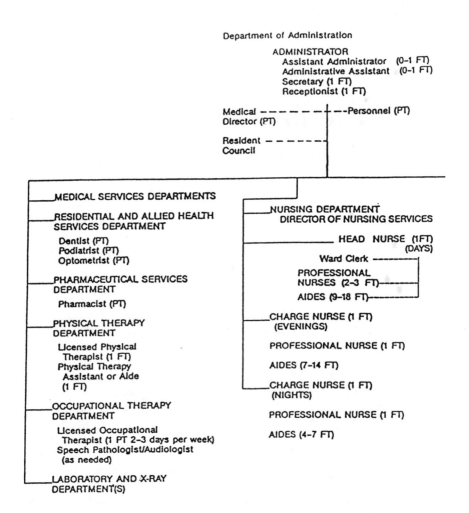

FIGURE 2-1. Organizational pattern for a 100-bed nursing facility.

BUSINESS DEPARTMENT
Business Manager (1 FT)
Bookkeeper (1 FT)
Secretarial Assistance
(1 FT)

MEDICAL RECORDS DEPARTMENT
Records Coordinator (1 FT)

ADMITTING DEPARTMENT (PT)

DIETARY DEPARTMENT

Food Service Director (1 FT)
Supervisors (2–3 FT)
Cooks (2–3 FT)
Salad Makers (2 FT)
Dietary Aides (3–5 FT)

SOCIAL SERVICES DEPARTMENT
Social Services Coordinator (1 FT,
BA degree)
Certified Social Work Consultant
(1 PT)
Social Work Assistant (1 FT)
Secretarial Assistance (PT)

RECREATION DEPARTMENT

Activities Director (1 FT)
Activities Assistant (1 FT)
Volunteers

HOUSEKEEPING DEPARTMENT

Housekeeping Director (1 FT)
Maids (4–8 FT)
Floor Custodians (1–2 FT)

LAUNDRY DEPARTMENT
Laundry Director (1 FT)
Laundry Assistants (2–4 FT)

MAINTENANCE DEPARTMENT

Maintenance Director (1 FT)
Maintenance Assistants (2–5 FT)

QUALITY ASSESSMENT
AND CONTROL COMMITTEE

AN INFECTION CONTROL
PROGRAM

A PHYSICAL PLANT
HEALTH AND SAFETY PROGRAM

Various Configurations

In actual practice, these 17 "departmental" areas can be, and routinely are, given different titles and combined variously. Nevertheless, however configured, these areas must be accounted for in the typical nursing facility organizational plan.

In Figure 2-1 each position within the 17 departments or functional areas (for instance, admissions) is depicted, along with the number of its staff and whether they are full-time or part-time.

The upper area in Figure 2-1 reflects the administrator, his immediate staff, and advisory roles (indicated by the dotted lines) of the medical director and resident council. The first column includes the medical and allied health professionals essential to the facility (for example, physicians, dentists, pharmacist, occupational and physical therapists). The nursing service with its three shifts is the second column. Areas in the third column are also necessary to the functioning of a facility (the business office, dietary, social services, activities, housekeeping, and maintenance). In the final column are activities mandated by the federal requirements.

Workable Variations

Numerous workable variations on the model exist. In this one, line authority is given to the administrator leading to the several functional areas or departments. The administrator has responsibility, directly or indirectly, for all the functions of the facility.

A variant of this model, more suited to a larger facility of perhaps 200 residents/patients, is to group several of these functions under middle-level managers who report to the administrator. One such arrangement is to appoint six middle-level managers (Johns & Saks, 2001; Miller, 1982; Noe et al., 2000) who are directors of

- Resident Services (volunteers, transportation, barbers, beauticians)
- Administrative Services (admissions, business office, clerical staff, and human resources)
- Therapy Services (physical, occupational, and speech therapy)
- Nursing Services (all nursing activities)
- Supportive Services (housekeeping, laundry, and maintenance)
- Dietary Services

The more common model is depicted in Figure 2-1 where all department heads report directly to the administrator. In the typical 100-bed nursing facility the administrator will have eight or nine department heads reporting directly to her.

We turn now to consideration of the organizational work to be accomplished by each department and consider their staffing requirements.

THE ADMINISTRATOR'S OFFICE

We have demonstrated that the administrator is responsible for ensuring that all work is accomplished according to policy at an acceptable level of quality.

Administration

To summarize briefly, consider the following as an initial description in no particular order of priority. It is the charge of administration to

- ensure a satisfactory quality of care and of life for residents/patients, staff
- advocate for the residents/patients and, as needed, staff and the facility
- monitor and control all the subsystems in the facility
- develop and manage the budget
- manage the interface between the facility and its many constituencies, the world outside
- monitor, manage the human resources functions
- coordinate or assure coordination of the work of all departments and functions in the facility
- lead, provide stimulus on a daily basis to activities that implement the facility's goals, and mission
- forecast and lead the facility to a successful future
- assist all staff and residents to understand the nature and value of change
- interface with owners, inspectors, ombudspersons, third-party insurers, hospitals, fire departments, and the myriad other persons, groups, and functions necessary to the survival of the facility
- communicate with staff, residents/patients, others
- empower department heads and staff to accomplish their work
- facilitate the functioning of the facility by walking around and similar management approaches
- set the tone for the facility in matters of dress, taste, compassion, and concern by word and behavior
- settle territorial and jurisdictional disputes among staff, residents, owners

The effective administrator does whatever it takes to have effective control of resident care in the facility. In recent years a number of facility administrators have utilized some variation of a daily department head meeting. Some call it "stand-up" and meet for 10 minutes or so each morning; others call it "stand-up" even though they sit down for about 30 minutes each morning and review every resident; others meet with department heads only once a week or less often.

In addition, more than any one else in the facility, the administrator is responsible for resident rights. Table 2-1 demonstrates 97%+ conform-

Table 2-1. Percentage of Nursing Facilities in the U.S. with Deficiencies for Resident Rights, 1993–1999

		Deficiency Group = Resident Right						
FTAG	Description	1993	1994	1995	1996	1997	1998	1999
F151	Exercise of Rights	1.4	1.6	1.3	1.2	0.8	1.3	1.1
F152	Free of Reprisal	1.7	1.1	0.7	0.7	0.7	0.9	0.9
F153	Access to Records	0.6	0.4	0.3	0.1	0.2	0.2	0.1
F154	Informed of Condition	2.6	2.8	1.7	1.3	1.0	0.9	1.1
F155	Refuse Treatment	1.5	1.6	1.2	1.1	0.9	1.1	1.0
F156	Notice of Rights and Services	12.5	11.0	7.0	4.1	3.4	3.1	3.1
F157	Notice of Changes	6.2	6.4	5.6	5.5	5.7	6.9	7.9
F158	Resident Manage Financial Affairs	0.2	0.2	0.2	0.1	0.1	0.1	0.1
F159	Facility Manage Personal Funds	8.7	5.6	3.9	2.4	2.4	2.4	.2.4
F160	Convey Funds	1.5	1.5	1.2	0.5	0.6	0.8	0.8
F161	Financial Security	3.1	2.4	2.3	1.2	0.9	0.9	0.7
F162	Limit on Charges to Funds	0.7	0.7	0.5	0.6	0.5	0.4	0.4
F163	Choice of Physician	0.2	0.2	0.3	0.2	0.2	0.2	.0.2
F164	Privacy and Confidentiality	7.7	7.0	7.4	7.2	6.9	7.1	7.2
F165	Voice Grievances	0.5	0.5	0.4	0.3	0.3	0.2	0.3
F166	Resolve Grievances	3.6	3.7	3.8	3.1	2.9	3.1	3.5
F167	Survey Results	6.8	7.1	6.1	4.0	2.7	3.4	3.6
F168	Information	0.2	0.2	0.2	0.1	0.1	0.2	0.2
F169	Work	0.3	0.2	0.1	0.0	0.0	0.0	0.0
F170	Mail	0.4	0.4	1.0	0.9	1.1	1.4	1.3
F171	Stationary	0.0	0.0	0.0	0.0	0.0	0.0	0.0
F172	Visitors	0.3	0.3	0.2	0.2	0.1	0.1	0.2
F173	Ombudsman	0.0	0.0	0.0	0.0	0.0	0.0	0.0
F174	Telephone	4.1	2.9	3.1	2.1	1.7	1.6	1.4
F175	Married Couples	0.1	0.1	0.1	0.0	0.0	0.0	0.0
F176	Administer Own Drugs	3.3	3.4	3.1	2.3	2.1	2.4	2.5
F177	Refuse Transfers	0.4	0.3	0.3	0.3	04	0.2	0.2

Nursing Facilities, Staffing, Residents and Facility Deficiencies, 1993-1999
Department of Social & Behavioral Sciences
University of California San Francisco

**Table 2-2. Percentage of Nursing Facilities in the U.S. with Deficiencies for
Other Activities, 1993–1999**

FTAG	Description	Deficiency Group = Other Activities						
		1993	1994	1995	1996	1997	1998	1999
F514	Clinical Records	-	13.5	10.7	10.0	9.1	9.4	10.2
F516	Records Safeguarded	-	0.6	0.5	0.4	0.6	0.5	0.6
F517	Plans for Emergency	-	0.7	0.5	0.3	0.4	0.4	0.4
F518	Emergency Training	-	3.3	2.9	2.2	1.8	2.2	2.4
F519	Transfer Agreement	-	0.0	0.1	0.0	0.0	0.0	0.0
F520	Quality Assurance Committee	-	0.7	0.9	0.8	0.7	0.6	1.0
F521	Quality Assurance Activities		3.1	2.5	2.1	1.9	2.0	1.9
F522	Disclosure of Ownership	-	0.0	0.1	0.0	0.0	0.0	0.0

Nursing Facilities, Staffing, Residents and Facility Deficiencies, 1993-1999
Department of Social & Behavioral Sciences
University of California San Francisco

ance in the area of resident rights with the exceptions of being able to provide F157, the 30-day notice of changes and F167, the subjective areas of privacy and confidentiality.

In Table 2-2 shows deficiencies for other activities, an area of general concern to the administrator, and 97.6% to 100% compliance was achieved with the exception of 89.8% compliance for clinical records. This is a difficult area as records are increasingly being transitioned from 100% paper to 5% paper and 95% electronic.

Assistant Administrator/Administrative Assistant. An assistant administrator has line authority to represent the administrator, can make decisions on the administrator's behalf, and is usually assigned some area to oversee. An administrative assistant, on the other hand, has no line authority, cannot make decisions for the facility, and does not represent the administrator except in an information-gathering or processing manner. The administrative assistant is a staff position.

In the typical nursing facility of 100 beds, there tends not to be enough organizational room for an assistant administrator; 300 or more beds would call for an assistant administrator. The appointment of an assistant administrator and administrative assistant depends on the personality of the administrator.

Secretary and Advisory Functions. Generally, the facility secretary works in the administrator's office, in an area shared with the receptionist/telephone operator/manager. The receptionist needs to know all the employee application procedures if applicants are to feel welcome and needs to be in the communication loop. The receptionist is key. If relatives were to walk in at 11:00 a.m. and the receptionist cheerily asked, "Are you here to see Uncle Don?", it would reflect badly on the facility if "Uncle Don" had died an hour earlier.

As a rule, the administrator has several advisory persons or groups, represented in Figure 2-1 by dotted lines. The medical director and resident council often fit into this slot. Other consultants, such as the pharmacist or dentist, and any other advisory committees might appear here. The administrator's office is responsible for keeping on file the original of several types of information, for instance, reports of the state facility inspection teams, department reports, and other important documents.

MEDICAL AND ALLIED HEALTH FUNCTIONS

Patterns of Physician Care

As a rule, the typical 100-bed facility does not require the services of a full-time medical director. The medical director is normally paid a contractual monthly fee to provide medical supervision. Federal requirements for the role of a medical director are vague, stating only that the medical director is responsible for (a) implementation of resident care policies, and (b) coordination of medical care in the facility.

The Open Medical Staff. The predominant pattern for nursing facilities of approximately 100 to 200 beds is to allow any physician licensed to practice in the state to admit patients/residents to the facility and to provide their medical care while they reside there (no one can reside in a nursing facility without physician admitting orders and continuing physician supervision). Under this pattern the part-time medical director tries to ensure that the medical needs of the patients/residents are met as they arise. The medical director often substitutes for the personal physician who fails to visit the patient on a timely basis or to perform the annual physical periodically as required by federal or state regulations. As we noted earlier under communication behaviors, people prefer to talk with those of equal rank, thus a vital role played by the medical director is to visit on a peer basis with physicians who are not meeting the actual care needs or making the required visits to patients in the facility. Because there is normally no organized medical staff, the medical director advises the administrator of the facility concerning the quality of its physician and nursing care and assists the director of nursing to ensure that a good quality of resident/patient care is delivered. The medical director may or may not admit and care for patients/residents in the facility, but usually does so for some of them. This has the functional value of allowing the medical director to be in the facility frequently walking around, seeing his/her patients.

The Closed Medical Staff. A second model of medical direction is the *closed medical staff.* This means that only physicians who have been approved by the organized medical staff of the facility may admit or treat its patients. An organized medical staff is the closed group of physicians who provide all the primary care to the patients. Initially, the board or governing body appoints one or more physicians to organize a medical staff, elect a medical director, and write bylaws to govern the medical care given in that facility, functioning much like in an organized hospital medical staff.

Closed medical staffs are more feasible for larger facilities of perhaps 300 or more patients/residents. In this situation the physicians, usually five or six for a facility of 500–600 patients/residents, divide care of the patients/residents among themselves. Numerous variations are possible. A closed medical staff has several advantages. One of them can be on duty (or immediate call) at all times and can attend to patients needing medical care but whose assigned physician is not immediately available. Some or all of the physicians may be full-time, but most are part-time. Continuous care is thus available and, because the staff physicians have some economic dependency on the facility, the administrator has available the required services. Under the open staff model considerable energy must often be devoted to gain conformity of medical services on the timely basis mandated by the federal (and state) requirements (Hogstel, 1983 pp. 27–28).

In a study of all New York State nursing facility administrators, Karuza and Katz (1994) found that on average they had 8.6 attending physicians, 32 residents per physician. Most medical directors were specialists in family practices (42%) or internal medicine (55%) and had a tenure of 7.5 years. Only 27% had an added certificate in geriatrics. Closed staff characterized 43% of facilities and were more likely in larger facilities with significant proportions of Medicaid patients. Closed medical staff had fewer physicians, more residents per physician. The investigators concluded that facility administrators should consider limiting practice privileges in nursing homes as a step toward improving quality of care (p. 787).

As demonstrated in Table 2-3 a 98% to 99.9% compliance rate is achieved regarding deficiencies for physician services.

Dental Care

Dental care is a major, often neglected, aspect of services delivered in the nursing facility. Local dentists normally do not own the portable equipment that costs from $2,000 to $15,000 or more, to give dental care

Table 2-3. Percentage of Nursing Facilities in the U.S. with Deficiencies for Physician Services, 1993–1999

		Deficiency Group = Physician Services						
FTAG	Description	1993	1994	1995	1996	1997	1998	1999
F385	Physician Supervision	1.0	0.6	0.5	0.5	0.3	0.3	0.4
F386	Physician Visits	4.2	3.3	2.0	1.8	1.3	1.4	1.5
F387	Frequency	2.1	2.1	1.6	1.5	1.5	1.8	1.9
F388	Physician Alternates	0.2	0.1	0.1	0.1	0.1	0.2	0.2
F389	Availability	0.1	0.1	0.1	0.1	0.0	0.1	0.1
F390	Physician Delegation of Tasks	0.2	0.1	0.1	0.1	0.1	0.0	0.1

Nursing Facilities, Staffing, Residents and Facility Deficiencies, 1993-1999
Department of Social & Behavioral Sciences
University of California San Francisco

inside a nursing facility. Beyond this lack is, perhaps, the dental practitioner's insecurity about functioning outside his office and dealing with the complex medical histories of patients. Finally, the dentist is reimbursed at approximately half the traditional office fee.

No one in the typical facility is trained in oral care. The mouth is not included in any significant way in the nursing curriculum; physicians do not focus on the mouth. Aides all to often practice poor oral hygiene themselves.

While the majority of current residents/patients in nursing facilities have dentures, the introduction of fluoride and other dental care efforts after World War II has resulted in increasingly larger proportions of residents/patients with teeth rather than dentures. So long as any patients/residents have dentures, the use of an inexpensive denture label kit will simplify life for the residents and staff of the facility. The need for periodic dental care does not change when one enters a nursing facility.

Solutions to this problem will vary, but any successful one will likely include appointing a local or area dentist who specializes in geriatric dental care as the dental director and paying her a monthly retainer fee of perhaps $2 to $4 per patient resident (just as one pays to have a part-time medical director). This dentist will make monthly visits, perform needed care and bill third-party payers for care given.

It is customary for the dental director to assist the facility in hiring a dental hygienist who will make rounds seeing patients/residents on a monthly or more often, and train the nursing staff to observe and meet the resident/patients' oral needs. One approach is to train oral care aides,

Table 2-4. Percentage of Nursing Facilities in the U.S. with Deficiencies for Dental Services, 1993–1999

FTAG	Description	Deficiency Group = Dental Services						
		1993	1994	1995	1996	1997	1998	1999
F411	Routine and Emergency Services (SNF)	0.4	0.4	0.4	0.3	0.4	0.5	0.5
F412	Routine and Emergency Services (NF)	0.0	0.3	0.2	0.1	0.2	0.2	0.4

Nursing Facilities, Staffing, Residents and Facility Deficiencies, 1993-1999
Department of Social & Behavioral Sciences
University of California San Francisco

a regularly employed nurse's aide who assumes responsibility for maintaining the daily oral health care of residents/patients in the facility.

Table 2-4 suggests a 99.5% compliance rate for dental services.

Foot and Eye Care

There is need for a *podiatrist,* a trained professional who is not a medical doctor, for care of the feet, including clipping of toenails for diabetics and others and for treating ailments such as corns and bunions.

As the nursing facility population becomes less and less able to make health care visits outside the facility, a periodic visit by a podiatrist (who usually brings an assistant) is becoming a routine part of resident/patient care. The podiatrist and assistant may arrange their work area in a room or even a secluded hallway on a monthly basis and provide care to a large portion of the residents/patients over the course of a morning or afternoon.

Eye care needs are similar to those for teeth and feet. As the population's mobility becomes more and more restricted, arrangements need to be made by the facility staff for a local optician to make periodic visits as part of routine health care.

Pharmaceutical Services

The consulting or the facility pharmacist is responsible at the minimum for assuring that

- all medications are available as ordered
- all medications are within the expiration date and properly labeled and handled
- all reorders and stop orders are implemented
- each resident/patient's medications are reviewed monthly for possible adverse reactions or interactions
- appropriate pharmacy policy and procedures are followed.

Additional information may be found at §483.60 in Allen (2000) *Nursing Home Federal Requirements and Guidelines to Surveyors.*

The consulting pharmacist is responsible for reviewing the drug regimen, including observing medication passes and recording and reporting drug error rates and any other problems observed. While the federal requirements call for the consultant to report to the attending physician and the director of nursing, the administrator would be wise to stipulate in the consultant contract that the pharmacist also keep the administrator fully informed either individually or at a meeting attended by the administrator and staff.

Besides receiving the required reports the administrator can talk with the pharmacist, nurses, physicians, and patients/residents to learn in greater depth how the system is functioning. If drug reorders are not arriving on time, the nurses will be ready to share this information with the administrator. If the patients/residents are not getting the medicines they believe they depend on, they will be quite willing to report it. But in this, as in every such case, both the resident and staff must be queried.

Table 2-5 suggests that in general a 97% to 99.5% compliance rate is achieved for pharmacy services, with the exceptions of 95% compliance

Table 2-5. Percentage of Nursing Facilities in the U.S. with Deficiencies for Pharmacy Services, 1993–1999

		Deficiency Group = Pharmacy Services						
FTAG	Description	1993	1994	1995	1996	1997	1998	1999
F425	Pharmacy	0.2	0.2	0.2	0.2	0.3	0.4	0.5
F426	Procedures	3.7	4.0	3.6	3.0	3.8	4.5	5.6
F427	Service Consultation	1.5	1.2	0.9	0.7	0.7	0.8	0.7
F428	Drug Regimen	2.4	1.9	1.1	0.9	0.7	0.8	1.0
F429	Report Irregularities	5.7	4.7	3.1	2.1	2.1	1.9	3.0
F430	Facility Action	0.0	4.7	2.7	1.3	1.2	1.5	2.0
F431	Labeling	2.3	2.3	1.9	1.6	1.6	1.8	2.2
F432	Storage	4.3	4.1	3.6	3.3	3.1	3.9	5.2

Nursing Facilities, Staffing, Residents and Facility Deficiencies, 1993-1999
Department of Social & Behavioral Sciences
University of California San Francisco

in the areas of procedures and storage. The computerization of medications is an area of rapid change.

Physical Therapy, Occupational Therapy, Speech Therapy

A facility of 100 patients/residents may or may not have in-house physical, occupational, and speech therapy services. A facility with a primarily long-term census (perhaps five to 10 new admissions per month) might contract for these services when prescribed by an attending physician. Where the focus is on rehabilitation with perhaps 30 new admissions per month these services will probably be provided in-house.

The therapist's work is not fully accomplished unless the nursing and other staff are involved in the process of helping the resident/patients achieve the desired level of function in their activities of daily living and not merely during the therapy period. This implies cooperation between the specialized rehabilitative staff and the regular staff who, in effect, are doing "habilitative" therapy for the patients/residents all the time.

A method of bridging the potential gap between the physical therapist's work and the nursing staff is to establish a restorative nursing program, usually undertaken by a nurse who specializes in this area. The restorative nurse works directly with both the therapy staff and the nursing staff to assure that efforts by the therapists are successfully integrated into the activities of daily living of the residents/patients.

The administrator may want to ensure that a rehabilitative team approach is being implemented. This can be accomplished by studying one or two resident/patients' rehabilitation plans, then casually observing the extent to which they are being implemented by the involved staff members.

As indicated in Table 2-6 a remarkable 99.2% to 99.8% compliance rate is achieved for rehabilitative services.

Table 2-6. Percentage of Nursing Facilities in the U.S. with Deficiencies for Rehabilitative Services, 1993–1999

		Deficiency Group = Rehabilitative Services						
FTAG	Description	1993	1994	1995	1996	1997	1998	1999
F406	Services	1.6	1.7	1.5	1.0	0.9	1.1	0.8
F407	Qualificallons	0.4	0.2	0.3	0.1	0.1	0.1	0.1

Nursing Facilities, Staffing, Residents and Facility Deficiencies, 1993-1999
Department of Social & Behavioral Sciences
University of California San Francisco

Table 2-7. Percentage of Nursing Facilities in the U.S. with Deficiencies for Laboratory Services, 1993–1999

		Deficiency Group = Laboratory Services						
FTAG	Description	1993	1994	1995	1996	1997	1998	1999
F502	High Quality, Timely Services	-	1.1	0.9	1.0	1.3	1.9	2.0
F503	Meets Lab Standards	-	2.6	1.1	0.4	0.3	0.3	0.4
F504	Services Ordered by a Physician	-	0.2	0.2	0.1	0.1	0.2	0.2
F505	Notifies Physicians	-	0.2	0.2	0.3	0.3	0.5	0.7
F507	Clinical Records	-	0.1	0.1	0.1	0.1	0.1	0.1
F508	Radiology and Other Services	-	0.1	0.1	0.1	0.1	0.2	0.2
F513	Records Signed and Dated	-	0.0	0.1	0.0	0.0	0.0	0.1

Nursing Facilities, Staffing, Residents and Facility Deficiencies, 1993-1999
Department of Social & Behavioral Sciences
University of California San Francisco

Laboratory and Other Diagnostic Services

On a physician's order, laboratory and X-ray or other diagnostic services must be provided. These may be on the premises or contracted for at a local hospital or private office. Portable X-ray and, increasingly, additional diagnostic services are generally available on an on-call basis to provide services when a fall or other event occurs that might have injured a resident/patient.

Delayed or inaccurate laboratory work is often a concern among nursing and medical staff. Telephone calls by frustrated nurses inquiring about results that should have been received may indicate a need to examine the current procedures and contracts to emphasize the need for timely communication.

Table 2-7 demonstrates 99.3% to 99.9% compliance for laboratory services in the less subjective tags and 98% compliance in F502 High Quality, Timely Services.

NURSING SERVICES

Nursing Department Tasks

The nursing service has the following responsibilities among others:

• providing nursing care to patients/residents as ordered by the physician

- completing the Minimum Data Set, any required protocols triggered by the Minimum Data Set, creating and implementing and updating the comprehensive plan of care
- administering medications to the patients/residents
- keeping patient records
- monitoring patients/residents for changes in condition and notifying the responsible physician—in short, serving as the physician's eyes and ears on a 24-hour basis
- achieving optimal quality of care and quality of life for patients/residents
- making certain that every resident/patient is functioning at the highest possible level
- playing a coordinating role with other staff, for example, assuring that planned physical therapy, activities, physician office visits, and the like take place

In short, nursing is involved in a myriad of activities such as • assessments • wound care • starting IVs • tube feeding • oxygen therapy • range of motion • toileting • feeding • counseling • friendship • comfort • ambulation • transfer • assistance with the activities of daily living • changing the diapers and sheets • turning patients • use of assistive devices • bathing • toileting • dressing • ambulating • cleaning up spills • washing hands • tidying room • ice water • hospice • discharge planning • recruiting • training • disciplining • evaluating staff • interfacing with the other departments • observing the universal precautions • interfacing with physicians, pharmacists, numerous health care professionals • reassuring families and significant others • coping with volunteers • cooperating with the police, the fire department • infection control • working short • conducting in-services • charting • bowel and bladder programs • fire safety • disaster preparedness • answering call bells • checking on the residents hundreds of times each day • participating in lengthy care-planning sessions • afternoon and evening snacks • getting food substitutes from dietary • settling battles among residents • coping with Alzheimer's, extensive dementia, learned helplessness, death and dying • emergencies • morticians, • endless admissions • lost clothing • lost teeth • lost jewelry • running out of bed pads • hazardous waste rules • inspectors from everywhere for days at a time • electrical outages • failing equipment • room transfers • roommate dissatisfaction • refusal to eat • broken bed rails • restraint issues • missing oxygen tank wrenches • snippy staff • arrogant physicians • dissatisfied residents • troublesome visitors • unresponsive decubitus ulcers • unresponsive medical directors • the on-call nurse or physician who doesn't return calls for 45 minutes • overflowing linen bins • broken wheelchairs • epidemics among staff and residents/patients • out-of-uniform staff • missing name tags • wan-

Table 2-8. Percentage of Nursing Facilities in the U.S. with Deficiencies for Resident Assessment, 1993–1999

		Deficiency Group = Resident Assessment						
FTAG	Description	1993	1994	1995	1996	1997	1998	1999
F271	Admission Orders	0.3	0.2	0.2	0.2	0.2	0.2	0.2
F272	Comprehensive Assessments	37.3	33.7	29.0	21.5	17.3	15.1	13.4
F273	Frequency	2.3	2.3	1.7	1.4	1.1	1.1	0.7
F274	Change in Condition	7.6	10.1	8.3	5.9	4.6	4.2	3.6
F275	Annual Assessment	1.5	1.0	0.8	0.8	0.7	0.6	0.6
F276	Review of Assessments	6.1	5.5	4.9	4.9	5.0	4.7	4.4
F277	Coordination	0.1	0.1	0.1	0.0	0.0	0.0	0.0
F278	Accuracy of Assessments	15.5	9.9	6.0	4.9	4.4	4.3	5.2
F279	Comprehensive Care Plans	30.5	29.1	24.6	19.9	17.1	15.2	16.1
F280	Plan Requirements	9.8	8.0	6.4	5.5	5.4	4.7	6.0
F281	Professional Standards	6.7	6.5	6.9	8.1	8.2	10.2	12.8
F282	Qualified Personnel	2.3	3.3	4.1	5.2	4.9	5.6	7.3
F283	Discharge Summary	7.5	4.6	2.4	1.2	1.1	1.1	1.1
F284	Post Discharge Plan	3.6	2.6	1.7	0.9	0.9	0.8	0.7
F285	Preadmission Screening	0.5	0.5	0.3	0.3	0.2	0.3	0.2

Nursing Facilities, Staffing, Residents and Facility Deficiencies, 1993-1999
Department of Social & Behavioral Sciences
University of California San Francisco

dering patients • pool (contract) personnel who don't know or don't care • misplaced charts • emergency carts that were used and not restocked • constant phone calls • late lab reports • physicians who don't sign orders or visit on a timely basis • And this is only the tip of the iceberg. Nursing is the quintessential embodiment of the reality that if it can happen it will.

With all these duties, it is not surprising that some things don't get done as acceptably as one would desire. In Table 2-8 indications are that while the vast majority of nursing duties are successfully carried out, achieving acceptable levels in the areas of performing comprehensive assessments and care plan remain a challenge in about 15% of the nation's facilities.

Subacute Care Nursing

When nursing homes admit subacute care patients, their nurses must become proficient in tasks previously considered within the expertise of hospital nurses. Additional high-tech nursing skills are required. Among them are the use of implanted ports (a vascular access that remains in

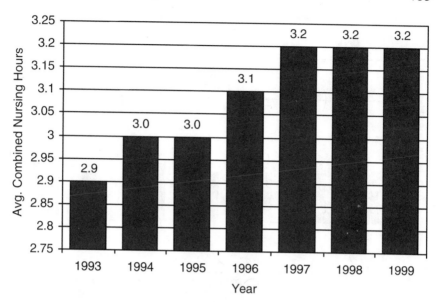

FIGURE 2-2. Total nursing hours per resident day in facilities with Medicaid and Medicare/Medicaid Beds, 1993–1999.
Nursing Facilities, Staffing, Residents and Facility Deficiencies, 1993–1999, Department of Social & Behavioral Sciences, University of California San Francisco.

place for an extended period of time); midline catheters (placed in the arm for a 3 to 4 week period of IV therapy); central line catheters (the area surrounding the heart); and epidural lines (just outside the spine usually to administer pain medicine). Most nursing facility nurses are skilled in administering epidural medications (that is, situated upon or outside the dura mater which is the outermost, toughest of the three meninges [membranes] of the brain and spinal cord), but are not skilled in what is known as category-two activities, which are more invasive.

Nursing service responsibilities are spelled out in some detail in §483.30 of the federal requirements. Figure 2-2 demonstrates nursing homes' response to the increasing acuity of residents being admitted during these years. The total nursing hours (RNs, LPN/LVNs, and NAs) per resident rose from 2.9 in 1993 to 3.2 by 1999. The total nursing hours varied across states from 2.6 in Illinois to 4.5 in Alaska in 1999 (Harrington, Carrilla, Tholaug, Summers, & Wellin, 2000).

Figure 2-3 breaks out the division of nursing hours among RN hours, LPN/LVN hours, and nursing aide hours. The main change over 1993 to 1999 was to add more RN time in response to the increasing acuity during those years.

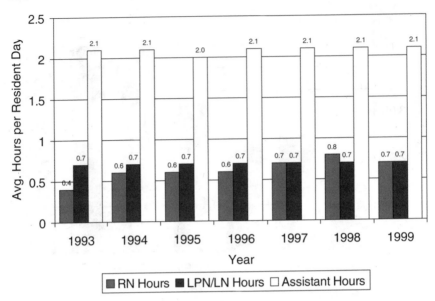

FIGURE 2-3. Average nursing hours per resident day in all certified U.S. facilities, 1993–1999.

Nursing Facilities, Staffing, Residents and Facility Deficiencies, 1993–1999, Department of Social & Behavioral Sciences, University of California San Francisco.

Quality of Resident/patient Life. There are unwritten dimensions to caring performed by the nursing service. It is not possible and perhaps not desirable, federal efforts notwithstanding, to set them all down, for many of the nursing acts that increase the quality of life cannot be fully spelled out in policy statements. The quality of life enjoyed is directly proportional to the quality of the effort given by the nursing staff.

Dr. William Thomas's Eden Alternative movement should cause alarms to sound. Dr. Thomas observes that today the majority of nursing home resources are spent on the war against disease when the real need is to address loneliness, helplessness, and boredom. The typical current nursing home is the creation of government regulations founded on a hospital model. "Edenizing" is the process of combining nature, hope, and nursing homes. A nursing home can be more nearly a human habitat when it is Edenized: that is, when it has birds, cats, dogs, fish, rabbits, chickens, children, and plants and gardens to walk in and eat from (Thomas, 1996). The Eden concept places an emphasis on intergenerational contact (Maddox et al., 2001).

Organizational Interdependencies. Organizational interdependencies between nursing and virtually every other area exist within the facility. Nursing is dependent on dietary, housekeeping, laundry, maintenance, the business office, the social worker, and the allied health professionals, to mention a few. In sum, for nursing to do its tasks properly, nearly every other department and functional area within the organization must also be doing its tasks in a cooperative manner.

Staffing. Three nursing shifts, 24 hours a day, 365 days a year offering a staffing challenge. The proportional ratios between registered nurses, licensed practical nurses, aides, and even geriatric nurse practitioners will vary with the staffing philosophy of the facility administrators and the patient profile. As acuity level increases in many facilities, the proportion of professionally trained nurses increases. Research by Patchner, and Patchner (1993) suggests that permanently assigning nurses and nursing assistants to sets of residents leads to improved care by enabling holistic care and becoming personally involved in and vested in their duties.

Administrative Observations. Just as the director of nursing services is expected to make daily resident/patient rounds, the administrator may decide to emulate nursing. The administrator must decide to what extent she wishes to receive daily reports on admissions, discharges, changes in resident/patient conditions, accidents, incidents, transfers, deaths, and the like as part of her information system. The reports are not a satisfactory substitute for the administrator's personal observation, on a daily basis, to learn by wandering around what is actually taking place in the facility. Also, one has to be on the scene to be the coach, energizer, and communicator of one's vision for the facility.

In 1999, administrators were 99.1% successful in providing the required number of registered nurse hours, but only 95% successful in providing sufficient nursing staff, as judged by the nation's surveyors (Harrington et al., 2000).

THE BUSINESS OFFICE

Part 3 of this text is devoted to finance, which includes the work of the business office where functions, human resources, and organizational interfaces of the business components are explored. In a typical 100-bed facility, one full-time and often an additional part-time employee staff the business office. Briefly, the business office

- keeps financial records
- manages accounts receivable, accounts payable

- maintains vendor files
- assists in monitoring the budget
- prepares the payroll
- keeps required records, makes financial reports
- deals with third-party payers, Medicare, Medicaid, and others
- safeguards and controls resident/patient funds
- often acts as receptionist, answers the telephone

MEDICAL/PATIENT CARE RECORDS

By federal requirements, a full-time employee must be assigned to keep the medical record service up to date. Usually this person is called a ward clerk. Facilities are required to keep a great number of records, among the most important of which is the medical record. If medical records are not complete and current, federal and state inspectors will normally issue a directive that it be corrected within a specified time period. Increasingly, medical records require a full-time person operating a computer. A professional therapist with 25 years' experience in several facilities in the same chain observes that within a 1-year period she worked in two facilities that actually provided equally good resident care. One facility kept excellent records and received very few deficiencies, the other kept poor records of the good quality care it was providing and received numerous serious deficiencies. Documentation truly does count.

ADMISSIONS

In states where first-come first-served rules do not exist, the person or persons in charge of admissions influence the case mix of the facility. Usually a person with social work background is employed as the admissions coordinator. Often a single employee will head both admissions and social work, and sometimes the director of nurses does admissions. In most cases, the admissions process is shared jointly by the director of nursing and the admissions director. In any case, admissions have a profound effect on the facility's work load, atmosphere, and ability to achieve its goals and provide appropriate care. Who is admitted from where and with what care needs and reimbursement rates are the lifeblood of the facility.

The admissions persons must find, screen, process, facilitate, and manage case mix, while balancing financial, light versus heavy care, the goodwill of the hospital discharge planners, and managed care or other source elements. They are important promoters of the facility, marketing to hospital discharge planners, the local physicians, third-party payers, managed care organizations, Worker's Compensation insurance, insurance companies, and the like. A daily fax to local hospitals showing bed availability can maintain a presence and lead to admissions.

Consider having an admissions application that can be filled out and submitted on your Web site. Your federal survey results are on-line for potential applicants to review, so let them also be able to apply on-line after they review your survey reports. The Web is becoming a major source of referral to facilities. Make sure that your listing is correct on such sites as www.seniorstreet.com, an on-line senior health-care facility directory where consumers search for long-term care facilities.

Make it Easy

- greet the customer
- listen to the customer
- identify the needs
- ask for the business: "In your opinion, do you believe we can serve your mother?"

Every "lost" admission can be a $90,000 loss to the facility.

Admission to a nursing facility is a major life transition for both the new resident and the significant others. A caring staff will always make sure that someone—the administrator, the head nurse, the admissions director-calls the significant others after the first night with a full report on how the resident is doing.

DIETARY DEPARTMENT

The Food Standard

Food is an essential ingredient in the quality of resident/patient life. Satisfaction with the facility is as often influenced by the food as by the quality of nursing care. Some families feel they may not have enough medical background to judge the adequacy of nursing care, but most do consider themselves experts in the matter of food. Tasty food is important to a satisfactory quality of life. Hospital food can be tolerated when eaten for a relatively short period of time. Nursing home food, consumed for much longer periods, sometimes forever, is subject to much greater scrutiny by both patients/residents and their families and significant others.

The Food Standard: Can it Be Met?

The dietary manager in the typical nursing facility (one with 70% Medicaid, 15% Medicare, 10% private pay, 5% other) is permitted to spend about $4 to $5 per day for raw food costs. The typical life care community (one with nearly 100% private pay) spends $12 or more per day for raw food costs. Although the nation's nursing facilities maintain good nutritional status for residents 90% of the time, there is some concern that surveyors believe that nutritional needs are not met 10% of the time (Harrington et al., 2000). A more realistic raw food budget for the nation's facilities would help. Surprisingly, the national surveyors believe that nursing facilities provide a well-balanced diet 99.8% of the time (F360).

The dietary department's influence extends 24 hours a day. The availability of bedtime snacks, or midnight snacks for insomniac patients/residents, is as much a part of the ambiance of the facility as the availability of continuous nursing services. This department is heavily interactive with nursing services (for example, providing refreshments at social activities) and with most other departments. The food service depends on other departments as well: on laundry for linens and on maintenance to keep the kitchen functioning. Some facilities contract for food service with outside vendors. In this situation, the head of dietary may be an employee of the food service contractor.

According to Table 2-9 the major area in need of improvement is sanitary conditions.

Table 2-9. Percentage of Nursing Facilities in the U.S. with Deficiencies for Dietary Services, 1993–1999

		Deficiency Group = Dietary Services						
FTAG	Description	1993	1994	1995	1996	1997	1998	1999
F360	Well-Balanced Diet	0.6	0.6	0.3	0.2	0.2	0.2	0.2
F361	Qualified Staff	1.5	1.1	0.7	0.4	0.4	0.4	0.5
F362	Sufficient Staff	1.6	1.3	1.0	0.7	0.6	0.6	0.8
F363	Menus and Nutritional Adequacy	15.0	10.1	7.1	4.3	4.3	3.8	4.8
F364	Food	14.0	11.5	9.9	8.2	7.3	7.7	8.4
F365	Individual Needs	2.2	2.0	1.8	1.6	2.0	2.4	2.4
F366	Food Substitutes	4.7	3.9	2.5	1.4	1.1	0.9	1.3
F367	Therapeutic Diets	1.8	1.3	1.5	1.5	1.1	1.3	1.8
F368	Frequency of Meals	5.7	6.4	5.0	3.8	3.5	4.2	4.7
F369	Assistive Devices	0.9	0.7	0.6	0.4	0.4	0.5	0.8
F370	Sanitary Conditions	0.2	0.1	0.6	0.0	0.0	0.0	0.0
F371	Food Sanitation	30.4	28.0	24.8	22.4	21.8	23.7	26.0
F372	Garbage Disposal	3.5	3.9	2.6	2.2	2.0	2.5	3.0

Nursing Facilities, Staffing, Residents and Facility Deficiencies, 1993-1999
Department of Social & Behavioral Sciences
University of California San Francisco

The administrator can monitor food services in a number of ways. Randomly timed walks through the kitchen, eating with residents in the dining hall, assisting with feeding in resident/patient rooms and in the dining rooms on a daily basis are productive ways to monitor. Much can be learned by getting a tray and eating its contents under circumstances similar to those experienced by the resident.

A few of the critical functions of dietary, achieving the nutritional diet prescribed by the physician and developed by the registered dietitian or registered dietitian consultant, ensuring tasty food at the right temperature, doing nutritional assessments, monitoring weight gains and losses, monitoring I/O (input and output), providing food substitutes as requested, catering for facility functions and its many visiting groups, maintaining the dietary area according to cleanliness standards.

SOCIAL SERVICES

Social services is concerned not only with the resident/patient's initial adjustment to the facility, but also his or her continuing accommodation to the environment. The social worker is also responsible for monitoring each resident/patient's socio-psychological experiences and orientation in the facility.

It is the social worker who is often most directly in contact with the resident/patient's family or significant others. This staff member is the one involved in assisting patients/residents who have current or impending financial needs that will be met by a public agency. In short, the social worker functions in the nursing home in a manner similar to social workers employed by the local social services agency. Maintaining the quality of each resident/patient's social well-being in a facility is a complex function.

Significantly assisting each resident to meet his or her various social, psychological, physical, environmental, family, financial and related needs in never achieved by the social worker alone. The social worker must stimulate the various other staff members to participate in this process. A typical problem to which the administrator must be attuned is a tendency for responsive patients/residents to receive the lioness's share of the social worker's time and attention. It must be remembered that the less responsive and unresponsive also have needs.

ACTIVITIES/RECREATION

Nursing services primarily address the medical needs of the patients/residents, and in the process partially meet their social and interpersonal requirements.

The activities coordinator's task is to ensure that the physical, social, and mental well-being of each resident/patient is included in each comprehensive resident assessment and the required comprehensive plan of care. For the nearly comatose, disoriented or agitated patients, this assignment is indeed a challenge. The activities director and the social services worker are assigned primary responsibility for attention to the quality of psychosocial life that exists within a facility. It is difficult to imagine a more complicated undertaking in shaping the quality of the resident/patient life.

In 1993, according to federal surveyors, 88% of facilities satisfactorily provided activities for residents. By 1999, 91% of facilities were meeting activities goals (Harrington et al., 2000).

HOUSEKEEPING

Not only do federal and state inspectors make intuitive value judgments about a facility based on its cleanliness and physical appearance, but so also will most of the resident/patients themselves and their significant others. Dirty floors and walls, empty toilet paper holders, yellowing toilets and lavatories and the offensive odors associated with them, communicate a message to the patients/residents, staff, and visitors that reveals what the facility thinks about itself. Inattention to housekeeping details leads inspectors and the public alike to wonder to what extent it carries over into resident/patient care, sanitation in food preparations, and cleanliness of the resident/patients themselves.

The head of housekeeping may have excellently designed job assignments for the four to eight housekeepers. The administrator can tell how effective these schedules are simply by walking around the facility. On these tours the administrator must be able to "see" dirt.

A surprising amount of regulation surrounds the housekeeping area, such as the required Material Safety Data Sheets for all chemicals, to which the head of housekeeping and the administrator must give attention.

In 1993, federal surveyors were satisfied that 80% of facilities were meeting housekeeping requirements. By 1999, 85% of facilities were satisfying federal surveyors that facilities were providing a sanitary, orderly, and comfortable environment (Harrington et al., 2000). A glance at Table 2-10 illustrates that what is considered good housekeeping varies markedly among states and over time within the same state.

LAUNDRY

Clean linens, clean resident/patient clothes, the availability of linens and clothes when needed, and safe, sanitary handling techniques for both

Table 2-10. Percentage of Nursing Facilities in the U.S. with Deficiencies for Housekeeping, 1993–1999

State	1993	1994	1995	1996	1997	1998	1999
AK	8.3	14.3	7.7	0.0	7.1	7.1	7.1
AL	8.2	6.4	5.1	5.3	0.5	3.7	6.1
AR	15.1	21.5	31.9	39.5	40.0	36.4	45.6
AZ	5.9	14.8	17.9	33.1	34.7	27.9	10.3
CA	38.0	34.9	23.6	26.0	25.1	28.8	31.3
CO	24.0	7.6	4.9	4.7	15.4	16.5	25.1
CT	4.5	0.0	0.0	2.6	2.4	4.0	4.2
DC	40.0	77.8	76.9	61.1	50.0	64.3	35.7
DE	81	4.7	6.1	0.0	0.0	0.0	11.8
FL	10.0	10.2	11.8	8.0	13.9	13.3	9.1
GA	15.9	23.1	16.7	17.6	16.1	24.3	25.8
HI	16.0	7.7	0.0	2.5	2.4	9.1	5.1
IA	8.5	9.3	4.4	7.7	9.8	8.1	7.2
ID	21.5	9.0	18.8	24.3	23.4	30.4	34.6
IL	23.4	24.0	27.8	26.1	25.7	23.7	24.1
IN	6.1	13.6	17.0	25.3	10.6	5.6	3.6
KS	63.1	40.7	38.2	30.2	16.8	13.5	16.1
KY	3.9	6.6	10.7	3.2	6.9	25.7	27.0
LA	33.2	22.3	20.5	6.7	7.4	7.4	5.1
MA	6.0	5.1	5.2	2.7	1.7	0.2	4.6
MD	2.1	4.5	5.4	5.8	6.0	3.5	3.7
ME	7.2	11.5	10.4	6.4	9.6	7.6	8.8
MI	45.3	42.0	43.2	30.2	30.3	33.5	34.6
MN	16.4	15.3	8.2	1.4	2.6	4.7	1.3
MO	17.1	9.5	12.5	10.7	10.4	5.4	3.7
MS	25.0	35.8	28.1	23.7	13.9	29.0	47.8
MT	13.7	18.8	11.0	4.3	3.2	4.3	3.1
NC	10.3	8.1	9.6	14.8	10.8	9.9	14.6
ND	5.0	4.9	10.8	23.0	16.0	14.8	2.3
NE	7.8	5.4	5.8	3.9	1.3	3.0	4.8
NH	3.0	4.5	8.3	10.0	5.3	6.7	7.6
NJ	7.6	10.5	11.2	6.3	3.8	2.9	1.9
NM	13.0	1.3	0.0	1.3	3.2	10.6	6.5
NV	25.8	30.0	33.3	25.6	31.6	19.5	7.5
NY	6.9	8.9	8.4	8.4	8.1	5.9	10.3
OH	17.8	21.9	23.0	14.1	6.2	10.2	12.4
OK	2.1	7.9	9.7	11.6	11.0	10.4	19.2
OR	16.7	12.7	10.0	5.2	8.6	3.2	2.1
PA	17.5	12.5	10.2	5.4	4.3	7.1	6.4
RI	3.9	16.3	8.5	5.8	12.0	21.3	16.3

Table 2-10. (Continued)

State	1993	1994	1995	1996	1997	1998	1999
SC	4.4	0.0	1.9	7.3	11.4	17.2	22.4
SD	8.3	3.8	2.7	4.0	5.9	15.1	24.7
TN	22.5	19.8	18.3	18.5	12.6	20.1	19.3
TX	30.8	31.8	27.9	24.0	22.8	22.4	21.0
UT	17.0	6.7	11.8	10.1	7.7	2.2	5.4
VA	16.0	12.5	7.6	7.9	2.1	0.9	1.2
VT	9.8	5.6	7.5	0.0	0.0	2.9	4.8
WA	43.0	31.2	25.3	25.8	25.7	33.2	40.8
WI	14.0	14.7	13.3	12.6	7.5	62	7.1
WV	72.5	35.2	28.4	-0.9	2.6	2.9	22
WY	10.7	2.9	21.1	5-4	8.3	6.0	2.8
US	19.5	18.3	16.9	15.1	13.3	14.4	15.3

Nursing Facilities, Staffing, Residents and Facility Deficiencies, 199321999
Department of Social & Behavioral Sciences
University of California San Francisco

soiled and clean linen are areas of responsibility of the head of laundry. Whether it is better to do laundry in-house or to contract with an outside profvider of linen service (which is known as outsourcing [Argenti, 1994]) is a subject of continuing debate. Whatever the decision, there will be procedures for handling linens that the administrator can observe for conformity to regulations and to facility policies.

MAINTENANCE DEPARTMENT

Distinguishing between maintenance and housekeeping responsibilities is often an issue. If a wall has a hole in it, it is clearly maintenance's job to fix the hole. If that same wall is only dirty and in need of washing, it is probably housekeeping's job. Each facility must designate through established policies the respective responsibilities of these two functions. The repair and upkeep of physical systems is clearly the responsibility of maintenance.

Preventive maintenance—anticipating when a machine will need servicing or risk ceasing to function—is a complex task requiring experienced judgment. A well-trained maintenance director can do much to anticipate troublesome, unnecessary breakdowns of equipment. The administrator can participate in the maintenance process by occasionally assuming a maintenance mind-set, then walking though the facility touching, feeling, and judging the state of repair of all she encounters.

TEAMWORK

Some areas requiring special teamwork attention from the administrator:

- patient care planning and implementation of resident/patient care plans
- successful billing, from recording supplies consumed to required wording for claims
- housekeeping versus maintenance
- dietary/nursing coordination in getting food to residents on a timely basis, at the right temperature, attractively presented with attention to accommodating resident/patient preferences
- differentiating between activities functions and the social worker function; dangers of resident/patient's needs falling between the cracks
- discharge planning
- resident advocacy to the staff and families
- nursing/housekeeping/laundry coordination

2.2 Identifying Human Resources Functions

HUMAN RESOURCES FUNCTIONS

Managers in organizations have always performed certain basic human resources functions, which are a range of activities that can include record keeping, employee recruitment and selection, training and development, compensation management, performance evaluations, and often labor relations (Chruden & Sherman, 1980; Noe et al., 2000).

- *Record keeping*—assuring that all necessary information is in the employee's file and that it is kept confidential; increasingly complicated as files are computerized
- *Recruitment*—assisting department heads in finding employees for vacant positions
- *Selection*—assisting department heads in interviewing and assessing job applicants
- *Training and retaining Employees*—assisting department heads in employee orientation, inservice training, and continuing education
- *Compensation management*—assisting department heads and payroll office in administering salary and the other benefits offered by the facility
- *Performance evaluation*—assisting managers in conducting employee evaluation in conformity with the facility's human resources policies
- *Labor relations*—assisting managers in creating a favorable work environment

• *Health and safety*—drug testing, monitoring employee health status (e.g., ensuring that hepatitis B and tuberculosis immunizations are provided as required and kept current.

HUMAN RESOURCES MANAGEMENT AS AN OCCUPATION

In his text *Personnel Management,* Chruden says that in its rudimentary state, human resources was the responsibility of each department manager. (In a 100-bed nursing facility, this tends to be true today. Usually, the department managers do initial interviewing, perhaps bringing the administrator in on the final selection.) Chruden speculates that historically, as the department supervisor's job became more complex, the responsibility for certain human resources activities (for instance, hours worked and payroll) were taken over by a clerical assistant. From this initial record-keeping activity, the responsibilities were gradually broadened until individuals began making a full-time career in what is now called human resources administration (Johns & Saks, 2001; Noe et al., 2000).

Human resources managers do not "manage" employees except for those who work under them in the human resources department, if there is more than one employee in that unit. Human resources management is a staff function; it has no line authority in the organization. All the employees in the organization are directly managed by their department supervisors, who hold line authority. It is the line managers in fact who are responsible for performing most of the human resources functions for the employees under them. The department heads do the actual hiring, require in-service training and development, give performance evaluations and promotions, award raises, and discipline, suspend, and discharge their staff.

The role of the human resources manager and staff is to assist the line supervisors (e.g., the department heads in the nursing facility) to carry out human resources responsibilities according to policies set by facility ownership. This staff makes an important contribution to overall employee satisfaction by assuring that human resources policies are carried out as consistently as feasible from one department to another.

In a facility of perhaps 100 to 150 residents/patients, no full-time human resources director is usually hired. However, some of the typical human resources department functions are usually given to one employee who, in effect, serves as a part-time personnel staff in the facility. This person is sometimes designated staff development coordinator or a similar title. Alternately, assisting the department managers with personnel matters such as record keeping, assuring that employees are tested for tuberculosis, and offering them Hepatitis B vaccinations (as required by the Bloodborne Pathogens regulations) may be assigned to an assistant administrator, an administrative assistant, a staff nurse, or an employee in the business office.

EMERGING HUMAN RESOURCE (HR) MANAGEMENT TECHNIQUES

Technologies now being utilized by HR staff include interactive voice technology, the internet, client-servers, relational databases, imaging, and specialized software (Noe et al., 2000).
   These technologies will facilitate

- employee control over their training and benefit package
- paperless employment offices
- computer access to employee records (no more 1-inch thick folders locked in a steel file)
- 24-hour access to files and changing files
- closer surveillance of employee performance
- a growing rash of privacy issues (Noe et al., 2000).

Interactive voice technology: Computer-based voice-activated systems will allow employees to access their files and accounts such as retirement accounts, vacation days, and the like.
   The Internet and the World Wide Web: Employees in any facility can communicate with employees in any other facility to compare opinions or open chat rooms.
   Networks and Client-Server Architecture: A network of desktop computers can share databases on employees and HR information. Employee data can be accessed by multiple users. A client-server can hold multiple data bases about employees; for example, financial, employment, and health records databases can be accessed singly or multiply. Relational databases with fields such as employee name, serial number, social security number, job classification, and immunization status can enable HR (and, unfortunately, other) personnel to quickly produce HR information, such as a list of employees needing to get retested for TB in the next month.

   Imaging: Using scanners allows for information like application, disciplinary actions, evaluations, health records to be stored electronically and printed on an as-needed basis. Paper will play a reduced role in HR management.

CD-ROM and laser discs: These devices are re-creating the training programs of facilities. A nurse's aide, for example, might complete a CD-ROM or laser disc course on infection control and document this in his required in-service record.

Groupware: Electronic-meeting software will allow multiple users to share and work on the same document simultaneously. Not everyone might have to come to a lengthy resident-care planning meeting to update an MDS form that is due.

Needless to say, accessing and using these databases creates privacy concerns. Just as nearly every American's debt status is instantly available to anyone in a computer-based credit report, complete information about every employee (and resident) may be only a keystroke away (Noe et al., 2000).

2.3 Planning Employment Needs: Writing Job Descriptions

In part 1 we indicated the need for each facility to break down all work to be accomplished (the processor portion of the systems model) into a set of activities that can be performed by one person. Several definitions provided by the U.S. Employment Service and the U.S. Office of Personnel Management may be useful to review at this point (Ivancevich, Szjlagyi, & Wallace, 1977).

• *Job Analysis.* The process of defining a job in terms of tasks or behaviors required and specifying the qualifications of the employee to be placed in that job (Noe et al., 2000).

• *Job Description.* Information about the job that results in a statement of the job to be done, usually including a list of duties and responsibilities in order of importance. Usually a job description includes (a) the title, (b) the qualifications, (c) to whom the worker is primarily responsible, and (d) the duties or specific expectations (Argenti, 1994; Noe et al., 2000).

• *Job Specification.* A statement of the skills, education and experience required to perform the work. This is derived from the job description.

• *Job Titles (or job classifications).* That which distinguishes one job from all others. Job titles may also indicate the occupational level of the job ("nurse supervisor" indicates a higher position than "registered nurse" administratively speaking) or the level of authority of seniority of job, such as registered nurse levels 1, 2, and 3.

• *Task.* A coordinated and aggregated series of work elements used to produce an output (such as, making beds).

• *Position.* The responsibilities and duties performed by one individual. There are as many positions as there are employees.

• *Job.* A group of positions that are similar in their duties, such as laundry, housekeeping, and grounds.

• *Job Family.* A group of two or more jobs that have similar duties, such as the duties of the registered nurse and licensed nurse practitioners (Ivancevich et al., 1977; Johns & Saks, 2001; Noe et al., 2000).

All the work to be accomplished in operating a nursing facility must be broken down into a series of tasks. Tasks are grouped together so that they can be performed by one individual. *Job analysis* is the process of grouping a series of related tasks into a position. Each position can the be described in terms of the tasks and behaviors involved and of the education and training needed to perform the job successfully.

POTENTIAL PROBLEMS WITH JOB DESCRIPTIONS

The federal government examines job descriptions and specifications for possible discriminatory effects. Each of the stated requirements for a job must be necessary for the adequate performance of that job. For example, if a nursing facility in an area with an unusually large number of available job applicants required 2 years of college for nurse's aide applicants, it must be able to demonstrate why this is essential to perform the job, that is, that the requirement has proven validity. This is a higher educational requirement than usual; therefore, the facility would be obliged to prove that it did not serve to discriminate against members of a particular group on the basis of sex or ethnic origins (Noe et al., 2000).

Once job descriptions have been written and the expected work load of the facility estimated, future employment needs can be forecast.

2.4 Forecasting Employment Needs

The planning process begins with a projection of the number of residents/patients and their expected levels of medical complexity that the facility expects to serve over a period of time, usually during the following 1 to 5 years. This forecast can then be translated into specific personnel requirements for the future (Noe et al., 2000).

TAKING A HUMANPOWER INVENTORY

Numerous factors must be taken into account in projecting the present and future availability of qualified personnel in sufficient number. This is the process of taking a humanpower inventory.

Several sources of employment information exist. The Employment Security Commission and the Department of Labor gather data that are useful in estimating the future availability of needed employees (Noe et al., 2000).

Identifying Trends

Data such as those mentioned help to identify trends, a number of which are of potential importance.

Competition for human resources. It is practical to take an inventory of present and planned health and related facilities that are or will be competing for similarly qualified personnel. For example, if no acute care hospital exists in the geographic area, but a large for-profit hospital is expected to be constructed within 2 years, competition may increase dramatically. Or, similarly, if the local hospital is one of the several local hospitals that are downsizing or closing their doors each year, the labor pool may be suddenly increased (Hitt et al., 2001). One result of worker shortages in various functional areas within the nursing facility is increasing dependence on outsourcing, such as having laundry done off-site (Noe et al., 2000).

Job Security. Companies no longer guarantee their employees job security. Over the past two decades employment has ceased to be a lifetime commitment by companies to their workers. Employees today increasingly perceive themselves as individuals who manage their personal career over their lifetime, which increasingly involves several employers. Companies are less committed to their employees, and employees to their companies (Noe et al., 2000).

Migration Patterns in the Labor Supply. Knowledge of whether the worker pool from which employees must be chosen is shrinking or enlarging is important. Statistics are usually available on the local unemployment rate. Unfortunately, for the nursing facility a low local unemployment rate can produce a noticeable reduction in the quality of applicants, level of job interest, and longevity for positions such as nurses' aide, housekeeper, and groundskeeper (Noe et al., 2000).

Wage Scale Movements in the Area. An growing worker pool may reduce wage scales, while a shrinking worker pool may cause the wage scale to rise. The widespread nursing shortage of the late 1980s and early 1990s resulted in rapid increases in nursing salaries during those years. As the nursing shortage eased in the mid-1990s, nurses' wages began to trend slightly downward. Nursing shortages are increasingly cyclical.

Expected Impacts of Educational Institutions. Educational institutions such as local community colleges are becoming major sources of training for humanpower needed by nursing facilities. Any expected increase or decrease in training activities, such as, the addition or closing of a licensed-practical-nurse program in the local community college, could dramatically affect the availability of labor, especially trained nurse's aides.

Knowledge of these trends can assist planners in taking action before an anticipated employment crisis. If a shortage is foreseen, the facility might join with other local health care providers in a program to attract additional health-related personnel to the area.

2.5 Recruiting

Once the forecast of the resident/patient profile has been translated into specific personnel requirements for the facility, they become the basis for the recruitment and selection program. The forecast assists the facility in determining the number and types of employees it will need to recruit as well as the sources for recruitment. (Noe et al., 2000).

FACTORS INFLUENCING RECRUITMENT

Affirmative Action and The Americans with Disabilities Act

Since the passage of the Civil Rights Act in 1964, the process of seeking new employees has become more public. Prior to 1964, facilities could choose employees without scrutiny by government agencies with regard to possible job discrimination based on age, sex, race, marital status, religion, national origin, or disability (Miller, 1982).

Today government agencies can review for possible legal violations by examining the following: (a) the facility's list of recruitment sources for each job category; (b) recruitment advertising; (c) statistics on the number of applicants processed by personal category (e.g., sex, age, race), level and type of disabilities, and by job category and level (Ivancevich et al., 1977; Johns & Saks, 2001).

The government may require a nursing home chain or an individual facility to recruit qualified employees whose group is not proportionately represented in their present staff. If, for example, there are no African American nurses on the staff and the government ascertains that the facility does not advertise its job openings at African American nursing schools or in newspapers or other sources normally used by African Americans seeking jobs, the government may require that a governmentally defined Equal Employment Opportunity program be used by the facility or chain.

Many employers are under governmental pressure to increase the number of minority members and women employed in the facility, especially at the higher levels from which these groups have traditionally been excluded (Chruden & Sherman, 1980). Requiring a facility to increase the proportion of minority persons is called *ratio hiring*.

While it has not been a matter for the Office of Civil Rights enforcement, disproportionately few male nurses tend to be hired, probably out of deference to the mostly female nursing facility population (usually about 75%) and availability of male nurses. In general, it is functional to seek a workforce that is diversified and representative of the community that the facility serves.

The Americans with Disabilities Act has also influenced the hiring process in a number of ways. This is explored in greater depth in part 4.

The Labor Market

The *labor market* is the geographic area from which applicants are to be recruited. Recruitment for a new administrator or director of nurses may be national in scope and today may be done via Web searches, as the population has become increasingly mobile. When staffing for jobs that require little skill, the scope of the labor market will tend to be a relatively small geographic area surrounding the facility. The new janitor or nurse's aide is unlikely to be willing, or economically able, to move in order to accept a position at the facility. In today's employment arena each facility needs its own Web site with an employment application that can be filled out over the Internet.

If there is a surplus of labor at recruiting time, the facility may be flooded with applications. If there is a shortage, such as during the nursing shortage, it may take considerable initiative to find and hire well-trained staff.

Transportation

The ease with which employees can commute to the facility will have a direct impact on the geographic area from which the facility can recruit. The absence of an efficient public transportation system, especially for evening and night workers, will oblige the facility to hire only persons who have access to automobiles or can walk to work.

Nursing facilities in the cities face special problems in finding suitable employees. Migration to the suburbs traditionally leaves less-qualified people in the center city, and suburbanites are less inclined to commute there. Some larger institutions have arranged special transportation to and from work for suburban employees in an effort to attract competent staff.

RECRUITMENT SOURCES

A number of sources for recruitment exist, both within and outside the facility. Present employees may be an excellent source.

Present Employees

The current employees of the facility can be a primary source for filling vacancies. Hiring from among present employees is a policy decision to promote from within, and there are a number of advantages to such a policy (Noe et al., 2000).

Career Ladders. *Career ladders* are paths along which the employee can hope to progress. They constitute a major source of employee incentive and satisfaction. Those entering the facility are encouraged to stay if there is reasonable expectation that when openings occur, there will be advancement possibilities from within the organization. This practice stimulates employees to develop skills that will be necessary to qualify for promotion (Noe et al., 2000).

Job Posting and Job Bidding. A job that becomes available is posted on appropriate bulletin boards and Internet, and employees are encouraged to bid or apply. Through this device employees become more aware of the actual requirements of positions and the selection processes for filling vacancies. Such information can also be placed on the facility's Web site. Advancement of present employees has the obvious advantage of recognizing and rewarding successful workers. It also benefits the facility by placing a person who already has some understanding of the organization and is loyal to its policies.

However, hiring exclusively from within may measurably slow the process of introducing persons with new ideas and fresh approaches into the facility. There are times when management may purposely seek to bring in an outsider who will be expected to reorganize or reengineer a department or work area.

Outside Sources

Unless it is planned to reduce the size of the staff, every vacancy presents the organization with an option to promote from within or hire from without.

A promotion from within might trigger a series of promotions. If the nursing supervisor is promoted to director of nursing, the charge nurse may be moved up to nursing supervisor, and the senior registered nurse to charge nurse, thus creating an opportunity for several moves up in seniority or level and eventually opening a beginning registered nurse position (Noe et al., 2000).

If filled from within, any vacancy will eventually result in hiring a new person from an outside source, some of which are now discussed.

Referrals. Satisfied employees, resident/patients, and their significant others are good sources of referrals and constitute a valuable asset for the recruiting effort (Noe et al., 2000).

Employee referrals can be especially beneficial. When a staff member's recommendation is accepted, he is receiving special recognition by the facility. In addition, the employee will have a vested interest in assisting the recruit to adjust to the environment and to be productive. However, the facility must be careful to avoid referrals that lead to nepotism (favoring one's family members) or to the formation of closely knit groups or cliques composed of persons who have close outside ties and tend to exclude others. Employee, resident/patient, and family referrals are, in essence, word-of-mouth recommendations that reflect the reputation of the facility in the facility.

Advertisements. Advertisement in appropriate media, such as newspapers and professional and trade journals, and on the Web is one of the most common methods for contacting prospective applicants. For registered nurses, the professional journal may be an appropriate medium; however, local newspapers are the most used source. For nurse's aides and maintenance staff, the local newspaper will also be an appropriate medium (Noe et al., 2000).

Public Employment Agencies. State governments operate local public employment agencies, using federal payroll tax rebates from the U.S. Employment Service (USES). Public employment agencies can provide lists of individuals who are unemployed and currently drawing unemployment insurance benefits (Noe et al., 2000).

Private Employment Agencies. Agencies in the private sector offer specialized services, more closely matching the needs of the potential employer and employee. Fees are charged, and most often the employee pays the agency. However, the employer sometimes shares in the fee and occasionally pays it altogether. The facility may also sign a contract with a private employment agency over a period of time. In this case, the contract should be carefully reviewed to avoid unwanted or unintended commitments, such as having to pay a fee to the agency for all new employees, whether found by the agency or the employer (Noe et al., 2000).

Search Firms. Search firms generally focus their efforts on middle-and upper-level management positions. Clients for search firms usually are employers who agree to pay the search firm for finding a suitable candidate. The search firm operates in a wider geographic area than is possible for the employer (although the Internet is changing even this), and it is able to offer a nationwide inventory. These firms can save the employer time and energy by providing extensive screening before any candidate is recommended.

Professional and Industry Organizations. Many professional and industry groups, such as health-care-facilities associations and nurses associations may maintain rosters of their members who are seeking employment, which they publish in their journals and post at meetings. Much interviewing, both formal and informal, occurs at association meetings for job openings. For nursing home administrators, the American College of Healthcare Executives publishes *Career,* a monthly employment newsletter. The American College of Healthcare Administrators offers its members access to employment openings through Job Bank USA. Company Web sites may also list job openings.

Educational Institutions. Accredited schools are an increasingly important source for nursing home personnel. Community colleges and technical institutes are training students not only to be licensed practical nurse positions but also to be nurse's aides (Noe et al., 2000).

Unsolicited Applications. A number of unsolicited employment inquiries will arrive at the facility by mail or in person. Although the proportion of such applicants who are suitable may be low, there are important reasons for paying careful attention to them. It is good public relations practice to extend courteous treatment to applicants who approach the facility on their own initiative and to deal with them candidly about the likelihood of employment with the organization.

Some administrators report a tendency for long-term care and hospital employees to seek a change of job every few years. They may be entirely competent people who periodically look for a new work situation while remaining within their field. Such individuals may submit unsolicited applications simply to let a facility know of their availability.

Electronic Recruiting and Screening

Computer recruitment networks and videoconference interviews allow employers to search for employees over a wide geographical area without having to leave the facility (Noe et al., 2000). Search firms often use a video interview as a first step in screening people for positions, and the facility can do likewise.

2.6 Hiring Staff

Recruitment is the process of locating prospective staff. *Personnel selection* is the process of deciding which of the applicants best fits the requirements of the job for which they are being considered (Owen, 1984). Often, however, this prospective staff member is evaluated not only for one of several positions the organization has open at that moment, but for anticipated slots in the near future. Nurses with extensive acute-care experience, for example, will be interviewed and kept in mind by a facility moving toward offering subacute care.

Through experience, employers have learned that when individuals are carefully selected for clearly defined positions, the result may be faster adjustment to the position, greater job satisfaction, and a minimum number of poor fits between applicants and job needs in the organization (Chruden & Sherman, 1980; Johns & Saks, 2001).

MEASURING THE IMPACT OF LEGISLATION

Employers are directing greater attention to the job selection process. This is because of the often intense scrutiny given employers by the government enforcers of the Civil Rights Act of 1964, the Equal Employment Act of 1972 and the Americans With Disabilities Act which was passed in 1990 (see part 4 for a discussion of the latter).

The Civil Rights Act of 1964 prohibits discrimination in employment practices on the basis of race, color, religion, sex, or national origin. This act created the Equal Employment Opportunities Commission (EEOC) to implement the provisions of the act. A later amendment, known as the Tower Amendment to Title 7, permitted the use of ability tests in employee selection procedures. Subsequently, the courts and the EEOC have made numerous rulings that determine the construction and use of ability tests (Maddox et al., 2001).

The Equal Employment Act of 1972 is an amendment to Title 7 of the Civil Rights Act of 1964 and is intended to cover all employers of 15 or more persons and numerous other groups such as educational institutions. Enforcement machinery was authorized and subsequently set up. Today human resources policy is shaped by these acts as well as by court decisions and regulations instituted by authorized governmental agencies. They affect such employment practices as retirement rules and considerations during pregnancy; and are discussed at greater length in part 4 under the section on management and labor legislation and regulations.

In 1987, four federal agencies jointly published a far-reaching document entitled *Uniform Guidelines on Employee Selection Procedures* (EEOC, 1978), establishing the standards by which federal agencies determine the acceptability of validation procedures used for written tests and other selections

The guidelines require the employer to be able to demonstrate that the selection procedures used are valid in predicting or measuring employee performance in a specific job. The define discrimination as follows:

> The use of any selection procedure which has an adverse impact on the hiring, promotion or other employment or membership opportunities of members of any race, sex, or ethnic group will be considered to be discriminatory and inconsistent with these guidelines, unless procedure has been validated in accordance with these guidelines. (EEOC, § 3A)

"Adverse impact" is defined as whenever the selection rate for any racial, ethnic, or group is less than 80% of the rate of the group with the highest selection rate.

For example, 200 of 1,000 White applicants are selected (a selection rate of 20%), at least 16% of the minority applicants must be selected. Several court rulings, such as Griggs v. Duke Power Company (which we discuss in detail in part 4), have already clearly established the principle that all human resources tests and activities must avoid having any discriminatory effect, whether intended or unintended (Noe et al., 2000).

The *Uniform Guidelines* have, in effect, become a handbook for decision making in human resources matters. The human resources selection process must now be reported to state and federal compliance agencies, usually on EEOC forms that require accurate data on the actual hiring results of the nursing facility. As Chruden and Sherman (1980) and Noe et al. (2000) have observed, what used to be the exclusive concern of the facility administrator and human resources officer can now be carried into the courtroom.

The Federal Equal Employment Opportunity (EEO) poster should be prominently displayed in an area accessible to both staff, applicants, and residents/patients. All advertising must announce the facility's position as an Equal Opportunity Employer. For facilities that receive revenues through Veterans Administration contracts, all job openings for positions of more than 3 days' duration and with a starting salary of $25,000 annually or less must be listed with the local state employment agency.

MATCHING HUMAN RESOURCES NEEDS WITH APPLICANTS

Taking on the right person for a position is a complex task. The employer understandably wants to find out as much as possible about the applicant to determine his or her likelihood of success if hired for a position in the facility (Johns & Saks, 2001; Matheny, 1984).

Methods of Obtaining Information

There are several methods for learning about applicants. Most organizations use written application forms, interviews, and background checks. The search for a new administrator or director of nurses may involve appointing a committee, lengthy exploration, extensive interviewing, obtaining departmental employee input, and the final selection. Filling a vacancy for a nurse's aide is much less complicated, but in both cases it is important that all the information solicited be demonstrably job-related or predictive of success in that position (Noe et al., 2000).

Reliability and Validity of Information

Information that is valid and reliable is necessary for making an informed decision about an applicant's skills, knowledge, aptitudes, level of motivation, and likely fit with the organization (Johns & Saks, 2001; Noe et al., 2000).

Reliability of the tests, interviews, and other tools used in selecting applicants refers to the consistency with which the same results are obtained over a period of time and when used by different testers (called interrater reliability).

In measuring applicants' abilities, reliability means that an applicant will achieve the same or nearly the same score or results when taking the test at different times, say a week or two apart. If a test were to give differing results from week to week it would be unreliable. Reliability also requires that different applicants with the same skills score the same on the test. If word-processing skill is being measured, applicants with the same level of skill must score the same on the test.

A test or selection procedure provides *validity* when it actually measures what it is intended to measure and does it well. In essence, *validity* is a measure of how effectively an instrument does its job (Chruden & Sherman, 1980; Noe et al., 2000). Personnel experts have relied on at least two types of validity for several years: *content validity and construct validity.* Both are used by governmental agencies in judging the results of a facility's hiring program (Noe et al., 2000).

Content Validity. Content validity is the degree to which a test, interview procedure, or other selection tool measures the skills, knowledge, or performance requirements actually needed to fill the position for which the applicant is applying. As more and more facilities begin to offer medically complex care, a nursing position may require the ability to administer drugs intravenously. A test establishing that the applicant can perform IVs skillfully has content validity.

Construct Validity. The extent to which a selection tool measures a trait or behavior that is perceived as important to functioning in a job is construct validity. Intelligence is an abstract construct, or trait, that is established putting together answers to a series of different questions that together yield a measure of the theoretical construct called intelligence.

The following is an example of construct validity: a nursing home administrator's requirement of a "friendly facial expression" toward patients/residents is an example of a construct (trait) that the administrator believes is needed for the position.

To validate a friendly facial expression as a job requirement, the administrator would have to identify the work behaviors required for the position; identify the constructs (e.g., smiling) that are required; and then show by empirical evidence that this selection requirement is truly related to the construct.

It is of real importance for a nursing facility to require that all staff treat patients/residents in a cheerful or friendly manner, although this directive may be difficult to achieve. In a Fort Worth, Texas, case a federal judge ruled that American Airlines had the right to discharge an otherwise good flight attendant because he did not smile enough. The flight attendant had sued the company, contending that he was a good employee and met all requirements of the job except for the smile. The federal judge upheld American's policy of requiring a friendly facial expression as "essential in the competitive airline industry" ("Now We Know Why They're So Friendly," 1985).

APPLICATION FORMS—PREEMPLOYMENT QUESTIONS

Employers must avoid questions that might be construed as violating the Civil Rights Act, Title 7, or the Americans With Disabilities Act. These include questions that relate to age, sex, race, national origin, education, religion, arrest and conviction records, marital status, and credit rating (Title 7) or disabilities (Americans With Disabilities Act and Title 7). The interviewer must review any unsolicited requests for reasonable accommodation under this Act. If the applicant is under 18 years of age, federal and state child-labor laws may specify hours of work, type of work, machinery to be operated, and supervision requirements. In recent years, about 1,500 complaints based on religious discrimination alone were filed annually (Noe et al., 2000).

Table 2-11 shows a list of subject areas that one is permitted and not permitted to ask questions about on application forms or in the preemployment interviews under Title 7.

DISABILITY-RELATED QUESTION

On May 19, 1994, the Equal Employment Opportunities Commission issued a 49-page notice (915.002 on May 19, 1994) with the goal of clarifying which questions employers are permitted to ask that might be related to disability as viewed under the Americans With Disabilities Act. This notice made it clear that handicap only after making a job offer may an employer ask about the nature of any need the applicant may have for adjustment to a disability. It is only at this point that the employer may consider what a reasonable accommodation might be. Prior to offering a job it is unlawful to ask such questions as, "Do you need a reasonable accommodation to perform the essential functions of the job? If so, what kind?"

In an attempt to clarify what preemployment interview questions are permissible and which are not, the EEOC Notice offered the following as examples:

Lawful	*Unlawful*
Do you drink alcohol?	How much alcohol do you drink per week?
How well can you handle stress?	Do you ever get ill from stress?
Are you currently using illegal drugs?	Have you ever been treated for drug problems?

Table 2-11. Suggestions for Interviews

Inquiries before hiring	Lawful	Unlawful*
1. Name	Name	Inquiry into any title that indicates race, color, religion, sex, national origin, handicap, age or ancestry.
2. Address	Inquiry into place and length of current address	Inquiry into foreign addresses that would indicate national origin
3. Age	Any inquiry limited to establishing that application meets any minimum age requirement that may be established by law	a. Requiring birth certificate or baptismal record before hiring b. Any other inquiry that may reveal whether applicant is at least 40 and less than 70 years of age
4. Birthplace or national origin		a. Any inquiry into place of birth b. Any inquiry into place of birth of grandparents or spouse c. Any other inquiry into national origin
5. Race or color		Any inquiry that would indicate race or color.
6. Sex		a. Any inquiry that would indicate sex b. Any inquiry made of members of one sex but not the other
7. Religious creed		a. Any inquiry that would indicate or identify religious denomination or custom b. Applicant may not be told any religious identity or preference of the employer c. Request pastor's recommendation or reference
8. Handicap	Inquiries necessary to determine applicant's ability to substantially perform specific job without significant hazard	Any other inquiry that would reveal handicap.

Table 2-11. (Continued)

Inquiries before hiring	Lawful	Unlawful*
9. Citizenship	a. Whether a U.S. citizen b. If not, whether applicant intends to become one c. If U.S. residence is legal d. If spouse is citizen e. Requiring proof of citizenship after being hired	a. If native-born or naturalized b. Proof of citizenship before hiring, c. Whether parents or spouse are native-born or naturalized
10. Photographs	May be requijred after hiring for identification purposes	Requiring photograph before hiring
11. Arrests and convictions	Inquiries into conviction of specific crimes related to qualifications for the job applied for	a. Any inquiry that would reveal arrests without convictions
12. Education	a. Inquiry into nature and extent of academic, professional or vocational. training b. Inquiry into language skills such as reading and writing of foreign languages	a. Any inquiry that would reveal the nationality or religious afffflation of a school b. Inquiry as to what mother tongue is or how foreign language ability was acquired
13. Relatives	Inquiry into name, relationship and address of person to be notified in case of emergency	Any inquiry about a relative which would be unlawful if made about the applicant
14. Organizations	Inquiry into organization memberships and offices held, excluding any organization, the name or charac~ter of which indicates the race, color, religion, sex, national origin, handicap, age or ancestry of its members	Inquiry into all clubs and organizations where membership is held
15. Military service	a. Inquiry into service in U.S. Armed Forces when such service is a qualification for the job b. Requiring military discharge certificate after being hired	a. Inquiry into military service in named service of any country but U.S. b. Request military service records c. Inquiry into type of discharge

Table 2-11. (Continued)

Inquiries before hiring	Lawful	Unlawful*
16. Work schedule	Inquiry into willingness to work required work schedule	Any inquiry into willingness to work any particular religious holiday
17. Other	Any question required to reveal qualifications for the job applied for	Any nonjob-related inquiry that may reveal information permitting unlawful discrimination
18. References	General personal work references not relating to race, color, religion, sex, national origin, handicap, age or ancestry	Request references specifically from clergymen or any other persons who might reflect race, color, religion, sex, national origin, handicap, age or ancestry of applicant

I. Employers acting under bona fide Afffimative Action Programs or acting under orders of Equal Emploympnt law enforcement agencies of federal, state, or local gpvernments may take some of the prohibited inquiries listed above to the extent t hat these inquiries are required by such program or orders.

II. Employers baying Federal defense contracts are exempt to the extent that otherwise proldibited inquiries are required by Federal law for -security purposes.

III. Any inquiry is prohibited which, although not specifically listed above, elicits information as to, or which is not job related and may be used to discriminate on the basis of, race, color, religion, sex, national origin, handicap, age or ancestry in violation of law.

*Unless bona fide occupational qualification is certified in advance by the State Civil Rights Commission.

Note: Long Term Care Administrator's Desk Manual, by Dulcy B. Miller, Ed. Greenvale, NY: Panel Publishers, Inc., 1982, Exhibit 203.H, pp. 2059–2061. Reprinted with permission.

Do you regularly eat three meals per day?	Do you need to eat a number of small snacks at regular intervals throughout the day in order to maintain your energy level?
How did you break your leg?	How did you come to use a wheelchair?
Do you have a cold?	Do you have AIDS?

INTERVIEWING APPLICANTS

Interviews are used extensively in evaluating job applicants. Each organization will develop its own style and identify its varying information needs as it conducts interviews (Noe et al., 2000).

Preliminary Interviews

One approach is to use a preliminary approach that generally consists of having the applicant fill out a short questionnaire, after which there is a brief conversation with the applicant based on the questionnaire. This serves to screen out unsuitable candidates, using a minimum of time and organizational resources.

Telephone and Video Interviewing/Screening

While setting up interviews with candidates the person who will do interviewing, can elicit and convey a good deal of information such as

- present employment
- why the candidate is looking for a position, what kind of next position is being sought
- candidate's salary requirements
- why the candidate left previous positions, past salaries
- persons supervised, if a manager, and their job functions
- information about your facility
- set up an interview if mutual interest exists after the above explorations

Interviewing Methods

Interviewing methods vary, but can be generally classified by three types according to the degree of structure: nondirective, in-depth, and patterned.

In the *nondirective interview* the interrogator refrains from influencing the applicant's remarks. This allows the applicant maximum freedom to ask questions and give information. The interviewer's task is to pay special attention to attitudes, values, or feelings that the candidate may exhibit (Johns & Saks, 2001).

This approach maximizes the amount of information the applicant may reveal and is often called an open-ended interview technique. The interviewer asks only broad general questions such as, "Tell me about how you did and how you liked your last job," or, "What is it about working in a long-term care facility that attracts you?" or "Where do you want to be in your career in the next 5 years?" There is no prescribed set of questions.

An *in-depth* interview provides more structure in the form of specific question areas to be covered. (This is sometimes called a directed interview.) Examples of questions appropriate to the in-depth interview are

- What do you consider your most important skills for this job?
- Tell me about your last job.

- Under what type of supervision techniques do you function best?
- What did you like most about your last job? What are your feelings toward older people? What do you like most and dislike most about older people?

The *patterned interview* allows the least amount of freedom to both the interviewer and the applicant. All questions are sequential and highly detailed. Generally, a summary sheet must be filled out by the interviewer interpreting the results of the encounter.

In every case, do anything you can to make the interviewee comfortable. And be on time for the interview.

Approaches

- Avoid forming strong impressions during the early minutes of the interview.
- Allow the candidate to do most of the talking.
- Don't clue the candidate into precisely what you are looking for early in the interview.
- Ask specific questions about past job behavior.
- Probe for all the information needed.
- Take notes, but not on the application form.
- Use second and third interviews when appropriate.

One major nursing home corporation suggests the following areas as appropriate general areas for questioning.

Professional Maturity

- What has been the toughest assignment you have ever had and how did you handle it?
- What would you do if [name an adverse situation that an employee in that job might encounter]?
- What actions have you taken if you disagreed with a supervisor's decision?
- What is the impact or role of your department on your current facility's objectives?

Skill Level

- What are your present job responsibilities?
- What results were achieved in terms of successes and accomplish?
- What do you feel you can learn from this position?
- What are your greatest strengths? What areas need improvement?

- What was the biggest contribution you made to your current position?
- How would your references rate your technical competence?
- The ability to solve problems is critical to this position. Please provide an example of how this ability has been important to your success.
- What important trends to you see in your profession?

Character

- What do you consider the most important aspects of a job?
- Where do you see yourself in two years? five years? ten years?
- What have you liked best about your present (recent) supervisor(s)? What have you liked least?
- Why should we hire you?
- How successful do you think you have been so far in your career?
- How long would it take you to make a meaningful contribution to this facility?

Research Findings on the Use of Interviews

A good deal of research has been conducted on the reliability and validity of interviews as a tool for judging job applicants. Chruden and Sherman (1980) report some of the major findings:

- Structured interviews are more reliable than unstructured interviews.
- When there is a greater amount of information about a job, interrater reliability is increased, that is, several interviewers are more likely to come to the same decision.
- Interviews can explain why a person would not be a good employee, but not why they would be a good one.
- Factual written data seem to be more important than physical appearance.
- Interpersonal skills and level of applicant motivation are best evaluated by an interview.
- Allowing the applicant time to talk provides a larger behavior sample. Also, one can learn more from listening than by talking.
- An interviewer's race affects the behavior of the person being interviewed.

Responding to the Market

While the above processes may serve well when there is a large applicant pool for jobs in the facility, the reality is that nurses, nurses' aides, and other facility employees often change jobs. An applicant may have taken the afternoon off to find a new job. Making such applicants feel welcome and offering an interview at the point of application may increase a facility's ability to have first choice in obtaining needed new hires.

BACKGROUND INVESTIGATIONS

If the interviewer decides the candidate is of interest to the organization, background information can be sought.

It is advisable to obtain from applicants a signed request for references. Increasingly, former employers are reluctant to put any recommendations into writing for fear of lawsuits. Many will only provide information about the date of hire, position held, and date of separation.

Background Checks

Background checks are increasingly important. Grant and Kemme (1993) recommend perseverance despite most employers' adoption of a neutral policy on employment (e.g., say revealing only name, job, title, and dates of employment). They recommend a screening process consisting of (a) background checks (trustworthiness, honesty, gaps in employment, required licenses, relevant background such as for a driver); (b) drug tests (the Americans With Disabilities Act does not protect drug users); and (c) criminal background checks (which may be mandatory). In the matter of criminal background checks, here the so-called business necessity rule applies. Employers must consider all job-related circumstances around a conviction to determine if the person would be a safe employee in the facility. Some allowable considerations are time of conviction, nature of conviction, number of convictions, facts of each case, job-relatedness, length of time between conviction and application, and efforts at rehabilitation (Grant & Kemme, 1993). Generally, any person convicted of substance abuse becomes a high risk for the facility. Reference requests should be obtained on at least two jobs, preferably the two most recent or for the past 3 years, whichever is longer. For applicants with no work experience, school, volunteer, or personal references can be used. For nurse's aide applicants two basic checks need to be made: (a) Verification through the state registry that certification is current and that the applicant has met training and competency requirements; and (b) determination through the substance abuse registry in every state in which the facility has reason to believe the applicant has worked as a nurse's aide to establish whether any record of resident abuse or neglect or misappropriation of resident property has occurred. Sometimes criminal background checks must be made.

The Privacy Act of 1974 (Public Law 93-579) gave federal staff the right to examine their human resources records, including letters of reference unless they waived this right when they requested said letters. Although not mandated by federal law, the Privacy Act of 1974 seems to have led to a trend among employers to permit staff to review and change their human resources files (Chruden & Sherman, 1980).

Lawsuits for negligent hiring can be minimized by gathering as much pertinent information as possible about applicants. Discrimination charges can be minimized by focusing on job-related criteria.

Credit Reports

Under the federal Fair Credit Reporting Act (Public Law 91-508), the employer must advise applicants if credit reports will be requested. If the candidate is rejected because of a poor credit report, he or she must be so informed and given the name and address of the reporting credit agency. The Internet makes credit checks nearly instantaneous.

Physical Examinations

All facility staff must have periodic health examinations to ensure freedom from communicable disease. The practical impact of this stipulation is to seek a preemployment physical. There is some debate as to whether requiring a physical before offering a job is permitted or whether one must offer the job first and then require a physical before the employee begins work. In essence, all applicants must be informed that a condition of employment will be the preplacement health exam following the conditional job offer.

There are several practical reasons for a physical examination. It establishes the physical capability of the applicant to meet the job requirements (a delicate proceeding given the tenor of the Americans With Disabilities Act), and it provides a baseline against which to assess their later periodic physical exams. The employment-related physical examination is especially valuable in determinations of claims of work-associated disabilities under Workers' Compensation laws (discussed in part 4). The laboratory analyses that are part of the exam also can detect the presence of illicit drugs in the applicant (Noe et al., 2000).

If the physician determines that the new employee cannot perform the essential functions of the job due to a disability under the definition of the Americans With Disabilities Act, the facility must follow policy on reasonable accommodations for individuals with disabilities. If the physician determines that the employee cannot perform the essential functions of the job but does not have a disability under the definitions of the Americans With Disabilities Act, the employee is notified that he or she is not qualified for the position.

Normally the health file is not considered part of the human resources file due to its confidential nature; only authorized persons may have access to the employee's health record on a need-to-know basis.

Family and Medical Leave Act of 1993 and the Americans With Disabilities Act are discussed further in part 4. The Immigration Reform and Control Act of 1986 determines which individuals are legally eligible to work in the United States, and is also discussed in part 4.

THE DECISION TO HIRE

Who should decide which applicant to hire? Generally, the final decision to hire is given to the head of the department in which the recruit will work, not to the human resources staff. The administrator of the facility can define a role for herself in the final decision making or leave it entirely up to the department head.

Approaches to the Hiring Decision

The hiring decision itself is complex, but two basic approaches have been identified in the literature: clinical and statistical.

In the *clinical approach,* the decision maker reviews all the information in hand about the match of the applicant and the job, and then decides.

In the *statistical approach,* the decision maker identifies the most valid predictors, then weights them according to complicated formulas. This method has been shown to be superior to the clinical approach (Meehl, 1954). However, few facilities will normally have enough staff time available to make this approach practical. One compromise is for the decision maker to rate each applicant for a position on several dimensions—such as test score results, education, experience, apparent interest level—and assign numerical scores on each dimension to each candidate. The results can provide a systematic set of comparison data for reaching the final decision (Jauch, 1976).

The Passion Index

It is not enough to establish that an applicant has the technical skills needed for a job. Staff must realize that successful caring for frail, elderly nursing-home patients is often less dependent on the technical knowledge of the staff than on their compassion for others. Knowing the technique for gait training for a disabled person is useless if the staff member cannot encourage the person to leave the chair. As the nursing home population becomes more medically complex, *both* caring and technical skills becomes increasingly important. Sensitivity, compassion, and caring constructs, as well as technical competence, will increasingly have validity as hiring criteria in the nursing home setting of the 21st century.

In part 1 we discussed the need for the administrator to have a passion for the tasks necessary to operating a cheerful nursing facility. It is not just the administrator or director of nursing who needs passion: All staff in the facility need to be passionate in carrying out their tasks. A sales vice-president of a large U.S. camera firm explained who makes the best sales people, translated here for the nursing facility. Drawing a vertical line down his flip chart on the left side, he listed basic skills and competencies such as knowledge of the tasks to be performed, being well informed about what competing facilities were doing, having a good employment record, experience in long-term care—all the usual requirements.

On the right side of the chart he wrote "Fire in the heart" (Kriegel, 1991), commenting that if he had to he would chose someone with fire rather than one well trained and well recommended. Staff who have fire, he felt, are more motivated, will work harder, will go the extra mile, and are more resourceful at meeting resident or facility needs. Nurses and nursing assistants who have drive and enthusiasm in caring for the resident/patient can be taught any technical skills they lack. Applicants who lack fire in their hearts or passion for their work are not so easily taught.

Counting Grades

How much do grades count? Do the highest grade point averages in nursing-school or the nursing-assistant test point consistently to the best candidates? Consider the following findings. More than half of the Fortune 500 companies' chief executive officers had a B- or C-average in college. Two thirds of U.S. Senators come from the bottom half of their class, and three-fourths of U.S. presidents were in the lower half of their school classes. More than half of millionaire entrepreneurs didn't finish college (Kriegel, 1991).

OFFERING THE JOB

Once the successful candidate is chosen, he or she should be informed. Information such as proposed salary, job title and level, starting date, and any other relevant information should be communicated. Normally, a period of time during which the offer may be considered is specified. In every case, the candidate needs to be informed about starting date, pay rate, where and when to report, and the name of the supervisor, at the very least.

It is useful to include the human resources handbook with the offer if the applicant has not yet received one. The handbook (discussed later in detail) describes facility policy on a number of matters about which the prospective employee should be made aware as part of evaluating the proposed offer and position. It is useful to set a 3-day time limit for the newly hired staff member to complete all paperwork. Unsuccessful applicants should be informed by letter as soon as the job is filled.

2.7 Training

ORIENTATION

First Day on the Job

Orientation is the foundation for employment. An employee who is not given orientation is a serious liability.

The first day on the job will potentially leave a lasting impression (Chruden & Sherman, 1980; Johns & Saks, 2001; Noe et al., 2000) and is an opportunity for the facility. Enthusiasm and anxiety characterize the first day, and the new employee traditionally brings an initial reservoir of goodwill toward the facility. A sensitively managed orientation program can help reduce new-employee anxiety and begin to build positive images of the new work environment.

Typical first day activities can include

- official welcome to the new employee
- introduction to as many of the staff as is appropriate
- tour of the facility, including location of lockers for safekeeping of personal effects, staff lounges, restrooms, parking arrangements
- instructions on use of any time clock
- safety rules, such as infection control and emergency procedures, especially those concerning fire and staff assignments in case of fire
- explanation of resident/patients' rights
- discussion of contents of the human resources handbook (Rogers, 1980).

There is only one "first day on the job" for an employee. Whether the orientation is for the new director of nurses or nurse's aide, it is equally important to the success of the organization. If the place is organized to take notice of the new employee and attempts to meet his needs on the first day, this latest member of the staff will be more likely to assist the facility in meeting its needs during the following months and years (Bryan, 1984).

Facilities of 300 beds are as capable of a personalized orientation program as those with only 80. In practice, by having a properly constituted human resources process, the larger organization may have a functional advantage over the smaller, where orientation may be left to chance and good intentions without assigned responsibility for this introduction.

Using a Checklist

Precisely because orientation is both an important and complex task, the use of a checklist is valuable. Those charged with familiarizing the new staff member with the organization are thereby less likely to overlook any element of the employee's new responsibilities as they review each item on the list (S. Scott, 1983). One researcher suggests that the use of a checklist may help reduce employee turnover by assisting each new employee in gaining an initial realistic and clear set of expectations about the new positions (R. Scott, 1972). Turnover is always expensive (Johns & Saks, 2001). Estimates vary from $1,000 or more, depending on the position and the length of training needed before the person is functioning efficiently.

Others consider it advisable that both providers and receivers of the orientation be required to sign each activity on the checklist (Davis, 2000; Rogers, 1980). This maximizes the probability that the orientation will be successfully completed. When this document is placed in the employee's human resources file, the signed orientation form becomes a legal basis for establishing that the information was received. Rogers (1980) and Davis (2000) suggest that responsibility for the orientation and its documentation be vested in a single staff member, who is thus accountable for its successful completion from introduction to signed checklist.

THE HUMAN RESOURCES POLICY HANDBOOK

The human resources policy handbook, often called the employee's handbook or the staff manual, is a compilation of the facility policies that directly relate to work conditions. Whereas a job description relates to only one job, the human resources policies are general in nature and cover the entire staff.

Each facility will have its own handbook. Chains generally have sets of policies that apply to all their staff, allowing local facilities to add

their own policies within the broader policy guidelines and any requirements specific to a state or local government regulations.

The main elements most often included in such a handbook are a
statement of general policies, followed by details of benefits and general
information relevant to the conditions of employment. The human resources handbook can be considered the rules, or terms, under which
staff are hired and carry out their work.

A. Introduction Welcome to the Facility

B. History of Background of the Facility/Mission Statement/ Handbook Disclaimer

C. General Employment Policies

1. Equal opportunity employment (conforming to the Civil Rights
   Act), sexual harassment policy, age discrimination policies (Argenti, 1994; Johns & Saks, 2001).
2. Classification of staff into full-time and part-time by number of
   hours worked per week; working hours of the facility.
3. Confidentiality of information about patients/residents and facility
   matters.
4. Resident/patient's rights statement.
5. Employee's records: confidentiality, employee access policy. Usual contents: (a) application for employment, (b) pre-employment
   checks, letters, records of phone calls; (c) credit checks; (d) performance evaluations, promotions; (e) federal and state withholding certificates; (f) correspondence; (g) disciplinary actions; (h)
   grievances; (i) attendance; (j) signatures for receipt of human resources policy manual, orientation activities, and inservice attendance records (k) health related materials such as annual physical
   results, hepatitis B vaccination records (bloodborne pathogens
   requirements), annual tuberculosis tests results, records of injuries
   or other medically related matters; (l) license or certificate verification, (m) other relevant materials.
6. Reporting policies: required call-in times prior to shift if unable to
   come to work.
7. Discipline system: whether a progressive system and, if so, a listing of each rule with a statement of disciplinary action (i.e., the
   number, if any, of oral or written warnings before dismissal). For
   example, failure to follow a dress code may allow an oral warning
   and one or more written warnings before dismissal, whereas physical abuse of a resident/patient could bring immediate suspension
   and investigation and, if appropriate after investigation, dismissal.

8. Uniforms and appearance.
9. General conduct: respect, vulgarity, courtesy, attendance and punctuality, working quietly, absenteeism, visitors to staff, outside work.
10. Gifts (not permitted from patients, their families, or significant others or sponsors).
11. Eating, drinking, smoking, kitchen traffic rules.
12. Use of alcohol and illegal drugs.
13. Parking, mail, rest breaks, meal breaks, lost and found, phone calls to staff, smoking and use of tobacco, employment of relatives, searches of staff (package and purse inspection).
14. Destruction of nursing home property.
15. Suggestion box, permitted uses of bulletin boards, solicitation and distribution of literature.
16. Probationary period, use of anniversary or other dates for human resources reviews, seniority policies.
17. Health requirements and physical examinations.
18. Employee debts, garnishment of wages.
19. Performance ratings, promotion policies and interdepartmental transfer policies, job posting.
20. Wages and salaries, time cards, pay plan, date procedures for determining payroll calculations, payrolls, deductions, overtime policy, severance pay.
21. Grievance procedures.
22. Hospitalization and first-aid treatment.
23. Facility position on unions.
24. Resignation notice and procedures, exit interview (Argenti, 1994).
25. On-the-job injuries policies.
26. In-service education requirements.
27. Reimbursement for specified expenses, e.g., travel, meals, memberships.
28. Confidentiality of company affairs/nondisclosure of information.
29. Family and Medical Act leaves, Worker's Compensation insurance.
30. Fire, disaster, evacuation plans.
31. Incident reports.

D. Benefits

1. Holidays
2. Vacations, accumulation of leave
3. Leaves of absence: sick leave, funeral leave, military leave, maternity leave, jury duty, extended leave
4. Health benefits, dental benefits
5. Tax deferred savings plans (401K plan; Keogh plan, etc.)

6. Stock purchase plan (if any) known as ESOPs (Employee Stock Option Plans) (Argenti, 1994)
7. Retirement benefits
8. Insurance: life insurance, unemployment compensation, occupational disease insurance, workers' compensation insurance, disability insurance (Noe et al., 2000), long-term care insurance, other
9. Shift differential (if paid)
10. Other benefits such as child care, meals at work, etc.
11. Group rates: facility-negotiated reduced rates on a variety of items such as accident insurance, life insurance, liability policies, if any

It is important to note that employee handbooks have been a subject of concern to management in recent years because some courts have held the handbooks to be an enforceable contract between the employer and the employee. Entering disclaimers in the handbook has not prevented staff from successfully suing in court.

TRAINING

As we have noted, directing is the task of ensuring that each work role is successfully communicated to the employee. Directing is the process of communicating what is to be done to the staff, then assisting them in performing their roles successfully (Givnta, 1984). Directing involves the communication and organizational analysis skills discussed in part 1.

Purpose

The purpose of the orientation program is to provide an initial introduction to the new employee. The purpose of training is to communicate the organization's needs to the staff and assist them in meeting those needs. This is a continuous process, beginning formally the first day on the job, but extending for the duration of the employee's association with the facility. Each employee will have his/her own learning curve (Argenti, 1994; Noe et al., 2000).

Steps in Establishing Training Needs

Staff members responsible for establishing the nursing facility's training program normally analyze three elements in planning for this course: (a) the organization, (b) the tasks, and (c) the person carrying out the work (Chruden & Sherman, 1980; Johns & Saks, 2001; Noe et al., 2000).

Organizational analysis consists of examining the facility's goals, resources, and internal and external environments to determine where training efforts need to be focused. A number of in-service topics are mandated for the various departments over the course of each year. These can form the initial framework for training needs (Noe et al., 2000).

Task analysis involves the review of job descriptions and activities essential for performing each job. The emphasis of training programs can then be placed on certain tasks that are judged to be inadequately carried out or simply in need of reinforcement because of their importance to the facility, such as fire drills and disaster preparedness. Additionally, whenever a facility begins accepting more medically complex patients/residents, training for new techniques for the nursing staff is often in order.

A person or employee *skill analysis* can be made to arrive at the skills, knowledge, and attitudes required in each position. It means interpreting each position in terms of the personal attributes or behaviors necessary for performing the job acceptable (Maddox et al., 2001).

Once the goal of a training program has been determined, the following steps can be taken:

1. Formulate instructional objectives,
2. Develop instructional experiences to achieve theses objectives,
3. Establish the performance criteria to be met, and
4. Obtain evaluations of the training effort (Chruden & Sherman; Johns & Saks, 2001).

On-the-job training is conducted by a staff member assigned to assist a new or continuing employee in acquiring the abilities needed in a position in the facility. Ideally, on-the-job training permits the trainee to be an additional or extra worker for the first few days, allowing observation and progressive involvement in performing the tasks and behaviors required (Noe et al., 2000).

In-service training refers to employee education offered throughout the career of the employee. Normally, in-service education consists of small seminars for groups of staff. All types of educational techniques are used including flip charts, films, lectures, videos, role-playing, case discussions, and the like (Ruhl & Atkinson, 1986). In many busy facilities, three or more in-service training programs occur every week.

The nursing facility is a training site for numerous educational programs. Most facilities participate as training sites for nursing schools, physical therapy programs, pharmacy programs, and similar allied health-training programs in nearby colleges and training programs (Noe et al., 2000).

New Methodologies

Increasingly, videos covering many training needs are available along with web-based training being offered by the national long-term care associations (Noe et al., 2000).

EVALUATING TRAINING

Evaluating training efforts can be difficult. While it is true that tests can be devised to measure memorization, the nursing home is seeking to assess something more complex: changes in employee behavior. To quantify behavioral changes, it is useful to state learning objectives as behavioral objectives (Johns & Saks, 2001).

Behavioral objectives can be measured by observing whether staff exhibit the behaviors sought as the objective of the training, in carrying out their duties. Usually the goal is to have the employee acquire a skill or change of an attitude (Noe et al., 2000; Wehrenberg, 1983). Using performance-centered behavioral objectives can assist evaluation.

For example, performance-centered objectives in a nurse's aide training program might be (a) to be able to demonstrate proper procedures for turning a resident/patient who is suffering from decubitus ulcers (pressure sores) (Maddox et al., 2001); and (b) to consistently greet any patients encountered in the hallways using a pleasant tone of voice.

Both of these are performance-centered objectives. Proper techniques for turning a resident/patient who has a decubitus ulcer can be physically demonstrated by the aide in training, and the aide's demeanor toward patients/residents encountered in the hallways can be monitored by the trainer or other staff members (Noe et al., 2000).

Diversity Training

The composition of the nursing facility staff reflects the changing demographic landscape. Diversity training is designed to change employee attitudes about diversity and developing skills needed to work in teams with employees of differing values, gender, ethnic, racial and religious backgrounds, and sexual preferences. Employees can gain an appreciation and acceptance of cultural differences among themselves (Noe et al., 2000).

2.8 Retaining Employees

2.8.1 What the Facility Needs from the Employee

We have argued that the facility needs employees who have a passion for their jobs and who will consistently make decisions in conformity with its policies. This is possible to the extent that each staff member can be characterized as having the following:

- a high degree of interest in the job—a willingness to make every effort
- a genuine dedication to the well-being of the patients/residents and their quality of care and quality of life—passion for the work
- a strong positive self-image, permitting employees to see beyond their own needs and to be concerned instead with those of the patients/residents and their significant others
- skills, both technical and interpersonal, in communication and human relationships
- the capacity and willingness to make decisions in accordance with the best interest of the facility, every act contributing toward providing the highest quality of life for the patients/residents, their significant others, the facility staff and the community
- the ability to be self-starting, reliable, creative, and to exercise positive appropriate leadership—a fire in the heart
- career commitment to the facility

Obviously, this is the description of an ideal employee, and few staff members will be able to embody fully all of these qualities. However, if these characteristics can be constantly encouraged and developed among the employees, the quality of life enjoyed by the residents/patients and staff should be high.

2.8.2 What Employees Need from the Facility

What employees require of the facility can be divided into five areas: (a) social approval; (b) self-esteem; (c) security; (d) use of power, accomplishment, service, and exercise of leadership; and perhaps most important, (e) working for an organization with a vision that allows the employee to participate in a larger meaning, giving them a sense of purpose and pride in their accomplishment (Johns & Saks, 2001).

The degree to which any one individual might seek satisfaction from employment will vary among the entire staff and within the same member as his or her personal situation changes over time.

SOCIAL APPROVAL

Most people rely on a network of approval and satisfying social interrelationships. Whether or not they express it openly, many of them enjoy engaging in activities sanctioned by significant others—persons to whom an individual looks for favorable regard of behavior patterns, ideas, and values. Family, members of the community, and one's social group are typical examples of *significant others.*

If the community or significant others disapproves of the employee's working at the facility, he or she will not have positive feelings about the job itself or feel that being a good employee is worth the effort.

SELF-ESTEEM

Adequate self-esteem is essential in order to function. Individuals need a positive self-image, that is, to feel good about themselves, what they are doing, and the world about them. Each person has a need for status. Most people want to be part of an organization that has a sense of purpose to which they can dedicate their energies with pride.

ECONOMIC SECURITY

In this case we define security as the financial benefits provided by the facility. Without income sufficient for maintenance, health insurance for eventualities, vacations for renewal, and funds to meet future retirement expenses, an employee may remain insecure.

HYGIENE FACTORS

Hygiene factors are those such as salary, company policies, basic working conditions. In theory, when hygiene factors are adequate they do not bring about appreciable levels of employee satisfaction. Hygiene factors, then, are the minimum work conditions (Argenti, 1994; Noe et al., 2000).

ADDITIONAL INTRINSIC NEEDS

Some employees expect even more of the work situation. Their intrinsic needs arise out of the essential nature of their personality (Johns & Saks, 2001). Wielding power and having authority in certain situations are intrinsic needs. Satisfaction from the process of completing their tasks, of achievement, is another such need, as is leadership. Giving service can be fulfilling behavior.

PARTICIPATION IN A VISION

Employees want to work for a corporation that stimulates their dreams and aspirations and touches their hearts. They enjoy collaborating with highly motivated people who are accomplishing work that matters, that has purpose and meaning beyond just striving to being the largest or the best known or the highest income company. The staff need the administrator to take a personal interest in them and to be recognized as an essential member of the team (Riter, 1993).

2.8.3 Strategies to Meet the Facility's and the Employees' Needs

Retaining high-performing employees over an extended period of time is economically desirable for the facility. The financial costs of training each new staff member can be high, especially if the employee participates extensively in in-service training programs offered by the facility and takes advantage of any additional on-the-job training for skills improvement (Johns & Saks, 2001).

In the nursing home setting, employee continuity is critical for the patients/residents themselves, providing an important element of stability and continuity in their lives. More than in most work settings, employees in nursing homes tend to form personal relationships with the patients and are often regarded as friends by residents who have lost family members and other cherished ones.

A motivated, contented staff, capable of contributing significantly to the quality of resident patient life, consists of employees who are enjoying a high level of job satisfaction and are thus enabled to provide a high level of patient care.

An administrator in a large California chain facility says he is successful because he concentrates his energy primarily on the staff. He believes only highly motivated, happy staff give loving care to residents. His zest and enthusiasm, and evident concern about staff enable them to treat residents and coworkers in the same manner.

A FACILITY PHILOSOPHY OF HUMAN RESOURCE MANAGEMENT

What motivates employees? Every day the administrators of more the 16,000 U.S. nursing homes make decisions based on their assumptions of what motivates their staff. These decisions reflect the administrator's beliefs about human resource management and may be consciously or unconsciously held. We will explore one general theory about employee motivation (Argenti, 1994; Noe et al., 2000).

Theory X and Theory Y

In 1960, Douglas M. McGregor, a management theorist, published a book expounding what he called Theory X and Theory Y. McGregor wrote that the behavior of administrators is strongly influenced by their beliefs. He asserted that most business managers are Theory X types, those who believe the employee naturally dislikes work, prefers to receive extensive direction from superiors, wishes to avoid taking responsibilities in the organization, has little ambition, and is motivated more by a need for security than any other factor. This approach requires that managers use fear or punishment to motivate employees, all of whom must be closely watched if the work is to be accomplished.

McGregor (1960) insisted that Theory X is not valid and that managers should be guided instead by what he called Theory Y, which is based on the following assumptions (pp. 33–35):

1. Using energy to work is as natural as using energy to play or rest. The administrator can control working conditions so that work is either a source of satisfaction and voluntarily performed, or a source of punishment and therefore to be avoided.

2. If individuals are committed to the organization's goals, they will exercise self-direction and self-control without the need for threat of punishment or external behavior controls.

3. Rewards for achieving organizational objectives result in employee commitment; employees can achieve personal self-satisfaction in achieving organizational goals.

4. The average employee, when properly motivated, will accept and also seek responsibility.

5. A preponderance of employees have the capability to exercise imagination, ingenuity, and creativity in assisting the organization in achieving its goals.

6. Most jobs underutilized the capabilities of employees.

McGregor's theory caused considerable discussion in management circles. One researcher doubted that most managers were Theory X types. To test this, he surveyed 259 managers in 93 companies and found that managers did not completely accept Theory X *or* Theory Y (Allen, 1973). In their opinion, reality is more complicated than either theory. Not surprisingly, this led a few years later to Theory Z.

Theory Z

Several writers proposed that, on balance, Theory Y is correct, but what motivates employees is dependent on shifting societal values and changes over time. They argue that administrators must constantly come up with new strategies for motivating employees. In their view a straightforward productivity-reward system is overly simplistic. A satisfactory quality of life, both for the individual and for the group, while more complex and abstract, is the appropriate focus (Argenti, 1994; Thierauf, Klekamp, & Geeding, 1977; White, 1984).

PERSONALITY TESTS

Some facilities utilize a variety of tests to evaluate applicants and employees. The most widely known is the Myers-Briggs Type Indicator personality test (Noe et al., 2000). As many as 2 million people take this test each year in the United States (Noe et al., 2000), which consists of 100 questions about how respondents feel or act in a variety of situations. The test categorizes respondents as introverted or extroverted, sensing or intuitive, thinking or feeling, and perceiving or judging. These characterizations are then used to place a person in one of 16 personality types. Someone whose test results show her to be extroverted-intuitive-thinking-perceiving is classed as a conceptualizer (Argenti, 1994). This and other tests are sometimes used to classify persons into "Left-brain" and "Right-brain" categories, the theory being that left brained persons are systematic, thorough, balanced, and ask detailed questions about each situation, whereas right-brained persons are more intuitive, quick, and less complex in their approach to decision making.

MEETING THE EMPLOYEE'S NEED FOR SOCIAL APPROVAL

Individuals have a need to be part of an enterprise that is regarded by their significant others as successful. Hence, approval of the nursing facility by significant others is important to nursing home employees.

In the community, the word-of-mouth reputation of the facility is important. Persons and groups regarded as experts in the field (the local hospital, home health agency, hospice, the local physicians, the case managers at the local health maintenance organizations (HMOs), Independent Practitioner Organizations (IPOs), Professional Provider Organizations (PPOs,) Workers' Compensation, and similar groups) can be considered significant others as well, whose approval is sought by the staff. Newspaper, radio, and television reports about their workplace shape employee feelings.

To cite an example, in one large city a nursing home operated by the county was attacked in the news media for 4 years and threatened with decertification for Medicare and Medicaid by federal and state officials because its sanitation and resident/patient care were regarded as significantly substandard. During that time it was difficult to hire staff. Nurses, janitors, physical therapists, nurse's aides, and maintenance people who worked there were harangued by friends and neighbors and workers in other health care facilities. Why were they willing to work under such conditions? After a succession of three administrators in the course of 4 years, during which the home suffered constant public attacks both by the media and individuals, an improving level of care became apparent.

Employees do care about the reputation of their organization.

MEETING THE EMPLOYEE'S NEED FOR SELF-ESTEEM

Why does one nurse's aide strive harder than another? Why does one registered nurse look for additional responsibilities while another seeks to avoid taking any? Why do wage incentives stimulate some individuals and not others? Why does a career advancement track within the facility stimulate some employees to strive while others ignore the opportunities offered?

What motivates employees varies not only for the individual employee but, over time, for the same employee. Motivation is a difficult concept to define. It has been described as the factor that energizes employee behavior, directing or channeling such behavior, and sustaining it (Johns & Saks, 2001; Steers & Porter, 1979).

An individual's needs, desires, and expectations change. When one need or desire is met at a satisfactory level, the salience or strength of others is modified. For a nurse who has just been licensed to practice, being accepted by the other nurses may be a priority until this recognition is achieved (Lorsch & Takagi, 1986). At that point other needs, such as maximizing income, may take precedence.

Understanding Motives

The complexity of motives has been described by Dunnette and Kirchner (1965) and Johns and Saks (2001), who attempted to apply motivational psychology to the work situation. They point out the following:

1. Identifying motives is complex. Some employees will work hard to obtain more money, but why? A strong need for additional money may reflect a desire for the increased status more money brings, meeting a need for a sense of economic security, providing a symbol of power, or simply a willingness to work harder until the car is paid off, at which point time off from work may replace the desire for more money as a primary motivation.

2. Motives are always mixed. Every individual experiences a wide range of motives that strengthen and weaken as circumstances change, and some needs are met while others are frustrated.

3. The same incentive (increased health insurance benefits, as an example) may generate different responses. Individuals also differ in the ease with which their needs are satisfied.

4. Some motives may recede when satisfied, for example, hunger and thirst. Others, such as a desire for increased status or more salary, may intensify when, as an example, more status or more income is achieved.

The process of giving employees increased roles in the decision-making processes of the facility is known as *job enrichment*. A nurse supervisor and aides, for instance, may be assigned complete responsibility for the care of a set of patients, rather than special responsibilities (i.e., some nurses doing medications, others doing range of motion exercises) (Argenti, 1994; Johns & Saks, 2001). *Job depth* refers to the extent to which an employee has power to influence decisions. When the director of nurses consults the aides on a floor about whether they are prepared to receive a proposed admission, these aides have increased job depth (Argenti, 1994).

A. H. Maslow's hierarchy of need is perhaps the most frequently cited human-need model in the literature (see Figure 2-4) (Argenti, 1994; Johns & Saks, 2001). He theorizes that needs become salient, that is, powerfully motivating, at each successively higher level, mainly after the needs at each lower level are satisfactorily met. In other words, until the individual has met the needs for survival and basic security (lower level), these needs will dominate.

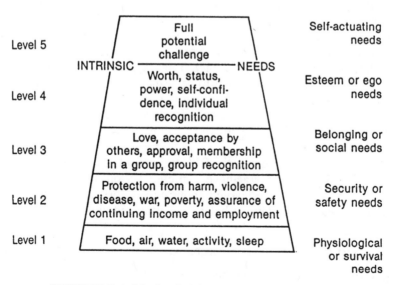

FIGURE 2-4. Maslow's hierarchy-of-need concept.

Once lower-level needs are met to a satisfactory degree, the individual's motivation may be dominated more by social, self-esteem, and self-actuating needs (levels 3, 4, and 5). Maslow's model is widely used. In our view, it seems to be a functional and useful explanation of some of the more basic dynamics of employee motivations.

One author has pointed out that while the lower-level needs may decrease in strength when achieved, the higher-level needs, especially the need for self-actualization, tend to continue growing stronger as they are being met (Lawler, 1973). Examples of these types of needs or motivations are those cited earlier as "additional intrinsic needs," such as being in authority, wielding power, accomplishing goals, and exercising leadership.

A word of caution: Every individual has a unique ever-changing pattern of need. In our view, what motivates an individual depends on a combination of life experiences and—as scientists are suggesting more and more—on individual genetic and chemical makeup.

Childhood experiences such as economic deprivation may cause an employee to be anxious about financial security, no matter how much income is earned. The social and economic class with which an employee identifies affects perceptions of "needs." Being raised as a male or a female can also influence the needs an individual will manifest on the job.

Personality Types A and B

Attempts have been made to identify basic personality types, and investigators who were focusing on the causes of heart disease described two. Type A is characterized as a hard-driving, achievement-oriented person who strives to the highest level in every area of activity, whether sports, job titles, or on-the-job productivity. Type A persons, especially those who are chronically angry, appear to be at increased risk of heart disease (Maddox et al., 2001).

Type B personalities are characterized as having only moderate achievement needs and as less competitive and more satisfied with moderation in their endeavors.

Type A employees come to the facility with a high internalized motivation level. They are overachievers in comparison to Type B persons. Why? Much has yet to be learned about motivation, genetic influences, and the influence of chemical balances within individuals.

Assessing Motivation: An Exercise

Supervisors' ideas about what motivates the staff often differ significantly from employees' ideas about what they find motivating. The reader can ask supervisors and employees in his or her facility to consider aspects of their jobs from the list that follows.

Ask participants to rank the items from 1 = most important to 10 = least important:

- to be treated fairly
- consistency from management
- job security
- interesting work
- full appreciation for work done
- good wages
- good working conditions
- feeling "in" on things
- promotion and growth within the facility/company
- sympathetic understanding of personal problems
- tactful discipline
- management loyalty to workers

In the following section, we discuss several areas available to an employer seeking to retain staff by meeting their needs for approval: leadership by vision, training programs, career paths, performance feedback and goal setting, recognition, power, respect for creative potential, teams, "Ninjas of joy."

Leadership by Vision

Most facilities have set goals. Meetings that exhort employees to meet those goals (such as making the month's budget, keeping census up) are, in the end, limitations. Goals limit unless they are part of, and remain part of, a vision. Organizations like nursing facilities need a vision to fire up the employees, to engage their spirits and set long-term directions for their efforts. Each department manager needs a vision of what her department can achieve, a vision to provide meaning to each employee's efforts. Kriegel (1991) argues that a vision or dreams are goals with wings. A dream or vision is an ideal state, a goal is more a realistic state. The dream supplies enthusiasm, vigor, and direction for the facility's efforts. Goals are short-term targets, such as assuring that all the paperwork for admissions are completed in a timely manner and all doctor's telephoned orders signed within the time permitted. Employees want to feel they are doing more than contributing to the profit ratio. They want to be part of a movement, a compelling vision that captures their imaginations. They want to be part of a facility that has a vision, a dream about the quality of life of each resident and staff member. Business is won (or lost) on the front lines (Maddox et al., 2001).

Training Programs

Training programs increase employee skills and simultaneously communicate to them that those skills are valued by the management.

The programs themselves serve numerous functions. They demonstrate management's interest in the staff and provide an additional arena for exchange among employees, as well as an increased opportunity for feedback to the administration about the degree of skills and understanding of facility goals among employees. As these dynamics occur, the level of employee satisfaction can improve. With the new skills or insights the employee experiences an increased feeling of being in tune with the performance expectations of the organization.

Career Paths

Offering a career path means providing upward mobility within the organization. In a freestanding nursing home, creating career mobility is more difficult than within a chain that owns and operates 400 facilities.

Making career paths available within the facility communicates to the employees that the organization wants to meet their desires to succeed and progress in job level and income. For the nursing aide, a career path might include facility support through released time or tuition assistance. This makes it more feasible to enroll at a local technical institute to become a licensed practical nurse or a registered nurse.

The charge nurse might receive support to participate in a program to become a geriatric nurse practitioner. The kitchen worker might be assisted in attending classes that lead to qualifying as a dietetic service supervisor.

The labor market can be an influencing factor. If the home is freestanding, in a rural area with a limited number of persons in the potential pool of nurse's aides or kitchen workers, career assistance may lead to an undesirable depletion of the worker pool.

On balance, however, providing career paths that create upward mobility appears to increase worker satisfaction and improve employee retention rates. Not all of the aides will aspire to become licensed nurses, since there are not all similarly motivated. However, the availability of a career program can improve workers' attitudes. Those who choose not to participate have the satisfaction of knowing the option is available and that they may choose to exercise it if they wish. In general, the mere presence of options is important to employees.

Performance Feedback and Goal Setting

Employees receive informal feedback on their job performance on a daily basis. Formal reaction and the formal process of goal setting for an individual employee occurs under more structured circumstances. This is known as the performance evaluation, which normally includes establishing goals for the employee to achieve until the next scheduled performance evaluation (Johns & Saks, 2001; Noe et al., 2000).

To Err Is to Learn. The facility administrators' attitude towards errors and failures is critical to success—as Kriegel (1991) has observed, failure is a good place to start. Failure itself is not a crime The problem, really, is failure to learn from failure. It is not a question of whether the medication nurse will make mistakes, it is what he/she does after making them that determines how good that nurse is.

Mistakes Are Inevitable. Mistakes are both inevitable and an opportunity to learn. If the facility's managers show that they understand this, the employees will respond with more openness about their mistakes. Covering up mistakes by employees takes a great deal of energy and usually leads to more lies to shore up the initial one. Someone who conceals mistakes is a problem for the facility. The employee who comes into the department manager's office and says, "I screwed up," is an employee with whom there is good communication, and an opportunity to learn has been created. In short, management needs a positive attitude toward mistakes. Employees prefer to work in an open, honest atmosphere in which management helps them to learn from their mistakes.

Recognition

Employees want to be thanked. Most employees seek recognition for their work. Much of their behavior can be interpreted through *expectancy theory,* pioneered by Victor Vroom in the 1960s (Argenti, 1994; Johns & Saks, 2001; Noe et al., 2000). This theory holds that the level of motivation to perform (make an effort at work) is a mathematical function of the expectation that individuals have about future outcomes multiplied by the value the employee places on these outcomes. Vroom defines expectancy as a "momentary belief concerning the likelihood that a particular act will be followed by a particular outcome" (Johns & Saks, 2001; Vroom, 1964).

The charge nurse who believes that working long hours and asserting herself on the job will lead to quick promotion to nurse supervisor is an example of an expectancy. It serves as a guideline for the charge nurse in seeking promotion to nurse supervisor. The charge nurse expects the behavior to be rewarded. Recognizing employees' expectancies can help a supervisor understand how they are motivated.

If the charge nurse's long hours and assertiveness lead to promotion, the expectation is reinforced. According to reinforcement theory, (Johns

& Saks, 2001) behaviors depend on reward. When rewards follow performance, performance improves (Johns & Saks, 2001). Conversely, when rewards do not follow performance, performance deteriorates. If the charge nurse had not been promoted, performance might have deteriorated (Noe et al., 2000).

In *reinforcement theory* the outcome reinforces the employee's response either positively, leading to repeating the response, or negatively, where it is not repeated. Influencing employee behavior through reinforcement is called *operant conditioning,* literally influencing working behavior by conditioning the employee's response through rewarding (or punishing) the behavior (Noe et al., 2000).

When employees perform in a desired manner and are given praise and recognition for that behavior, the manager is engaging in what may be called behavior modification (Johns & Saks, 2001; Maddox et al., 2001). Behavior modification involves operant conditioning, usually through rewards, praise, and positive recognition when an employee performs as desired by the facility.

One theorist (Rotondi, 1976) suggests the following as a pattern for modifying employee behavior to conform to facility goals:

- Maintain a consistent work environment.
- Consciously identify the desired behaviors of employees.
- Decide on the rewards to be used.
- Clearly communicate to the employees both the desired behaviors and the rewards.
- Reward desired behaviors immediately.
- Scale rewards to the behavioral achievement attained, that is, vary the rewards.
- Minimize the use of punishments.

Power and Control

Nursing facility administration needs to define policies to govern their decision making, thought this has both positive and negative results. The positive aspect is that the staff is given guidance and an appropriate framework within which to make decisions for the organization. The negative aspect is that deciding beforehand, through policy making, can substantially deprive the employee of a feeling of personal involvement in decision making for the organization. (Johns & Saks, 2001).

Powerlessness

Christopher Argyris is a behavioral scientist who has observed a tendency for organizations to overlook what he believes is the desire of most employees to function in a mature, adult manner. In the literature this is referred to as the *immaturity-maturity theory*, which holds that most organizational designs treat employees as if they were immature, thus frustrating their need to function as responsible adults.

Argyris (1972) believes that the typical organization tends to ignore individual potential for competence, for taking responsibility, for constructive intentions, and for productivity. He feels that in the typical lower-level job of the nurse's aide, the laundry worker, or the housekeeper, staff members are treated as immature. This he argues, alienates and frustrates these workers, leading them to feel justified in rejecting responsible behavior and tempting them to defy the organization by allowing the quality of their work to deteriorate.

He sees the same problems among managers who work within organizational structures that create environments hostile to trust, candor, and risk taking. In such situations, the attitudes actually encouraged are conformity and defensiveness, which tend to be expressed by producing detailed substantiation for unimportant problems and invalid information for critical issues. Argyris (1972) asserts that this leads to ineffective problem-solving, poor decisions, and weak commitment to any decisions that are made.

Argyris is pointing to the converse of a coherent set of policies to cover all decision making in the facility: little significant role in decision making is left to the employee, which may lead to a high level of frustration among those affected.

Some common reactions to frustration might be selecting an acceptable substitute goal that is attainable or engaging in behavior that is maladaptive (Chruden & Sherman; 1980). An employee who is barred from making any meaningful decisions at the facility may stop trying and may concentrate his energies on a leadership role in an outside voluntary organization. Or the employee may relieve his frustration through aggressive or abusive behavior toward other employees or the patients/residents (Chruden & Sherman, 1980).

Combating Powerlessness: Employees as "Owners." You don't wash a rental car, because you don't own it. A solution to the problem of powerlessness is to attempt to make everybody an "owner." Giving all employees a sense of ownership in the facility means treating each employee as a member of the team (Argenti, 1994). This can be accomplished by allowing them some control in their work and giving them information about what the facility is attempting to accomplish. Tom Peters advocates this approach in *A Passion for Excellence.* He calls the approach "all people as 'businesspeople' " (Peters & Austin, 1985).

Ownership implies that all employees exercise some real portion of control in the facility. Of course, each employee does exercise some fraction of control over the workplace. It is up to the individual staff member to decide whether to give care pleasantly or in an uncaring or disrespectful manner when alone with the resident/patient.

"Businesspersons." Tom Peters' belief is that if the organization treats every employee as a "businessperson," the employees will respond as "businesspersons," fully engaged in the facility's goal of giving quality care and adequate income and being committed to its success. A sense of ownership is accompanied by a feeling of control over what happens. This is sometimes accomplished by job enlargement, increasing the number of tasks an employee performs so that she finds increased satisfaction through involvement in a process from start to finish (Argenti, 1994). Peters cites examples from the experimental laboratory and from the field (Noe et al., 2000).

An industrial psychologist gave the subjects in a study some difficult puzzles to work and some boring proofreading to do. While they were attempting to accomplish these tasks, the psychologist played a loud tape recording of one person speaking Spanish, two speaking Armenian, and a copy machine in use.

Half of the subjects were given a button to push that would stop the noise, the other half had no control over it. Those with the buttons solved five times as many puzzles and had 25% fewer errors in proofreading, although ever pushed the button. Those who perceived that they had control over their situation clearly outperformed those who felt they had little or no control. In numerous repetitions the same results were obtained.

In the field, the same results were achieved: Workers who were given buttons to push achieved superior results for the company. The Ford Motor Company plant in Edison, New Jersey, gave every worker on the assembly line a button to push that shut down the assembly line. The workers shut down the assembly line 30 times the first day, and an average of 10 times a day thereafter. After the first day the shutdown lasted an average of 10 seconds—just enough time to make this or that small adjustment or turn a bolt (Peters & Austin, 1985).

What happened at the plant? Production remained steady, but three other factors changed significantly. The number of defects dropped from 17 per car to less than 1, the number of cars requiring rework after coming off the line dropped by 97%, and a backlog of union grievances plummeted. Why? Because the lineworkers felt they had some meaningful control over their jobs: They had a sense of ownership in the plant. Employees who have a sense of ownership in the facility will try to do what is best for it. The nurse's aide with this perception is more capable of meeting his social needs such as self-esteem, self-acceptance, and status.

How can nurses' aides be given ownership in the facility? One director of nurses accomplished it by consulting the aides before admitting a patient to their area. When the aides told the director of nurses that the care load was too great at one particular point, the director of nurses refused the proposed admission.

These aides had a sense of control over their work situation. They worked harder and exercised their control judiciously to make sure the quality of resident/patient care was not compromised by overadmitting. These nurses' aides had a "button to push," and they never pushed it without a good reason.

Nurses' Aide Ownership. Why should nurses' aides be involved in running the facility? Ford Motor Company has a practice of soliciting input from all hourly workers. The assembly line workers are asked to comment on the manufacture of parts and are members of advance design teams. Hourly workers offered 1,155 suggestions for changes in design or production for three small trucks. More than 700 of these suggestions were adopted (Peters & Austin, 1985). Techniques that involve nurse aides in the organization's decision making may provide personal fulfillment and growth, leading to higher staff retention.

The nursing home administrator is commonly conceived to have at least three immediate constituencies: the staff, the residents/patients, and the residents/patients' significant others. In part 5 we will argue that one of the administrator's major tasks is to create and enforce as many opportunities as possible for residents/patients to feel in control of their lives. Here we maintain that one of the administrator's major tasks is to create and enforce as many opportunities as possible for staff to feel in control of *their* work. Not an easy task for either group. The forces of institutionalization appear to move naturally toward removing control from the residents/patients. Similarly, the forces of regulations and the accompanying need for conformity in the workplace naturally move toward removing control over work from the staff members. In a study of staff's self-perceived influence on decision making (498 staff in 51 nursing homes), nurse assistant involvement in shift reports, frequency of unit staff meetings, and administrators' decision-making autonomy from the governing board were found the associated with increased levels of nurse's aide involvement in decision making (Kruzick, 1995; Maddox et al., 2001).

One administrator gives nurses' aides 50 cents an hour for each employee they get and *keep* at the facility. When the administrator asked an aide how she was doing, she replied, "My company's fine." She had six employees in her "company" and was now earning $3 more per hour. Creative incentives are endless.

Respect for the Creative Potential of Each Employee: Maintaining Passion

The "business" of every nursing facility is providing resident/patient care. We mentioned in part 1 that in *A Passion for Excellence* Tom Peters insists that there are only two ways to create and sustain superior patient care: first, by taking exceptional care of patients by providing superior services and quality of care; and second, by constantly innovating (Peters & Austin, 1985).

According to Peters, this is not accomplished by the genius of the administrator or by mystical strategic moves. Excellence in patient care comes from "a bedrock of listening, trust, and respect for the dignity and the creative potential of each person in the organization" (Peters & Austin, 1985).

High-patient care depends on whether the administrator has enabled the employees—the housekeepers, kitchen staff, laundry workers, maintenance persons, accountant, and secretary as well as the nursing staff— to "buy" into the facility.

Stow the Firehoses. Most individuals and organizations tend to resist change. It has been observed that the only people who really welcome change are patients with wet diapers and busy cashiers. There is a tendency to "firehose" employee's ideas for new ways to accomplish the facility's goals. Some common responses to the suggestions are, "It's not within the budget," "It'll never work," "We've already tried that," "Yeah, but, things are fine the way they are," and "We don't do it that way around here."

According to Kreigel, conventional wisdom holds that everything happens in cycles. The belief is that things will cycle back—back to normal, back to the good old days. Criticizing new ideas leads to sticking with the tried-and-true approach. Kreigel argues that the new reality is, change will be followed by change. The waves will not flatten out, but will continue to get bigger and come faster.

Membership on a Team

We have mentioned the team concept several times and will return to it in the discussion of resident/patient care planning in part 5.

Industries have repeatedly discovered that small groups produce higher quality, more personalized service, and more innovations than do larger entities (Johns & Saks, 2001; Peters & Austin, 1985). American companies like General Motors, Hewlett-Packard, and Emerson Electric now typically limit the size of the plant they will build to between 200 and 500 employees. The Japanese organize their largest industrial plants into small teams of 10 to 40 workers. Ask each worker, "What do you need to do a better job?"

A Natural Head Start. The nursing home enjoys a natural advantage over these companies. Federal regulations have demanded a small-team approach since 1973. Those who drew up the federal requirements already knew what industry is only beginning to realize: Employees perform better when they are part of a team (Noe et al., 2000).

Team membership is a valuable tool in efforts to retain employees because it helps meet the employee's need for social involvement, communication with other employees, and meaningful personal involvement in the real work of the facility.

As a matter of practical reality, the work of a nursing facility cannot be successfully accomplished without the departments functioning as a single team. Achieving and maintaining this necessary teamwork is one of the nursing facility's constant challenges.

Trying Easy. Ever more intense regulatory efforts and continuous squeezing of the funds made available to nursing facilities can lead to a faster-is-better mentality, what Kriegel (1991) refers to as the "Gotta's" (p. 53): I gotta make medication rounds quickly, gotta finish all the paperwork, gotta cut costs, gotta get the patient ready for that meal, gotta get the trays out fast.

A Lesson from Chaplin. Kreigel cites the Charlie Chaplain film *Modern Times,* in which Chaplin is happily decorating cakes on the assembly line, adding a rose here, a fancy frosting there. Then the assembly line speeds up, and in his haste the icing gets sprayed everywhere and the cakes begin falling off the end of the assembly line creating a growing mound on the floor. The more recent equivalent is known in Japan as *karoshi,* or death from overwork. Many Japanese workers have been obliged to work in perpetual overdrive leaving them frustrated, nervous, and irritated—a true Type A lifestyle requirement.

Because of low reimbursement levels the pressure to provide more service with fewer employees in the nursing facility can lead to reduced quality and service. Creativity and innovation lose to speed. The turnover rate among directors of nursing and the nursing assistants are testimony to this. Caudill and Patrick developed a 56-item questionnaire for nursing assistants, which was completed by 996 of them. Weekly and permanent resident/patient assignments were favored over rotating responsibilities. Aides responsible for larger number of patients/residents left more often. (Caudill & Patrick, 1992). Kreigel relates his experiences with athletes trying out for the Olympic team. After recording their times in the first round, he told them to run at 90% of their capacity, not flat out. Each ran faster the second time. An Arkansas study of long-term care nurse administrators by Vaughan-Wrobel and Tygart (1993) confirmed that most nurse administrators are ill-prepared by prior administrative training for their positions.

Turnover. Turnover rates are as high as 60%. The nurse administrator position normally requires a tremendous effort from people who are without adequate prior training. Conventional wisdom, Kriegel notes (1991), tells us to move at 110% capacity to get the necessary work done. The administrator can assist employees in giving a passionate 90% effort, which results in job satisfaction, rather than pressuring for a panicky 110% effort, which results in job dissatisfaction. Patients who hear the proverbial excuse, "We're working short today," know that the effort will lead to lower quality and care on that shift (Johns & Saks, 2001; Noe et al., 2000).

"Ninjas of Joy"

Work ought to be fun, and several West Coast firms in Silicon Valley have led the way toward this concept. Dress is California informal, life is laid-back, having fun is an important value. Aristotle once observed that pleasure in the job puts perfection in the work (Kriegel, 1991). If nurses who love nursing can be hired, if nursing assistants who love taking care of older people can be hired, if maintenance persons who love to tinker and repair and maintain can be hired, the facility will be a pleasant place to spend one's hours.

The Importance of Having Fun. It is perhaps more important to have fun in a nursing facility than in most work settings. As one writer observed, coal miners used to take birds into the shafts to serve as early warnings of danger. Laughter and good humor are the canaries of the workplace: When the laughter dies its' an early warning that life is slipping from the facility (Kriegel, 1991). The ice-cream manufacturer Ben and Jerry's appointed "joy gangs" whose responsibility was to bring more joy into the facility. Similar groups in nursing homes could devise activities and events that would encourage the employees and residents/patients to loosen up and have fun with each other. It is not necessarily an easy task in the nursing home environment, and is therefore all the more important.

Turnover and burnout are high among nursing facility staff. Kriegel (1991) observes that conventional wisdom says "play to win"; instead, Kriegel says, "play, to win" (p. 256). There is a saying that getting there is half the fun. Actually, winning must take place not at the end of the game but every day along the way. Work must be fun each day if employees and patients/residents are to experience quality living. He or she who laughs, lasts. This is true both of employees and patients/residents.

MEETING THE EMPLOYEE'S NEED FOR ECONOMIC SECURITY

For the purposes of this discussion, by the term *security* we mean the finance-related benefit package provided for the employees. This is explored further in chapter 2.9, "Paying Employees." Often employee behaviors are rewarded through incentive plans (any rewards that motivate employees) that are designed to achieve facility goals (Argenti, 1994).

A Simplified Model

The following is one way to view what employees need from the facility:

What:	knowledge of what the organization needs
How:	skills to do what the organization needs
Will:	the desire to do what the organization needs
Equipment:	the tools to get the job done to professional standards
Time:	enough staff to permit the desired behaviors

2.9 Evaluating Employees

JOB PERFORMANCE EVALUATION: A LINE MANAGER FUNCTION

Job performance evaluation is a task assigned only to line managers. Such responsibility distinguishes staff from line management functions: staff, having no line authority, should not be assigned line responsibility for human resources matters—hiring, evaluating, promotion, reprimanding, suspending or discharging employees—because to do so violates the concept that each employee should report to only one manager.

PURPOSE OF PERFORMANCE EVALUATION

In part 1, we cited W. Edwards Deming's third deadly sin: evaluation by performance, merit rating, or annual review of performance. These methods, Deming, asserted, destroy teamwork and nurture rivalry. Performance ratings build fear, leave people despondent, bitter, and beaten and encourage mobility of management. Having acknowledged this, what is a department manager to do? How is the facility to judge the performance of its employees over time? There are those like Deming who would argue that being a member of a productive team affords the facility managers sufficient evaluation and control over an employee's performance. Perhaps so.

Yet there may be problems with doing away with annual or other reviews of employee performance. The frequent change of staff, including department managers in the average nursing facility, means that the organization's "memory" can be short. If an employee is seeking to build a career at a facility and there are no records, her progress over an extended period is more subject to the impressions of department managers who are only passing through (Noe et al., 2000).

As a practical matter, all of us are judged by ourselves and our co-workers as we go about out daily work. The organization needs some method of creating a track record, both to reward the good employee and to identify employees who function at the margin of competence and for whom considerable documentation must be in place when the time comes for dismissal.

A basic purpose of the job performance evaluation is to focus the energies of the employee on the performance level expected of him (Johns & Saks, 2001; Smith, 1984). Whereas on-the-job and in-service training are part of the directing role of department heads, job performance evaluation is a function of comparing and controlling personnel performance quality. The goal of the performance evaluation, of course, is to nurture the performance needed for the success of the facility, and, so far as practical, to reward good work (Noe et al., 2000).

The EEOC and more recently the American With Disabilities Act have done a great deal to stimulate employers to keep accurate evaluation records of employees' work. Court hearings have also contributed to the desirability of carefully documenting worker performance (Chruden & Sherman, 1980).

THE PERFORMANCE EVALUATION

Three Basic Objectives

Three basic objectives of performance evaluations are (a) to give employees feedback about their work performance, (b) to provide a basis (plan) for directing future employee efforts toward organizational goals, and (c) to provide a basis on which managers will decide on promotions, compensation, and future job assignments (Johns & Saks, 2001; Locher & Teel, 1977; Noe et al., 2000).

The performance evaluation can force communication that might not otherwise occur concerning the manager's feelings about the employee's work. Setting up a performance evaluation system may simply be a needed formalization of the department managers impressions of the daily work of the employee. Most industries use the performance evaluation. A study by the Bureau of National Affairs revealed that among the industries studied, 84% had regular procedures for evaluating office personnel and 58% for evaluating line workers (Bureau of National Affairs, 1975). The majority of evaluations were given on an annual basis.

On balance, the absence of any written system for evaluation of long-term performance is more likely to expose the individual to the whim of managers who head the employee's department.

Outline of the Process

First, the manager defines the functions, tasks, demands, and expectation of the job and translates them into performance criteria (Baker, and Morgan, 1984; Bianco, 1984; Johns & Saks, 2001; Noe et al., 2000; Smith, 1985). To implement this, forms and procedures must be developed, including standardized methods of rating employees to be used by supervisors in conducting evaluations.

Approximately two weeks before an evaluation date, the manager completes the form and sends a copy to the employee, together with notification of time and place of the evaluation. This gives the employee time to prepare for the meeting.

At the evaluation the manager reviews the completed form and may modify sections, if appropriate. Performance goals for the next time period are reviewed and are modified if employee and manager concur.

At the end of the session employee and manager both sign the evaluation. Provision is normally made for any addendum the employee may wish to write or for the employee to indicate disagreement with the findings. In the event of such a difference of opinion, appeal procedures are normally available.

As Deming has been eager to point out, the performance evaluation process is not without its faults.

Possible Problems

Whatever the importance to the facility and however rational the evaluation process may seem, resistance to its effective utilization often arises, making the program difficult to implement (Johns & Saks, 2001; Snell & Wexley, 1985).

Evaluations often are given at the time the employee hopes for an annual raise, focusing primary attention on past performance rather than future performance goals. The managers are not usually rewarded when they take the time to give thorough evaluations. Most managers are uncomfortable with face-to-face judgemental roles, and employees are highly sensitive to negative evaluations, which leads managers to avoid conflict. Employees want the appraising manager to meet at least three criteria: The appraiser should (a) have had adequate opportunity to observe the employee's work (Johns & Saks, 2001; Smith, 1984); (b) thoroughly understand the employee's job and have clearly stated standards by which to judge the employee's efforts (Smith, 1984); and (c) judge the work from an informed viewpoint. Nurses' aides, for example, want someone trained as a nurse, who presumably understands the nature of their job, to write their evaluation.

Performance evaluations sometimes fail. One major nursing home corporation has identified the following contributing causes: (a) lack of previously agreed-upon objective, (b) poor skill of the manager, (c) lack of a defined evaluation process, and (d) managerial behavior that does not contribute to the self-esteem and self-image of the employee. Employees, the corporation points out, do not normally outperform their self-image: If their self-image is high, high performance can be anticipated, and the converse is true if their self-esteem is low. Performance evaluation, they point out, should not be the first time people hear about things. A major goal is, be a coach, not a critic. One point to remember: Evaluate performance, not the person. One can be candid and specific about performance without attacking the person.

METHODS OF RATING EMPLOYEES

Rating Scales

Rating scales are consistently used (Chruden & Sherman, 1980), which list a number of characteristics, traits, and requirements of the employee's position on a line or scale (Sears, 1984). The evaluator checks off the degree to which the employee is believed to meet a trait or requirement. For example, a scale recording degree of initiative might appear thus:

Initiative
Lacks initiative   Meets requirements   Highly resourceful

Work Quality
Needs to improve   Meets standards   Exceeds standards

Often the manager will be asked to provide a *global rating* for the employee. This normally is regarded as a summary score based on the components of the evaluation. Generally, each employer establishes a numeric or alphabetic scale for the facility. For example, 1 might represent the highest and 5 the lowest rating.

Inevitably, the scale comes to resemble the grading system everyone knew in elementary and secondary school. Whatever symbols are used, the person comes to understand that he is an A, B, C, or D performer— or an F, in which case a termination notice might be pending. However much or little the manager may write or discuss with the employee, the employee's real concern is whether he is a "1" performer, and if not, why. The employee knows that the "1" performers get first shot at whatever rewards the system has to give, be it a promotion, bonus, salary increase, or high status.

Errors Made by Managers Using Rating Scales

Rating scales, too, have their drawbacks. At least three types of errors can occur.

The Leniency Error. To avoid conflict, some supervisor give consistently high ratings. The lenient supervisor's ratings are difficult to compare accurately with those of a stricter and more demanding supervisor.

The Error of Central Tendency. Other supervisors consistently give only moderate scores to employees whether their performance is poor or outstanding (Johns & Saks, 2001).

The Halo Effect. The halo effect occurs when a supervisor who values one particular type of job behavior (punctuality, for example) permits the presence or absence of this trait to color several or most other traits ratings. A habitually late employee might be excellent in resident/patient care, but receive a low rating in most categories because the supervisor is irritated by the persistent tardiness.

Rating by Essay

The use of essays or paragraphs describing employee progress is less frequent than rating scales. It is especially difficult to compare employees when the essay method permits supervisors simply to write whatever evaluative comments occur to them. A brief essay at the end of a rating scale can be valuable, however.

Possible Outcomes from Evaluations

Evaluations are primarily intended to give feedback to the employee about performance to date and projected activities. Some of the possible results can be transfer, promotion, or demotion, or, in the case of the reductions in force, the basis for discharge.

Transfer. A transfer is the placement of an employee in another position that is approximately equivalent to the present position. A nurse, for example, may find that working on the medically complex hall is beyond his current level of technical skills and ask for a lateral transfer to a lighter-care hall.

Promotion. A promotion is the placement of an employee to a higher level within the facility or group of facilities (promotion to a job at the corporate level, for instance). There are at least two recognized bases for promotions: merit and seniority. Seniority is concerned with length of service and tends to be automatic. The merit system relies on the performance evaluations of supervisors for placement of a worker at a higher level. Under the seniority system a nurse who serves the required number of months or years at Level 1 is automatically promoted to Level 2. Under the merit system a nurse may or many not be promoted from Level 1 to Level 2, depending on evaluation decisions of the supervisor.

Demotion. Demotion is the change of assignment of an employee to a lower level in the organization, usually with less pay, fewer responsibilities, and reduced status. Demotions are often accomplished through "transfers" (Noe et al., 2000), whereby a formerly more productive employee may be transferred to a lower position, with pay and status intact. Another alternative to demotion is promotion to a position with little responsibility or power.

Layoff. Layoffs are usually temporary dismissals and are potentially demoralizing to the remaining employees as well as to those laid off. Unambiguous layoff policies can reduce anxiety among the remaining employees. However, such policies also tie the hands of management, who might, for example, seek to retain a recent but especially valued employee. Layoffs are carefully scrutinized by employees for fairness and equitability in their implementation.

Discharge. When companies downsize, some basis for deciding who is dismissed is exercised. Discharging those employees with the lowest evaluation ratings first is a frequently used approach.

COP VERSUS COACH

One of the reasons Deming advises against performance evaluation reviews is that it places the manager more nearly in the role of policeperson than of coach. The performance evaluation usually focuses on "areas in need of improvement," the negative side of the employee's work, on what the employee is not doing right, rather than on her strengths. The department manager is the employee's coach, and the coach's job is to bring out the best in the individual. When managers cite employees' weaknesses in the performance evaluation, the employee feels "more busted than trusted" (Kriegel, 1991). It is the employee's strengths, not weaknesses that will carry her through to success. As Kreigel observes, one can get by by improving upon weaknesses, one can become great by building on strengths.

Evaluation Do's and Don'ts, Lessons Learned by One Corporation

One major national nursing-home chain suggests the following useful ideas about evaluations:

- Evaluation information should be given only to those who have a definite reason and legal right to it.
- Evaluations should be conducted in private.
- It is unfair not to be frank with an employee in an evaluation interview and discuss areas of needed improvement.
- The evaluation form should reflect accurately the employee's performance.
- Effective evaluation interviews that produce results take time.
- Evaluations should be made only on those issues that are relevant to the job.
- A supervisor will find it difficult to follow up on the "I'll try harder!" solution from an employee.
- If policy permits, the employee has a moral and ethical right to see his or her evaluation form.
- Overrating all employees is a mistake in the long run.
- Recent events, both positive or negative, can unduly bias a performance evaluation interview.

2.10 Paying Employees

The nursing home is labor intensive. In most facilities wages and benefits make up more than half the operating costs. One writer estimates that about 65% of nursing home expenditures are personnel-related (Buttaro, 1980). Estimates are that in 1992 benefits made up 39% of employee compensation (Arnett, 1994). A 1997 survey revealed that employee compensation nationally was 55% of expenses in all industries and 62% of nursing industry costs (Noe et al., 2000).

Careful management of wages and benefits is one of the major sources of cost control available to the nursing home administrator.

TYPES OF COMPENSATION

Compensation is generally considered the reward given to employees in exchange for their work effort. How willing an employee may be to work hard and assist the facility toward its goals can depend on how justly the employee feels her wages and benefits fit her work effort (Belcher, 1974; Noe et al., 2000).

Money Is Liquid Value

The most liquid benefit a facility can give to its employees is the paycheck. Health insurance, sick leave, and the like, are important, but the benefit most highly regarded by the employee is the dollar value of the paycheck, which provides maximum control over the product of the work effort.

The wages paid the employees normally determine their standard of living (Johns & Saks, 2001). Wages also affect status in both the facility and in the community and are perceived as a statement by the facility about the relative worth of the skills of each employee.

For the typical nursing-home employee the wage rate is salient, and even a few cents more or less per hour can spell the difference between satisfaction or dissatisfaction with wages for an individual who is making comparisons with a similarly qualified coworker.

Benefits

Economic theory holds that employees prefer a dollar in cash to a dollar's worth of any specific commodity because the cash can be used to purchase the commodity or something else; in other words, cash is less restrictive. Nevertheless, benefits as a percentage of wages and salaries have increased from 17% in 1955 to 42% by 1997 (Noe et al., 2000). Government programs requiring certain benefits, such as Social Security, have partly caused this shift. Favorable tax treatment of certain benefits, tax-deferred 401k plan contributions, for example, have also contributed to this trend (Noe et al., 2000).

Equity Theory

According to equity theory, employees seek an exchange in which their wages and benefits are equal to their work effort, especially when compared to wages and benefits paid to similarly situated coworkers (Johns & Saks, 2001; WhiteHill, 1984). If the individual feels equitably paid, less tension may exist. However, if she suspects that others with similar skills and investment of effort receive more, a tension exists that most employees will seek to resolve.

Typical worker responses to perceived inequities are to ask for a pay raise, reduce their effort, file a grievance, or in some cases seek employment elsewhere. Alternatively, the employee may encourage those who are perceived to be similarly situated yet benefiting more to work less hard. Reactions to perceived inequities can take many directions (Ivancevich, 1977).

WAGE POLICES

Developing and administering compensation policies are important administrative duties. Policies should cover such areas as the following (Chruden & Sherman, 1980; Johns & Saks, 2001; Noe et al., 2000):

- the rate of pay, set below, at, or above the prevailing community practice
- the discretion supervisors can exercise in differentiating an individual's pay from the set scale

- the amount of spread between pay rates for employees with seniority and pay rates for new employees
- periods between raises and the weight given to seniority and merit in determining a new pay rate

Hourly Wages or Salaries?

Most facilities distinguish between hourly employees (wage earners) and those who are paid stated salaries periodically. Hourly employees generally are required to punch in and out on a time clock and are paid only for the hours worked as verified on the time card. Salaried workers are paid a set wage regardless of the hours worked, which may or may not be required to be recorded on a time clock. Usually, department managers in the nursing facility are paid a set salary. However, some department managers—perhaps the head of dietary who encounters numerous occasions for long days—may negotiate to work on an hourly basis.

HOW MUCH TO PAY: THE WAGE MIX

Determining wage rates and benefits is a complex task affected by a number of factors called the wage mix (Noe et al., 2000). These factors are the labor market, prevailing wage rates, cost of living increases, ability to pay (Noe et al., 2000), collective bargaining, individual bargaining, and the value of the job.

The Labor Market

Once governmental requirements for minimum wage rates are met (sometimes the influence of unions are also taken into account), supply and demand dramatically affect the wage rate. During the early decades of this century physicians were able to restrict their numbers and keep them lower than the demand; this resulted in favorable influences on their incomes, which now average well over $100,000 per year. Similarly, the nurse shortage of the early 1990s resulted in dramatic increases in the wages earned by nurses in the facility. In many cases the salary of the director of nurses increased beyond that of the administrator. Many administrators benefited when their own wage was pushed up to keep it above that of the director of nurses.

Prevailing Wage Rates

According to a government study, more than half of businesses surveyed indicated that the prevailing wage scale in their communities for comparable jobs was the most influential factor in determining wages actually paid (Noe et al., 2000).

This tends to be true for nursing facilities, which generally are viewed as paying somewhat lower salaries than do local hospitals to employee categories such as nurses. In general, the local hospital's wage rate sets the prevailing wage rate against which the other health care providers set their own pay scales ("Long-Term Care Employee Shortage," 1986).

Wage surveys for the community or region are taken by many organizations. They may be carried out by a single facility or through agreements with others to share this information (Brennan, 1984). In most communities nursing facilities share wage information with each other and with other health providers.

Cost-of-Living Increases

During periods of inflation, a cost-of-living adjustment may be made in wage rates. The purpose of these increases is to assist workers in maintaining their purchasing power. Often embodied in escalator clauses of labor contracts, cost-of-living increases provide for wage adjustments based on some index, usually the Consumer Price Index (CPI). The CPI is a government-defined measure of the cost of living compared to a base point, usually of a few years earlier, which is designated as 100. Any increase or decrease in the cost of living is then expressed as a percentage of the base figure of 100.

Collective Bargaining

Where employees are unionized (discussed in part 4), nursing homes are subject to union influences, regardless of wage rates paid.

Individual Bargaining

Individuals with especially desirable skills may be able to negotiate a higher wage than others in similar positions. When a highly qualified maintenance director or director of nurses is sought, the facility may bargain with such a person and offer a premium.

Key Job Comparisons

In the nursing facility the wages paid to the nurses tend to become the benchmark against which the earnings of other staff members are compared and established (Noe et al., 2000).

Wage Classes and Rates

To approach equity and achieve some flexibility for supervisors who are evaluating employees, wage classes, or grades, and wage rates are usually established (Brennan, 1984a). All jobs within that class are paid at the same rate or within the same rate range. A rate range is the variation permitted within a class or grade (Noe et al., 2000).

Merit Pay

The use of merit pay is a complex matter. Usually a merit-increase grid is developed for each merit pay position. The size and frequency of pay increases is tied to (a) the individual's performance rating, and (b) the position of that individual's pay in the merit-increase grid. Merit pay often increases individual competition among staff, thus reducing willingness to perform as a team. A fair and accurate performance system that is satisfactory to most employees is difficult to develop and administer, which leads to increased levels of employee dissatisfaction, and perhaps turnover (Noe et al., 2000). Group incentives are useful, but also have limitations inasmuch as they may pit groups against each other. This is undesirable in the intimate atmosphere of the nursing home setting where all departments (groups) must cooperate and work as a team with one another if quality of care is to be delivered (Noe et al., 2000).

2.11 Disciplining Employees

The following are some of the more common staff disciplinary problems faced by nursing facilities:

- excessive or unexcused absences or tardiness
- leaving the facility or work area without permission
- violation of rules about smoking, intoxication, narcotics, gambling, fighting, firearms
- failure to follow safety procedures, especially the Bloodborne Pathogens Act requirements
- failure to accept direction
- failure to report accidents
- failure to take resident/patient safety and welfare into account
- verbal, physical, or other abuse of patients/residents
- theft, punching another employee's time card, falsifying records
- insubordinate behavior or abusive language
- failure to report one's own condition of illness
- solicitation or acceptance of gratuities from patients/residents, their families or significant others
- immoral, indecent, or disorderly conduct

THE NEED FOR RULES AND CONSEQUENCES

Each facility should carefully state and consistently enforce policies regarding disciplinary actions, which is easier said than done. Employees must be made fully aware *before any infraction occurs* of the facility's rules and the consequences of disciplinary action for breaking them

(Cameron, 1984; Hill, 1984). Although policies and rules may have been clearly formulated, these policy statements remain confusing unless they are continually reinforced by positive (motivating) and negative (disciplining) actions (Discenza & Smith, 1984). Unless the facility can document that it had just cause for firing an employee, there is a significant chance that the employee will be able to collect unemployment benefits.

Grievance Procedures

Grievance procedures are an important safety valve for policies regarding disciplinary actions. Employees need to know that there are equitable procedures through which their reactions and views can be expressed when they feel they have been dealt with unfairly.

Progressive Discipline

For most offenses, progressive discipline—beginning with verbal warnings, followed by written warnings for any subsequent violations—makes the most sense. Progressive discipline may prevent repetition of the offending behavior after only a verbal warning, thus bringing about an early solution to the problem.

Employees who are dismissed have the right to present their case to the employment security commission, and many do. It is necessary for the employer to keep a well-documented record of having made every reasonable effort to persuade the employee to conform to facility policy before dismissal (Tobin, 1976). Administration must be able to demonstrate that disciplinary actions were based on rational judgments about the offending behavior, not on personal vindictiveness or the excessive emotional reactions of supervisors to employee behavior (Chruden & Sherman, 1980).

Each facility needs to define clearly its own policies governing suspension and discharge procedures. Several managers, including the administrator, usually participate in a decision to suspend or discharge an employee.

One major nursing facility chain recommends that the following conditions be adhered to strictly:

- The requirement reasonably relates to the operation of the facility and that the requirement has been properly communicated.
- Management has investigated the matter fairly, objectively and in a timely manner.
- The requirements and penalties are and have been administered fairly and objectively, without any form of discrimination.

- The situation is dealt with and a penalty determined in a manner consistent with past practice for similar situations.
- The penalty is appropriate to the seriousness of the infraction.
- Misconduct (e.g., patient abuse, theft, and substance abuse) is reported to the appropriate agency for investigation according to state or federal regulations.
- Where the penalty is discharge, employees have warning or knowledge of the probable consequences of their actions.

Discharging Employees

The process of terminating employees, especially executives, can be eased by helping that person find alternative employment. This is called disemployment, outplacement, or dehiring (Chruden & Sherman, 1980; Noe et al., 2000). The managers themselves may assist the employee in finding another position or hire an employment firm to do so. This is referred to as outplacement counseling or transferring problems (Noe et al., 2000).

REFERENCES: PART TWO

Allen, J. E. (2000). *Nursing home federal requirements and guidelines to surveyors* (4th ed.). New York: Springer Publishing Co.

Allen, L. A. (1973). M for management: Theory Y updated. *Personnel Journal, 52,* 1061–1067.

Argenti, P. A. (1994). *The portable MBA desk reference.* New York: Wiley

Argyris, C. (1972). A few words in advance. In A. J. Marrow (Ed.), *The failure of success.* New York: AMACOM.

Arnett, G. M. (1994, March 29). Pricing health care. *The Wall Street Journal,* p. A16.

Baker, H. K., & Morgan, P. I. (1984). Two goals in every performance appraisal. *Personnel Journal, 63*(9), 74–78.

Belcher, D. W. (1974). *Compensation administration.* Englewood Cliffs, NJ: Prentice-Hall.

Bianco, V. (1984). In praise of performance. *Personnel Journal, 63*(6), 40–50.

Brennan, E. J. (1984a). Everything you need to know about salary ranges. *Personnel Journal, 63*(3), 10–16.

Brennan, E. J. (1984b). Restraint of the free labor market. *Personnel Journal, 63*(5), 22–25.

Bryan, L. A. (1984). Making the manager a better trainer. *Supervisory Management, 29*(4), 2–8.

Bureau of National Affairs. (1975). *Employee performance: Evaluation and control,* (Personnel Policies Forum Survey No. 108). Washington, DC: Bureau of National Affairs.

Buttaro, P. J. (1980). *Home study program in principles of administration of long term health care facilities.* Aberdeen, SD: Health Care Facility Consultants.

Cameron, D. (1984). The when, why, and how of discipline. *Personnel Journal, 63*(7), 37–39.

Carter, M. F., & Shapiro, K. P. (1983). Develop a proactive approach to employee benefits planning. *Personnel Journal, 62*(7), 562–566.

Caudill, M. E., & Patrick, M. (1992). Turnover among nursing assistants: Why they leave and why they stay. *Journal of Long-Term Care Administration,* 29–32.

Chruden, H. J., & Sherman, A. W., Jr. (1980). *Personnel Management* (6th ed.). Cincinnati, OH: South-Western.

Cole, A., Jr. (1983). Flexible benefits are a key to better employee relations. *Personnel Journal, 63*(1), 49–53.

Davis, W. E. (2000). *Introduction to health care administration.* Bossier City, LA: Publicare Press.

Delaney, W. A. (1984). The misuse of bonuses. *Supervisory Management, 29*(1), 28–31.

Discenza, R., & Smith, H. L. (1985). Is employee discipline obsolete? *Personnel Administrator, 30*(6), 175–186.

Dunnette, M. D., & Kirchner, W. K. (1965). *Psychology applied to industry.* New York: Appleton-Century-Crofts.

Equal Employment Opportunity Commission, Civil Service Commission, U.S. Department of Labor and U.S. Department of Justice (1978). Adoption by four agencies of uniform guidelines on employee selection procedures. *Federal Register, 43* no. 166, 38290–38315.

Givnta, J. (1984). For good job training, you need a good beginning. *Supervisory Management, 29*(6), 19–21.

Gomez-Mejia, L. R., Page, R. C., & Tornow, W. W. (1985). Improving the effectiveness of performance appraisal. *Personnel Administrator, 30*(1), 74–82.

Grant, D. A. & Kemme, J. (1993). How to conduct security checks on prospective employees. *Nursing Homes,* 12–14.

Green, E. (1977, October 17). Heart disease: New ways to reduce the risk. *Business Week,* 135–142.

Harrington, C. H., Carrillo, M. S., Thollaug, S. C., Summers, P. R., and Wellin, V. (2000). *Nursing facilities, staffing, residents, and facility deficiencies, 1993 through 1999.* University of California at San Francisco: Department of Social and Behavioral Sciences.

Hill, N. C. (1984). The need for positive reinforcement in corrective counseling. *Supervisory Management, 29*(1), 10–14.

Hitt, M. A., Ireland, R. D., Hoskisson, R. E. (2001). *Strategic Management: Competitiveness and globalization* (4th ed.). Cincinnati, OH: South-Western College.

Hoff, R.D. (1983). The impact of cafeteria benefits on the human resource information system. *Personnel Journal, 62*(4), 282–283.

Hogstel, M. (1983). *Management of personnel in long-term care* (27–28). Bowie, MD: Prentice-Hall.

Ivancevich, J. M., Szjlagyi, A., & Wallace, M. (1977). *Organizational behavior and performance.* Santa Monica, CA: Goodyear Publishing.

Jauch, L. R. (1976). Systematizing the selecting decision. *Personnel Journal, 55,* 564–567.

Johns, G., & Saks, A. (2001). *Organizational behavior,* (5th ed.). Toronto, Canada: Addison Wesley Longman.

Karuza, J., & Katz, P. R. (1994) Physician staffing patterns correlates of nursing home care. *Journal of the American Geriatrics Society, 42,* 787–793.

Kriegel, R. J. (1991) *If it ain't broke . . . break it.* New York: Time Warner.

Kruzick, J. M. (1995). Empowering organizational contexts: Patterns and predictors of perceived decision-making influence among staff in nursing homes. *Gerontologist, 35,* 207–216.

Lawler, E. E., III. (1973). *Motivation in work organizations.* Monterey, CA: Brooks/Cole.

Locher, A. H., & Teel, K. S. (1977). Performance appraisal—a survey of current practices. *Personnel Journal, 56,* 245–247, 254–255.

Long-term care employee shortage taking shape nationwide. (1986). *Today's Nursing Home, 7*(10), 2–3.

Lorsch, J. W., & Takagi, H. (1986). Keeping managers off the shelves. *Harvard Business Review, 64*(4), 60–65.

Matheny, P. R. (1984). How to hire a winner. *Supervisory Management, 29*(5), 12–15.

McGregor, D. M. (1960). *The human side of enterprise.* New York: McGraw-Hill.

Maddox, G. L., et al. (2001). *The encyclopedia of aging* (3rd ed.). New York: Springer.

Meehl, P. E. (1954). *Clinical vs. statistical prediction.* Minneapolis, MN: University of Minnesota Press.

Miller, D. B. (Ed.). (1982). *Long-term care administrator's desk manual.* Greenvale, NY: Panel.

Noe, R. A., et al. (2000). *Human resource management: Gaining a Competitive Advantage,* (3rd ed.). Boston: McGraw-Hill.

Now we know why they're so friendly. (1985, July 22). *Fortune, 112*(2), 120.

Olian, J. D., Carroll, S. J., Jr., & Schneier, C. (1985). It's time to start using your pension system to improve the bottom line. *Personnel Administrators, 30*(4), 77–83,152.

Owen, D. E. (1984). Profile analysis: Matching positions and personnel. *Supervisory Management, 29*(11), 14–20.

Patchner, M. A., & Patchner, L. S. (1993). Essential staffing for nursing home care: The permanent assignment model. *Nursing Homes,* 39–40.

Peters, T. & Austin, J. (1985). *A passion for excellence: The leadership differ-ence.* New York: Random House.

Riter, R. N. (1993). Some practical advice for the new nursing home administra-tor. *Journal of Long-Term Care Administration,* 40–41.

Rogers, W. W. (1980). *General administration in the nursing home* (3rd ed.). Boston: CBI.

Rothberg, D. S. (1986). Part-time professionals: The flexible work force. *Per-sonnel Administrator, 31*(8), 29–32.

Rotondi, T., Jr. (1976). Behavior modification on the job. *Supervisory Manage-ment, 21*(2), 22–28.

Ruhl, M. J., & Atkinson, K. (1986). Interactive video training: One step beyond. *Personnel Administrator, 51,* 360–363.

Scott, R. (1972). Job expectancy—an important factor in labor turnover. *Person-nel Journal, 51,* 360–363.

Scott, S. (1983). Finding the right person. *Personnel Journal, 62,* 894–902.

Sears, D. L. (1984). Situational performance appraisals. *Supervisory Manage-ment, 29*(5), 6–10.

Smith, K. E. (1984). Performance appraisal: A positive management tool. *Col-lege Review, 1*(2).

Snell, S. A., & Wexley, K. N. (1985). Performance diagnosis: Identifying the causes of poor performance. *Personnel Administrator, 30,* 117–127.

Steers, R. M., & Porter, L. W. (1979). *Motivation and work behavior* (2nd ed.). New York: McGraw-Hill.

Thierauf, R. J., Klekamp, & Geeding, (1977). *Management principles and prac-tices.* New York: Wiley.

Thomas, W. H. (1996). *Life worth living: the Eden alternative in action.* Acton, MA: Vander Wyk & Burnham.

Tobin, J. E. (1976). How arbitrators decide to reject or uphold an employee discharge. *Supervisory Management, 21*(6), 20–23.

Vaughn-Wrobel, B. C., & Tygart, M. W. (1993). Management education needs of nurse administrators in long-term care. *Journal of Gerontological Nurs-ing,* 33–38.

Vroom, V. H. (1964). *Work and motivation.* New York: Wiley.

Wehrenberg, S. B. (1983). How to decide on the best training approach. *Person-nel Journal, 62,* 117–118.

White, E. (1984). Trust—a prerequisite for motivation. *Supervisory Manage-ment, 29*(2), 22–25.

Whitehill, A. M., Jr. (1976). Maintenance factors. *Personnel Journal, 55,* 516–519.

PART THREE

Finance and Business

3.1 The Administrator's Role As Financial Manager

An administrator's duties encompass nearly every aspect of managing the facility, from assisting in the recruitment of professional medical staff to assuring the efficient operation of the laundry department. Not surprisingly, the administrator is also finally responsible for the income and expenses of the facility. In reality, the administrator who is the one person who is held accountable for the entire financial operation of the facility.

SELECTING AND EVALUATING FINANCIAL PERSONNEL

Although we will explore their individual functions in more detail later, let us say here that it is the *bookkeeper* primarily who records the daily cash transactions of the facility, keeping track of all money going out or coming in. It is the *accountant* who uses the information compiled by the bookkeeper to generate reports on the financial standing of the facility. The bookkeepers and accountants record the financial transactions, but the administrator is de facto chief financial officer of the facility, not the bookkeepers and accountants or even the business manager or the chief financial officer (CFO).

The administrator must ensure that the business office process runs smoothly, that the bookkeeper is qualified for the job and has access to the information needed for recording all the facility's financial transactions. Thus, the administrator must have some knowledge of bookkeeping in order to know whether this important task is carried out as it should be.

The administrator may also have to select an accountant, either as an employee or as a consultant for the facility. If the administrator manages one of a chain of nursing homes, the accountant will probably be an employee of the corporate office. The administrator should therefore have some understanding of accounting in order to be able to assess the accountant's performance.

More important, however, the administrator must be able to interpret the financial reports developed by the accountant and the corporate office. The administrator's primary role as financial manager is to use the financial information to make informed decisions about the facility. The administrator needs to know how these reports are prepared.

"CORPORATE" PURPOSES: FACILITY OWNERSHIP PATTERNS

Corporate offices often use individual facilities for various purposes, for instance, to balance the cash flow and tax affairs of the corporation through the network of facilities rather than by individual facility performance. A single facility be carried on the books may be considered a high debt load while another, similarly situated facility may be considered a low debt load. The administrator must grasp the nuances of these matters to be able to compare her figures after debt service and taxes with those of a sister facility that is carried at a different debt load. They may vary, yet the level of success of staff performance may be comparable.

Nursing facility ownership patterns have been somewhat stable for a number of years. During the period 1993—1999 the percentage of for-profit facilities was 64.8%, nonprofits 28.6%, and government-owned facilities 6.7%—about the same as in the 1980s (see Figure 3-1). As seen in Table 3-1, ownership patterns vary widely across states. Alaska and Wyoming have a high percentage of government-owned facilities. Alaska, Minnesota, North Dakota, Pennsylvania, South Dakota, and Washington, D.C. have a high percentage of nonprofit facilities, and Arkansas, Oklahoma, and Texas have the highest percentage of proprietary facilities (Harrington et al., 2000).

MAINTAINING INCOME

In addition to bookkeeping and accounting, we will also take a close look at costs. There are many different types of costs, and we will

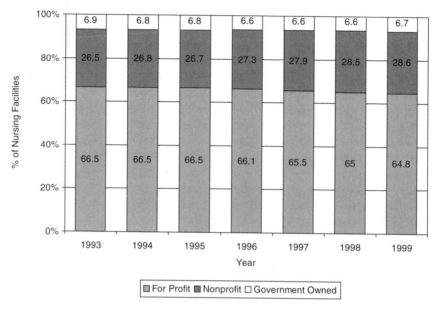

FIGURE 3-1. Percentage of distribution of U.S. nursing facilities by ownership, 1993–1999.
Nursing Facilities, Staffing, Residents and Facility Deficiencies, 1993–1999, Department of Social & Behavioral Sciences, University of California San Francisco.

explore how viewing costs in different ways can provide the administrator with information not included in the financial reports prepared by the accountants.

As the facility's ultimate financial manager, the administrator must ensure the availability of funds for conducting business: to purchase supplies and pay salaries and to meet the regular payments on any borrowed funds. Without these purchases and payments, the facility cannot operate. When money is not available to meet expenses, the facility cannot continue to operate for very long and may be obliged to close its doors.

SETTING RATES

How does the administrator (or corporation) guarantee that the facility will receive sufficient funds? The administrator needs to know how to set rates for the services offered and how to produce the number of residents/patients who will require these services. Appropriate rates for

Table 3-1. Percentage Distribution of U.S. Nursing Facilities by Ownership Type, 1993–1999

State	For Profit							Nonprofit							Government Owned						
	1993	1994	1995	1996	1997	1998	1999	1993	1994	1995	1996	1997	1998	1999	1993	1994	1995	1996	1997	1998	1999
AK	8.3	7.1	7.7	6.3	7.1	7.1	7.1	50.0	50.0	46.2	56.3	57.1	57.1	57.1	41.7	4?.9	46.2	37.5	35.7	35.7	35.7
AL	78.4	76.8	76.3	76.4	76.5	76.4	75.8	12.4	12.8	12.6	13.5	14.3	13.9	14.1	9.3	10.3	11.1	10.1	9.2	9.7	10.1
AR	81.2	80.2	81.9	79.7	78.8	80.1	77.4	14.2	14.5	13.1	15.2	16.1	14.8	16.6	4.6	5.4	5:0	5.1	5.1	5.1	6.0
AZ	62.7	63.0	67.0	62.0	65.3	63.6	65.5	34.8	35.6	30.4	36.6	33.9	34.1	31.0	2.5	1.5	2.7	1.4	0.8	2.3	3.4
CA	73.0	73.4	73.8	73.8	74.0	74.2	74.9	23.1	22.3	22.0	21.9	21.7	22.2	21.4	3.9	4.2	4.2	4.3	4.2	3.6	3.7
CO	60.0	63.5	62.1	62.6	63.0	62.3	63.9	29.5	27.4	26.6	26.3	26.9	27.8	25.6	10.5	9.1	11.3	11.1	10.1	9.9	10.5
CT	77.8	78.8	77.7	79.4	77.9	77.8	76.1	21.8	20.8	21.5	19.7	21.3	21.8	23.1	0.4	0.4	0.8	0.9	0.8	0.4	0.8
DC	40.0	33.3	38.5	33.3	31.8	14.3	28.6	40.0	50.0	46.2	61.1	59.1	71.4	71.4	20.0	16.7	15.4	5.6	9.1	14.3	0.0
DE	59.5	51.2	42.4	54.1	42.9	40.7	47.1	32.4	39.5	45.5	37.8	47.6	48.1	44.1	8.1	9.3	12.1	8.1	9.5	11.1	8.8
FL	78.2	77.9	76.4	75.9	77.7	77.4	76.3	19.4	19.6	21.3	21.6	20.5	20.8	21.9	2.5	2.4	2.3	2.2	1.8	1.8	1.9
GA	75.2	74.3	75.1	75.6	76.6	75.4	76.3	16.8	17.5	16.7	17.6	16.4	17.7	17.2	8.0	8.3	8.2	6.8	7.0	6.9	6.5
HI	40.0	34.6	38.1	37.5	42.9	43.2	46.2	36.0	34.6	33.3	35.0	33.3	31.8	28.2	24.0	30.8	28.6	27.6	23.8	25.0	25.6
IA	54.1	55.2	53.9	53.4	53.1	54.4	50.6	39.9	39.4	41.0	41.3	42.0	40.6	44.9	6.0	5.3	5.1	5.4	4.9	5.0	4.5
ID	58.5	59.0	57.5	59.5	61.0	58.2	60.3	16.9	16.7	18.8	14.9	15.6	17.7	16.7	24.6	24.4	23.8	25.7	23.4	24.1	23.1
IL	64.0	64.2	63.8	64.3	64.5	63.3	65.1	29.8	30.1	30.2	29.8	30.3	31.1	29.6	6.2	5.7	6.0	5.8	5.1	5.6	5.3
IN	77.9	77.4	77.2	74.9	74.8	73.7	72.2	19.9	20.2	20.5	22.3	22.3	23.5	24.6	2.2	Z4	2.3	2.8	2.9	2.8	32
KS	56.8	54.3	54.4	54.0	53.0	52.3	50.5	29.5	33.0	33.1	32.5	34.2	33.5	35.5	13.7	12.7	12.6	13.6	12.8	14.3	14.0
KY	68.3	68.3	68.4	67.1	64.2	64.8	63.5	282	28.6	28.2	28.9	31.9	32.2	33.0	3.5	3.1	3.4	3.9	3.8	3.0	3.5
LA	77.3	73.8	74.0	74.8	73.3	73.2	73.8	18.0	18.7	18.7	17.9	19.3	19.5	18.5	4.8	7.5	7.3	7.3	7.4	7.4	7.7
MA	79.6	77.8	76.4	74.5	71.1	68.6	71.8	17.7	20.0	21.3	23.0	26.5	28.7	25-6	2.7	22	2.3	2.5	2.5	2.7	Z6_
MD	67.2	63.0	62.4	57.5	57.7	56.7	52.2	29.6	33.5	34.4	39.6	39.1	40.9	43.3	3.2	3.5	3.2	2.9	3.3	2.3	4.5
ME	82.4	74.0	72.2	72.8	72.0	74.6	69.3	14.4	22.1	23.5	23.2	24.8	22.0	26.3	3.2	3.8	4.3	4.0	3.2	3.4	4.4
MI	62.1	62.6	65.0	62.8	63.5	61.9	63.2	27.4	27.2	25.1	27.7	26.6	27.9	27.1	10.5	10-2	9.8	9.5	9.9	10.2	9.7
MN	31.8	31.4	31.8	35.2	30.4	30.9	29.3	52-2	54.5	52.6	50.8	54.6	56.4	56.7	15.9	14.1	15.5	14.0	14.9	12.7	14.0
MO	64.6	64.4	65.0	64.7	65.3	63.2	65.T	27.0	26.8	26.8	26.0	26.3	27.8	25.0	8.3	8.8	8.2	9.3	8.4	9.0	9.3
MS	75.6	72.8	72.4	70.5	68.7	68.5	70.3	9.8	10.5	11.1	13.7	16.9	16.5	15.9	14.6	16.7	16.6	15.8	14.4	15.0	13.7
MT	43.2	40.6	73.8	37.6	36.8	35.9	35.1	372	38.5	41.0	43.0	45.3	46.7	46.4	19.0	20.8	20.0	19.4	17.9	17.4	18.6
NC	75.0	74.5	73.8	74.0	73.4	73.5	73.0	20.4	20.9	21.8	21.9	22.2	22.9	22.6	4.6	4.6	4.4	4.1	4.5	3.6	4.3
ND	11.3	9.9	12.0	11.5	13.3	11.4	12-6	88.8	87.7	85.5	86.2	84.0	85.2	82.8	0.0	2-5	2.4	2.3	2.7	3.4	4.6
NE	45.2	45.2	44.7	45A	45.1	45.7	45.2	30.6	30.8	32.7	32.3	32.6	31.7	33.5	24.2	24.0	22.6	22.3	22.3	22.6	21.3

Table 3-1. (Continued)

State	For Profit 1993	1994	1995	1996	1997	1998	1999	Nonprofit 1993	1994	1995	1996	1997	1998	1999	Government Owned 1993	1994	1995	1996	1997	1998	1999
NH	48.5	50.7	52.8	54.3	52-0	54.7	53.0	39.4	31.3	31.9	30.0	33.3	29.3	33.3	12.1	17.9	15.3	15.7	14.7	16.0	13.6
NJ	66.2	64.6	66.7	63.8	64.4	60.5	60.7	28.5	28.2	27.1	29.6	30.1	34.6	34.0	5.3	7.1	6.3	6.6	5.5	4.9	5.3
NM	59.4	57.1	58.4	582	58.7	65.2	61.0	31.9	32.5	29.9	32.9	30.2	28.8	32.5	8.7	10.4	11.7	8.9	11.1	6.1	6.5
NV	74.2	77.5	77.8	74.4	73.7	78.0	70.0	12.9	7.5	11.1	12.8	7.9	7.3	20.0	12.9	15.0	11.1	12.8	18.4	14.6	10.0
NY	46.2	47.8	47.9	46.2	47.2	48.0	46.3	44.5	43.2	43.3	45.0	42.7	43.1	45.6	9.4	9.0	8.8	8.8	10.2	8.9	8.1
OH	74.9	73.5	75.1	73.4	73.2	73.6	70.3	21.5	22.9	21.7	23.2	23.5	23A	26.3	3.6	3.7	3.2	3.3	3.3	2.9	3.4
OK	83.4	81.8	82.2	81.8	79.1	78.8	81.4	13.6	13.5	12.8	13.5	14.4	14.1	13.4	3.0	4.7	5.0	4.7	6.5	7.1	52
OR	75.6	76.7	74.0	77.3	75.0	74.8	74.6	192	19.3	21.3	18.8	21.7	21.9	21.1	5.1	4.0	4.7	3.9	3.3	3.2	4.2
PA	46.0	45.2	43.8	41.8	412	41.0	42.4	45.9	47.9	49.4	51.9	53.3	53.4	62.0	8.1	6.9	6.9	6.2	5.5	5.6	5.6
RI	76.6	78.3	78.0	74.4	77.2	77.5	75.0	23.4	21.7	22.0	25.6	22.8	22.5	25.0	0.0	0.0	0.0	0.0	0.0	0.0	0.0
SC	75.6	73.9	73.4	73.9	75.4	74.8	75.5	12-6	15.7	13.6	15.2	12.6	13.5	12.9	11.9	10.4	13.0	10.9	12.0	11.7	11.6
SD	31.5	34.9	32.4	36.0	36.6	34.9	38.8	63.9	60.4	63.1	60.0	59.4	59.3	55.3	4.6	4.7	4.5	4.0	4.0	5.8	5.9
TN	72.3	69.5	70.3	69.4	69.2	67.6	67.1	20.1	22.1	22.3	22.2	22-9	22.6	22.5	7.6	BA	7.3	8.3	7.9	9.7	10.4
TX	83.8	82.5	81.6	83.1	80.9	81.0	80.3	13.0	14.7	15.7	14.2	15.8	15.8	16.6	3.2	2.8	2.7	2.8	3.3	3.3	3.1
UT	75.0	77.8	80.3	79.7	81.3	77.5	75.7	17.0	16.7	14.5	16.5	14.3	18.0	18.9	8.0	5.6	5.3	3.8	4.4	4.5	5.4
VA	61.9	62.0	65.1	64.3	64.1	61.9	62.7	32.0	32.7	30.3	31.3	32.5	33.3	33.5	6.2	5.3	4.6	4.4	3.4	4.8	3.8
VT	70.7	72.2	75.0	75.7	73.0	64.7	64.3	24A	22.2	22.5	21.6	27.0	324	33.3	4.9	5.6	2.5	2.7	0.0	2.9	2.4
WA	71.1	70.6	70.6	70.0	68.1	68.3	68.7	22.0	21.6	21.6	22.1	23.9	24-O	22.6	6.8	7.8	7.8	7.9	8.0	7.7	8.7
WI	50-0	49.2	48.0	48.3	47.6	49.0	48.9	34.0	35.3	36.8	36.8	37.6	36.4	35.8	16.0	15.5	15.3	14.9	14.8	14.6	15.4
WV	68.8	66.4	64.2	65.5	61.5	65.2	64.9	22.5	23.4	23.9	23.6 -	28.2	30A	24.6	8.8	102	11.9	10.9	10.3	4.3	10A
WY	39.3	44.1	44.7	48.6	44.4	45.0	44.4	21.4	20.6	21.1	13.6	16.7	15.0	13.9	39.3	35.3	34.2	37.8	38.9	40.0	41.7
US	66.5	66.5	66.5	66.1	65.5	65.0	64.8	26.5	26.8	26.7	27.3	27.9	28.5	28.6	6.9	6.8	6.8	6.6	6.6	6.6	6.7

Nursing Facilities, Staffing, Residents and Facility Deficiencies, 1993-1999
Department of Social & Behavioral Sciences
University of California San Francisco

resident/patient care services must reflect their true full costs, so the administrator must be able to measure these costs.

Besides being available in sufficient amounts, funds must be received on a timely basis. The good financial manager understands the billing and collection procedures that keep money owed to the facility coming in regularly enough to meet financial obligations.

PLANNING AND BUDGETING

Financial management is important to planning and budgeting. To make a financial plan, or a budget, the administrator must be able to predict both the costs of running the facility and the money it can expect to earn in the coming year(s). Knowledge of the facility's past financial performance and insight into the reason for earlier budget shortfalls or successes are essential for preparing a realistic and useful budget. The administrator who is not familiar with the cost and earnings of all the departments cannot expect to guide the organization on a reliable path in the future.

RESPONSIBILITY TO OTHERS

By virtue of his/her position as director, the administrator is responsible for the effective operation of the nursing facility—responsible to its residents/patients and their significant others, to the employees, to the owners or stockholders, and to the governing body of the facility. When signs of ineffective financial management become apparent, these parties will turn to the administrator for explanation.

Because nearly every decision will have financial implications, an understanding of financial management is incumbent on the administrator, the person ultimately responsible for the performance of the facility, even in chain-operated homes.

However good the relationship of the manager with staff or however capable he/she may be in other aspects of administration, if finances are poorly or improperly handled, the administrator is likely to be judged ineffectual by the board or the facility owners.

3.2 Generally Accepted Accounting Principles: The GAAPs

The accounting system defines the manner in which financial records must be kept, and it is used by nearly every type of organization, including nursing homes. *Financial records* refers primarily to the books and financial statements of the facility. Books are a set of records that list, in a prescribed manner, each monetary transaction (all money earned or spent) of the facility.

Maintaining the books constitutes bookkeeping, and the books are used to prepare the financial statement. Financial statements are simply a summary of all the transactions recorded in the books, and they reflect the soundness of the organization's financial status.

The books and financial statements are prepared according to a series of rules known as Generally Accepted Accounting Principles (GAAPs). These are consistent standards of accounting that allow the financial records to be understood by the various parties who have an interest in the financial position of the facility and also permit the financial statements of different homes or other organizations to be more easily compared. A discussion of selected GAAPs follows.

ENTITY CONCEPT

Entity is a basic concept of accounting, under which the nursing facility is regarded as a whole, entirely separate from the affairs of the owners, managers, or other employees. This means that if the owner, for instance, withdraws from or adds to the funds of the facility, this transfer must be recorded in the books to reflect the effect on its finances.

ONGOING CONCERN CONCEPT

Another basic rule of accounting is the *consistency* or *ongoing concern* concept. This concept requires that the accounting reports for a facility be prepared in the same way from year to year, in order to compare accurately the reports between two or more different time periods. It does not require that the organization prepare reports in a manner that is not suitable to the needs of management, but suggests that the method of reporting be carefully selected and that changes occur infrequently, if at all. Clearly, financial statements that are prepared in a different format every year will make comparisons difficult.

CONCEPT OF FULL DISCLOSURE

The concept of *full disclosure* related to consistency. It means that all financial information—all money spent, earned, invested, or owed by the facility—must be shown in the financial records to represent accurately its financial standing. The concept of full disclosure has important legal implications, because failure to disclose all financial information may affect the amount of taxes a facility owes or the level of reimbursement it should receive from Medicare, Medicare, and other third-party payers.

TIME PERIOD CONCEPT

Also known as the accounting period, the *time period* is the interval covered by the financial reports, usually 1 year. The accounting period should be consistent from one year to the next; that is, the fiscal year (the 12-month period designated for financial record-keeping) should begin on the same date every year. Accounting records are frequently prepared more often than once a year, usually monthly, to provide management with current information. These shorter time periods should also remain consistent. Typically, monthly financial reports are prepared and distributed to the management while quarterly and annual reports are prepared and distributed to both managers and ownership.

OBJECTIVE EVIDENCE CONCEPT

The *objective evidence* concept requires accounting records to be prepared with documentable records that are kept by the facility. Every transaction should be accompanied by a documented record, that is, by a piece of paper that confirms the transaction. These papers (or equivalent electronic information) are the objective evidence of the transaction; they include receipts for bills that have been paid, bills (or invoices) for money owed by the facility, bank statements indicating interest earned periodically, or case receipts for money received by the facility each day or designated period These are called the *source documents* of the transactions. Objective evidence is necessary so that estimates need not be used. Instead of estimating the cost of supplies purchased during a month, for instance, all invoices are filed in an orderly fashion and used as objective source documents in determining the cost of supplies for the month. Estimates should be used as infrequently as possible, as this introduces an element of error and inconsistency in the accounting reports. When estimates are necessary, the process used in arriving at the estimated figure should be noted in the financial statement.

3.3 Cash Accounting and Accrual Accounting

There are two systems of accounting: cash and accrual. The difference between the two primarily, is, the time period in which expenses and revenues are recorded in the books. *Revenues,* the money coming into the facility, can be recorded for the period when, for example, the money from resident/patient care is earned or when the cash payment is actually received by the facility.

Expenses, which will be defined in more depth later, are the monies spent by the facility and can also be recorded in two ways. An expense can be recorded when payment is made for items purchased. In accounting terminology, money paid out is called an expenditure. An expense can also be recorded when the items purchased are actually used up by the facility.

The difference in the time of recording is the difference between the two systems of accounting and results in two very different ways of preparing the financial records.

CASH ACCOUNTING APPROACH

In cash accounting, expenses are recorded when the cash is actually disbursed, and revenues are recorded when the money from, for example, resident/patient services is received by the facility. Thus, the cash system of accounting simply records expenditures and receipts (the actual flow of cash out of and into the facility) as they occur. Organizations using the cash system of accounting, therefore, do not include in their accounting records "noncash expenses" such as depreciation because depreciation (the cost of wear and tear on equipment, for example) is a cost of providing services to residents/patients that does not involve a cash expenditure.

Cash accounting also does not recognize those expenses that are prepaid, such as insurance paid up months or years ahead. If the premium for a 3-year insurance policy is paid in the first year that the facility is covered by the policy, an insurance expense would be recorded in the month it as paid and would be listed only as an insurance expenditure for that 1-month time period. The fact that it was a prepaid expense and would last over several accounting periods is not acknowledged. In the same way, money that is owed to the facility for services already provided would not be recorded as accounts receivable, but would be counted as revenue only after the facility received payment. The chief advantage of cash accounting is simplicity; it is similar to one's personal checking account.

Cash accounting, however, has several disadvantages. One is that expenses and revenues for a single time period are not attributed to that same period. For example, medical supplies might be paid for in August but actually be used over the next 4 months. The cost of providing medical services in September would not include the cost of the medical supplies, as that expense would have been recorded in August. Thus, the total cost and revenues, and therefore the real profit or loss for those months, would not be accurately measured.

As already mentioned, the cash accounting system does not recognize the very real cost of depreciation of the facility's building, or plant, major equipment, or other capital items. It also does not recognize money that is owed to creditors by the facility (known as accounts payable, a deferred expense) or money that is owed to the facility by residents/patients for services provided (accounts receivable, a deferred revenue).

Last, since the only means of recording expenses and revenues is when cash changes hands, the accounting records are subject to mismanagement by those involved in the accounting process. For these reasons, the cash system is used infrequently. Perhaps 99% of all nursing facilities use the accrual accounting approach.

ACCRUAL ACCOUNTING APPROACH

Under the accrual system of accounting, revenues are recorded when they are earned and expenses when they are incurred, regardless of the time the cash transactions take place. The previous definition of expense can now be more precisely stated as a cost that is used up, or expensed.

Using the example of the medical supplies, the cost of the supplies purchased in August is expensed over the next several months. The accounting records for September would show a medical supplies expense equal to the cost of the supplies used in September, and so on. This should help the reader realize why understanding the accounting and record-keeping procedures discussed in the next sections is necessary. The accrual system requires that every expense incurred by the nursing facility be attributed to the period, usually the month, in which it is incurred and all revenues to the month in which services are rendered.

Its complexity is the main disadvantage of the accrual basis of accounting, but it has numerous advantages. Most important, it allows the facility to measure the revenues earned after expenses have been paid, or losses incurred, by matching revenues and expenses for each time period. It also includes depreciation, accounts payable, accounts receivable, and prepaid expenses in the accounting records, providing a more accurate picture of the facility's actual financial position. It is less subject to tampering because expenses and revenues are usually backed by several forms of objective evidence. The following discussion of accounting and record keeping will be based on accrual accounting.

3.4 The Accounting Process: Recording Transactions and Preparing Financial Statements

RECORDING TRANSACTIONS IN JOURNALS AND THE GENERAL LEDGER

The accounting process involves two main steps: keeping the books and preparing the financial statement. *Bookkeeping* is a system of recording all revenues and expenses and matching those revenues to expenses during the same time period. This process is necessary for the preparation of the *financial statements,* which are a summary of the nursing facility's financial well-being within a time period.

The accounting process is fairly universal and will be described here in chronological order, from the chart of accounts to the preparation of the financial statements.

Chart of Accounts

The chart of accounts is simply a list of every account in the facility. The accounts are organized into six main groups:

- assets—things owned by the facility
- liabilities—things owed by the facility, or its obligations

- capital—money invested in the facility, also known as the facility's net worth
- revenues—earnings from operations or other sources
- expenses—costs of salaries, supplies, etc., that have been used up, usually through the provision of services
- fund account—any funds that have been established for restricted or unrestricted uses

As can be seen from the sample chart of accounts in Table 3-2 each account has a number. The first digit indicates the categories into which the account falls; the second digit usually is a subcategory. For example, RN (registered nurse) salaries are an expense (category 5) in the nursing department and have an account number 5201.

Note that the salary expense account number for every other department ends with 1 also. This system of classifying accounts is useful, as it identifies every account of the facility and thus is a means of control; expenses, for example, are automatically applied to a specific source so that random or unauthorized expenses cannot accumulate unnoticed. The numbered system also saves time by recording a number rather than a long title on many documents. It is especially convenient for a computerized bookkeeping system.

THE JOURNALS

Any transaction that takes place will affect some account. The journals are the first place that transactions are recorded; they are the books of original entry. Each facility will have its own system of journals, but generally there are six journals:

- *The cash receipts journal* records all cash received for services provided, for example, sales refreshment machines.
- *The billings journal* lists all bills sent for services rendered.
- *The accounts payable journal* (purchase journal) records all purchases made that will be paid within the next few months.
- *The cash disbursements journal* records all payments made for services and supplies used for resident/patient care and for all other operations of the facility.
- *The payroll journal* summarizes all payroll checks distributed during the pay period.
- *The general journal* is a record of nonrepetitive entries.

The journals are characterized by another concept of accounting: double-entry bookkeeping. For each transaction, two entries are made in the appropriate journal, a debit and a credit.

Table 3-2. Chart of Accounts, Old Well Home

Assets		Liabilities	
	Current assets		Current liabilities
1101	Cash-petty	2102	Accounts Payable-supplies
1103	Cash-payroll account	2104	Notes Payable-short term
1106	Cash-operating fund	2107	Mortgage Payable-short term
1112	Investments-money market fund	2109	Debts Payable-current
1114	Investments-C of D	2111	Emp. Benefits Payable
1117	Investment-depreciation fund	2113	Emp. Health Ins. Payable
1122	Accounts Receivable-Medicare	2115	Salaries Payable
1123	Accounts Receivable-Medicaid	2201	Taxes
1124	Accounts Receivable-Private	2204	Taxes Payable-state
1126	Accounts Receivable-other	2205	Taxes Payable-municipal
1131	Interest Receivable	2207	Taxes Payable-federal
1163	Unexpired Liability Insurance	2221	Interest Payable
	Non-Current Assets		Non-Current Liabilities
1302	Land	2303	Notes Payable-long term
1305	Land improvements	2313	Mortgage Payable-long term
1402	Building-Main	2323	Bonds Payable
1414	Building-Welsh Hall	2401	Pensions Payable
1426	Building-garage/storage		
1430	Building Improvements		Capital
1502	Fumiture-Main	3001	Owner's Equity
1504	Furniture-Welsh Hall	3101	Net Income (Loss)
1512	Equipment-Main		
			Revenue
1514	Equipment-Welsh Hall		Nursing Care
1516	Equipment-office	4001	Medicare
1518	Equipment-kitchen	4003	Medicaid
1519	Equipment-laundry	4005	Private
1521	Equipment-transportation		
1524	Equipment-land maintenance		Ancillary
		4212	Physical Therapy
	Contra Assets, Accum. Depr.	4214	Occupational Therapy
1602	Accum. Depr.-main bldg.	4216	Social Services
1604	Accum. Depr.-Welsh Hall	4218	Speech Therapy-contract
1606	Accum. Depr.-garage/storage		
1636	Accum. Depr.-bldg. Improvements		Uncompensated Care
1642	Accum. Depr.-furn., main	4311	Contract. DiscQunt-Medicare
1644	Accum. Depr.-furn., Welsh	4313	Contract. Discount-Medicaid
1651	Accum. Depr.-equip., main	4315	Contract. Discount-Other
1654	Accum. Depr.-equip., Welsh	4332	Donated Care
1666	Accum. Depr.-office equip.	4341	Bad Debts
1668	Accum. Depr.-kitchen	4351	Patient Refunds
1669	Accum. Depr.-laundry		
1671	Accum. Depr.-transportation		
1674	Accum. Depr~-land maintenance		
1680	Accum. Depr.-bldg. Improvements		

Table 3-2. (Continued)

Assets		Liabilities	
	Current assets		Current liabilities

Assets		Liabilities	
	Administration	5411	Payroll tax
5001	Salaries-administration	5432	Supplies
5002	Salaries-clerical.	5442	Repairs
5003	Consultation fees	5461	Contract services
5006	Health Insurance		Housekeeping
5011	Payroll tax	5501	Salaries
5013	Taxes-income	5506	Health Insurance
5015	Taxes-property	5511	Payroll tax
5022	Insurance-liability	5532	Supplies
5026	Pension fund	5542	Repairs
5032	Supplies		
5034	Telephone		Rehabilitation
5035	Travel		Physical Therapy:
5037	Postage	5601	Salaries
5039	Licenses and Dues	5606	Health Insurance
5042	Repairs	5611	Payroll tax
		5632	Supplies
	Plant Operation	5642	Repairs
5101	Salaries		
5106	Health Insurance		Occupational Therapy:
5111	Payroll tax	5661	Salaries
5122	Utility-electricity	5666	Health Insurance
5124	Utility-gas	5671	Payroll tax
5126	Utility-water	5682	Supplies
5128	Utility-sewage	5692	Repairs
5132	Supplies		Social Services
5142	Repairs	5701	Salaries
	Nursing	5706	Health Insurance
5201	Salaries-registered nurses	5711	Payroll tax
5202	Salaries-licensed practical	5732	Supplies
5203	Salaries-aides	5742	Repairs
5206	Health Insurance		Activity
5211	Payroll tax	5801	Salaries-beautician
5222	Pharmacy	5802	Salaries--crafts
5224	Laboratory	5806	Health Insurance
5232	Supplies	5811	Payroll tax
5237	Uniform	5832	Supplies--beauty
5242	Repairs	5833	Supplies-crafts
	Dietary	5835	Transportation
5301	Salary-dietician	5837	Special Events
5302	Salary-food service	5842	Repairs
5306	Health Insurance		Capita_!l Expenses
5311	Payroll tax	5904	Interest-mortgage
5332	Supplies	5907	Interest-long term debt
5342	Repairs	5914	Debt Se~rvice-mortgage
	Laundry	5917	Debt Service-long term debt
5401	Salaries	5934	Dep~eciation-plant
5406	Health Insurance	5936	Depreciation-equipment

Table 3-3. Transactions Recorded as Debits and Credits

Debit	Credit
(+) Increase m assets	(−) Decrease in assets
(+) Decrease in liability	(−) Increase in liability
(−) Decrease in capital	(+) Increase in capital
(−) Decrease in revenues	(+) Increase in revenues
(−) Increase in expenses	(+) Decrease in expenses

A *debit* in accounting simply means the left side of the journal account; *credit* refers to the right side. When all debits and credits are totaled at the end of each month, they should be equal. Thus, for every debit entered, one or more credits are entered that equal the debit, and vice versa. Table 3-3 indicates which transactions are recorded as debits and which as credits.

Journal entries are set in the shape of a *T* as in Table 3-3 and thus are often called T-accounts. Data from the journal entries are the source documents, the objective evidence referred to at the beginning of this section.

An example of the billings journal is used to illustrate the process of journalizing. When a bill is sent to a resident/patient or to that person's payer, the bill represents revenues earned by the facility that it expects to receive. This account receivable is an asset because it is cash to which the facility is entitled. Thus, a bill to Ms. Jones for $1,000 would be recorded in the debit column as an increase in assets. On the credit side, $1,000 would be recorded as in increase in revenue. This journal entry is illustrated in Figure 3-2. The source document for this entry would be a copy of the invoice sent to Ms. Jones.

			Debits	Credits
3/02	Acc't Receivable – Jones, F.		1 0 0 0 00	
3/02	Revenue			1 0 0 0 00
3/02	Acc't Receivable – Ross, M.L.		2 0 0 00	
3/02	Revenue			2 0 0 00

FIGURE 3-2. Old Well Home billings journal.

When the billings to all service recipients for the month are entered in the journal in this manner, the sum of debits should equal the sum of credits at the end of the month. Notice that the billings journal is used only for the billing of a service; the service recipient's payment of the bill will be recorded in the cash receipts journal. The complete transaction would be recorded as follows:

Billings Journal
	Debit _____	Credit _____
3.02	Acc/Rec $1,000.00 (account receivable)	
3/02		Revenue $1,000.00

Cash Receipts Journal
	Debit _____	Credit _____
4/22	Cash $1,000.00 (account receivable)	
4/22		Acc/Rec $1,000.00

The credit in the cash receipts journal would not be due to an increase in revenue, but to a decrease in accounts receivable. As mentioned, under the accrual system of accounting, revenue is recognized when the services are provided, rather than when the cash is received.

Role of the General Journal

The *general journal* records transactions that do not properly fit into any of the other journals. Note that the first five journals all record cash transactions; the general journal is used to make adjustments in the books to conform to the accrual system of accounting.

As with medical supplies, the supplies purchased in August will be only partially consumed in that month, but the cash disbursements journal would record the cash expenditure for the supplies purchased in August. Under the accrual method of accounting, only the costs of supplies used in August would be included in the August financial reports, so the total cost of providing services can be compared with the revenues earned in the same period. Therefore, an entry must be made in the general ledger to adjust the medical supplies expenditure in the cash disbursements journal to the cost of medical supplies used up in August. This is known as an *adjusting entry.*

If an expenditure of $300 for medical supplies is made in August, and the inventory records compiled at the end of August revealed that $75 remained in inventory, the adjusting entry in the general journal would be as follows:

General Journal

Debit _____   Credit _____

8.29   Med Supp $225.00
           (increase in expenses)

8/29   Inventory $225.00
                                         (decrease in expenses)

8/29   Inventory $75.00
           (increase in assets)

8/29   Med Supp $75.00
                                         (decrease in expenses)

In addition to adjustments for inventory, entries for depreciation and prepaid expenses are also recorded in the general journal to reflect the cost of using the plant or equipment over the time period, as well as the amount of prepaid expenses used up.

Finally, the general journal can be used to correct errors made in the other journals. The general journal accounts are usually repeated from month to month and therefore should be standardized to the extent possible. This prevents omission of unapparent, but very real costs.

The General Ledger

At the end of each month, when all adjusting entries have been made in the journal accounts, the financial information in all journals is *posted* (written or entered in) to the General Ledger.

The *general ledger* can be thought of as a summary of all debits and credits contained in the journals for the time period. It usually has a page for each account in the chart of accounts.

The purpose of the ledger is twofold. First, it keeps a continuous balance of the amount in any account for each month. It also enables a *trial balance* to be run. Before the financial statements can be prepared, the total of all debit columns in all journals must equal the total amount from all of the credit columns. By accumulating all journal entries in one book—the ledger—debits and credits can be easily added up and compared. When total debits equal total credits, the books are said to balance, and thus a trial balance has been calculated. If total debits do not equal total credits, then there is an error in one or more of the journal entries.

Under the double-entry concept of accounting, each debit recorded in a journal must be matched by a credit of an equal amount. The trial balance, therefore, indicates whether or not an error has been made in recording transactions.

With so many accounts, there is ample opportunity for error. Thus, accuracy in preparing the journal and ledger entries will save a great

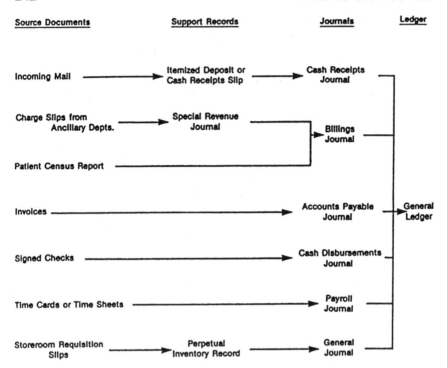

FIGURE 3-3. Source documents, support records, journal, ledger.
Adapted from Catholic Hospital Association, p. 14.

deal of time in a search for possible mistakes. The relationship between the journals and general ledger is shown in Figure 3-3 and Figure 3-4.

The general ledger should be arranged in the order that the accounts will appear in the financial statements. Once the trial balance and gain/loss statements are prepared, the ledger is closed. This process will be discussed in the following description of the financial statements.

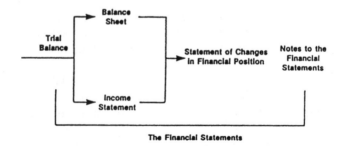

FIGURE 3-4. The financial statement.

PREPARING THE FINANCIAL STATEMENTS: THE INCOME STATEMENT AND THE BALANCE SHEET

The financial statements are the summary of all transactions made during a particular time period and their effect on the finances of the facility. The GAAPs require that the financial statements include four reports.

1. Income statement or profit/loss statement
2. Balance sheet or statement of financial position
3. Statement of changes in financial position
4. Notes to the financial statements

The income statement and balance sheet are prepared directly from the general ledger (Figure 3-4) and will be described below. The statement of changes in financial position and the notes to the financial statements are prepared from the income statement and balance sheet, and they will be discussed in less detail.

Profit and Loss: The Income Statement

The income statement shows whether revenues were sufficient to cover expenses, whether the facility made or lost money during the time period.

In accounting, income does not refer to the funds coming into the facility, but to revenues minus expenses, or the profit or loss experienced by the facility (or, in not-for-profit operations, income compared to expenses). Net income indicates that the facility made money or had some revenues in excess of expenses, and a net loss indicates the facility lost money in the time period covered by the income statement. A net loss, or any negative figure on the financial statements, is usually shown in parentheses.

The income statement in Table 3-4 shows a net income of $833 for the month of July and $35,625 for the year until then. Revenues are listed first on the income statement, usually starting with the largest source of revenues. From the general ledger, all of the revenues earned from providing room and board and other services are calculated as routine services, separated by the level of care or type of service.

When all revenues earned from providing services, or operating revenues, from the general ledger have been computed, any deductions from revenue are subtracted from the gross operating revenues. Deductions from operating revenues might include money owed to the facility that cannot be collected (known as bed debts or charity care), or they might be due to contractual discounts.

In the process of setting rates at which they will reimburse the facility for care, Medicare, Medicaid, or other third-party payers sometimes pay

Table 3-4. Old Well Home Income Statement

Revenues	July 'X1	Year to date	Vertical analysis percentages (YTD)
Operating revenues			
Nursing	357,603	.2,207,814	
Total nursing	357,603	2,207,814	
Ancillary			
Physical therapy	9,974	61,839	
Occupational therapy	9,890	59,340	
Social services	2,866	16,909	
Total ancillary	22,730	138,088	
Gross operating revenues	380,333	2,345,902	
Less deductions	45,640	281,508	
Net operating revenue	334,693	2,064,394	
Non-operating revenue			
Miscellaneous			
Meals	430	2,494	
Concession	1,358	8,691	
Beauty shop	790	4,819	
Total miscellaneous	2,578	16,004	
Interest	2,640	15,312	
Non-operating revenue	5,218	31,31 6	
Total revenues	339,91-1	2,095,710	
Expenses			
Operating expenses			
Salaries			
Nursing	135,192	833,151	68%
Dietary	15,582	93,492	8%
Administration	9,551	54,441	49%
Laundry	3,409	20,454	2%
Housekeeping	13,435	81,282	7%
Maintenance	5,287	32,145	3%
Physical therapy	9,652	.60,808	5%
Occupational therapy	3,450	20,735	2%
Social serv	2,146	13,305	1%
Total salaries	197,705	1,209,812	100% 59.0%
Supplies	31,393	189,928	9.2%
Activity	2,065	12,390	0.6%
Capital equipment	200	1,600	0.1%
Utilities	8,764	52,584	2.6%
Telephone	163	1,043	0.1%
Insurance	4,000	24,018	1.2%
Taxes (real estate)	3,313	19,878	1.0%
Capital costs			
interest	27,816	166,896	30% 8.1%
Mortgage payment	24,029	144,174	26% 7.0%
Depreciation	39,627	237,762	43% 11.5%
Total capital costs	91,472	548,832	100%
Total expenses	339,078	2,060,085	100%
Net income (loss)	833	35,625	
Income tax (@ 45%)	375	16,031	
Profit after tax	458	19,594	

the nursing facility somewhat less than the facility's full charges. This discount from the regular price of providing care is known as a *contractual discount*. This discounted rate is the price at which the facility has agreed to provide care when it admits the insured resident/patient. Contractual discounts are therefore deducted from operating revenues instead of included as an expense. Today, most hospitals are forced by competition to offer contractual discounts to large groups such as HMOs. Nursing facilities are similarly affected by competition and the desire to admit residents/patients from such large third-party payers.

Total deductions are subtracted from the gross operating revenue to get the new operating revenue. In Table 3-4, net operating revenues for the Old Well Home in July are $334,693. Nonoperating revenues, income from sources other than direct resident/patient care, are listed next. In July the Old Well Home earned $900 in interest on funds invested in a local bank and $4,318 from a certificate of deposit. Miscellaneous sources of revenue are also included directly from the appropriate page in the general ledger. Miscellaneous revenues for Old Well Home are from guests' meals, the beauty shop, or concession income.

Expenses are listed next, starting with the largest item, which is usually salaries. All salaries are listed by department, and the salary expense generally includes any employee benefits and payroll taxes paid by the facility.

Supplies, which are separated by department in the ledger according to the chart of accounts, are combined into one expense item in Old Well's income statement. A capital expense of $200 was incurred in July by the purchase of equipment.

Capital equipment is assets that will be used by the facility to provide services for more than 1 year and will not be sold in the course of operations. In addition to equipment, capital items also include such assets as the building, beds, and furniture. If we were to look at the general ledger under the chart of accounts number for capital equipment expenses, we would discover that the $200 was used to purchase office equipment for Old Well.

Further down on the income statement there is an expense called capital costs. A capital cost is an expense related to the use of capital items. At some earlier time the Old Well Home had borrowed money for new dining and lounge furniture and money to purchase the building, both at an annual interest rate of 14%. For the month of July the total interest expense was $27,816. Interest expenses, then, are one cost of using capital.

A mortgage payment expense of $24,029 for July is a second source of capital costs. Another cost of using capital is depreciation; the cost of wear and tear on old Well's depreciable assets was estimated to be $39,627 for 1 month. (See section on depreciation for estimation of this expense.)

To compute the net income, or profit or loss, the total expenses are subtracted from total revenues, which results in the net income before taxes. Subtracting percentage for income tax shows that Old Well's profit after taxes is $458. Although depreciation is a real cost of providing services, it does not represent an actual cash outflow, and depreciation may be added to the after-tax profit to give the actual cash standing of the facility.

The income statement, then, shows the operating performance of the facility for a period of time, and it is usually prepared on a monthly and annual basis.

Closing the Books

Because revenues and expenses must be measured for finite periods of time, these accounts must be brought to a sum of zero so that they can be recorded over again for a new time period. Closing the books means bringing the expense and revenue accounts to zero.

To close the general ledger:

1. For all revenue and expense accounts with a credit balance, add a debit equal to the credit to bring the account to zero.
2. For all revenue and expense accounts with a debit balance, add a credit equal to the debit to bring the account to zero.

According to the double-entry accounting, compensation must be made for these new debits and credits in some other account.

1. Add up all the newly added debits
2. Add up all the newly added credits.
3. Subtract the debits from the credits
4. Enter the difference in the retained earning account, as follows:
   (a) If the difference is a profit, enter it as a credit.
   (b) If the difference is a loss, enter it as a debit.

Thus, all revenue and expense accounts have been brought to zero, and the books are balanced and ready for a new time period.

Statement of Financial Condition: The Balance Sheet

Unlike the income statement, which summarized operating performance over a period of time, the balance sheet records the financial position of the nursing facility at one point in time. Whereas the income statement shows the ending balance of the revenue and expense accounts, the balance sheet summarizes the assets, liabilities, and capital accounts of the facility. This document is called a balance sheet because the asset accounts must balance with the liability and capital accounts. This relationship can be expressed as an equation, called the accounting equation:

$$\text{Assets} = \text{Liabilities} + \text{Capital}$$

The balance sheet for the Old Well Home for the year is shown in Table 3-5. Assets are listed on the left in order of liquidity

Current assets refers to those possessions of the facility that will be or theoretically can be turned into cash within 12 months. Prepaid insurance is considered an asset because the coverage is something owned by the facility. The income statement (Table 3-4) records the proportion of the prepaid insurance that was used in the month of July ($4,003), and the balance sheet (Table 3-5) shows the amount of insurance that remains ($2,400).

Noncurrent assets, refers to those assets that will not be liquidated within the year; they usually include plant (the building), property, and equipment. These are also called fixed assets and are recorded as their cost at the time of purchase, rather than their current market value.

The *historic cost* concept is another basic tenet of accounting and relates to the ongoing concern concept: Because capital assets will not be liquidated any time soon, their current market value is of little relevance. The value of these assets to the facility, however, must include the depreciation on plant and equipment over the years, and so this accumulated depreciation is subtracted from the historic cost of the depreciable assets. Although land usually appreciates in value over time, it does not do so simply through the operations of the facility and is therefore recorded at historic cost, with no depreciation from its value.

Depreciation, therefore, is an expense associated with the use of an asset, so depreciation is included both as an expense on the income statement and a *contra asset* (literally, "against an asset") on the balance sheet. Note that employees are not included as an asset. This is because assets are those things owned by the facility; an organization cannot own its employees.

Liabilities are the obligations of the facility. Current liabilities are those obligations that must be met within the next 12 months, such as bills from suppliers of foodstuffs and medical or office supplies, and short-term bank loans.

On this particular date according to its balance sheet, Old Well owes its suppliers $2,852. If this debt were paid the next day and a balance sheet made up then, Old Well would have no accounts payable on its balance sheet. Notes payable refers to loans that must be repaid within 12 months. Old Well owes $33,625 to a local bank for interest on its borrowed funds, as well as a portion of a long-term debt due within the

Table 3-5. Old Well Home Balance Sheet

Assets	July 31, 'X1	'X0
Current assets		
Cash	60,700	2,834
Accounts receivable		
(Less Bad Debts of $9,032)	53,517	61,397
Securities	225,275	10,500
Inventory	62,006	54,880
Prepaid insurance	2,400	3,600
Total current assets	403,898	133,211
Noncurrent assets		
Equipment	1,983,000	1,981,200
Plant	5,767,004	5,767,004
Less Accumulated Depreciation	2,772,192	2,362,300
Plant and Equipment	4,977,812	5,385,904
Property	2,650,000	2,650,000
Total fixed assets	7,627,812	8,035,904
Total assets	8,031,710	8,169,115
Liabilities		
Current liabilities		
Accounts payable	2,852	24,606
Notes payable	33,625	355,271
Benefits payable	24,843	630,388
Current portion of		
Long term debt:		
Mortgage	230,680	192,233
Long term debt	75,000	75,000
Total current liabilities	367,000	1,277,498
Noncurrent liabilities		
Mortgage payable	3,460,202	3,690,883
Debts payable	675,000	750,000
Total non-current liabilities	4,135,202	4,440,883
Total liabilities	4,502,202	5,718,381
Net worth		
Retained earnings		
Year to date	35,625	27,507
Total	370,956	335,331
Owner's equity	3,122,927	2,087,897
Total net worth	3,529,508	2,450,735
Total liabilities and capital	8,031,710	8,169,115

year. The noncurrent liabilities sections shows which debts these are. Old Well has a payment due on its debt for new furniture, and a portion of its mortgage payment is due also.

Capital accounts, or new worth, are recorded below the liabilities. This section is also called owners' equity, shareholders' equity, fund balance, or retained earnings, depending on the origin of the funds that make up this section. It includes funds that the owners have put into the facility, whether the owners be one person, a partnership (two or more unincorporated owners), a corporation, or a charitable organization. Net worth also usually includes retained earnings, or the net income that has been put back into the facility over the years.

If the facility incurs a net loss, this amount is subtracted from the net worth. The Old Well net worth includes the retained earnings of the year to date and the retained earnings from its earlier years of operation. It also shows that the owners have invested $3,122,927 in the facility over the years. If this amount was from stockholders, it would be called shareholders' equity; if from a charitable organization, it would be a fund balance.

The most important thing to remember about the net worth is that it is not a pool of cash. The funds recorded as net worth are monies that have been put into the facility at some time; it is merely a record of these funds, not cash available for operations or investment.

To summarize, the balance sheet shows the financial position of the facility for only a given point in time. Its relation with the income statement is the retained earnings, which usually include the net income in the net worth.

Thus, the basic accounting equation can be expanded to

$$\text{Assets} = (\text{Liabilities} + \text{Owner's Equity}) + (\text{Revenues}—\text{Expenses})$$

Additional Financial Statements

Statement of Changes in Financial Position. Also simply called the statement of changes, this financial report shows the major transactions that occurred over the period covered by two balance sheets, or the way that working capital was used during that period. Working capital simply refers to the current assets and current liabilities from the balance sheet. The amount of working capital available is

$$\text{Current Assets}—\text{Current Liabilities}$$

The statement of changes shows the transactions that caused the amount of working capital to change over a time period. It is therefore a very useful document for those interested in knowing how the facility acquires and uses its funds.

Sources of funds are generally an excess of revenues over expenses of operations, interest income, and contributions to the facility (or owners' equity). Noncash items, such as depreciation or money designated for repayment of debts, are added as a source of funds because this is still cash (a current asset) owned by the facility.

Uses of funds would include nonoperating expense such as repayment of a portion of a debt or additions to property. The uses of funds are subtracted from the sources of funds to give the change in working capital over the time period. This difference should equal the change in working capital calculated from the balance sheets at the beginning and end of the time period covered.

Notes to Financial Statements. The notes to financial statements are included to explain the accountant's interpretation or calculation of figures or variation in the books due to a change in the organization, which may not be readily understood by those reviewing the financial statements. The financial statements are not considered complete without each of these notes.

Staff Functions in the Accounting Process

The number of staff persons in the business office and their degree of specialization will vary with the size, complexity, and ownership of the facility. In general, however, those responsible for the accounting functions will be the bookkeeper, the accountant or comptroller, and the administrator.

The bookkeeper maintains the journals and ledger and performs the trial balance. An accountant or comptroller may also check the trial balance, but her primary task is the preparation of the financial statement.

For all practical purposes, it is legally mandatory that a nursing facility have its books officially audited, that is, audited by a person who is a certified public accountant. It is almost impossible to do business without having the facility's books audited by a CPA, who, in effect, serves as the public's representative.

Administrators of a chain-owned facility will generally send the data from the books to a regional or corporate office, where the financial statements, as well as a variety of other schedules, will be compiled and returned.

3.5 Putting Financial Statements to Work: Working Capital, Ratio Analysis, and Vertical Analysis

The net income is an important and readily identifiable item of interest on the financial statements, but what other information can be gleaned from these reports? There are several tools the administrator can use to extract this information. Three tools are discussed below.

WORKING CAPITAL

Current assets minus current liabilities equals the working capital available. This can also be considered the funds available to the facility.

Suppose the administrator of the Old Well facility wants to learn if enough funds are available to purchase $60,000 worth of capital equipment for the nursing department. Where can this information be found?

As Table 3-5 shows, the net income for the month of July—and for the entire year—has been reinvested in the facility, as indicated by the net worth section of the balance sheet; these funds may or may not still be available. Although the net worth shows the funds that have been invested in the facility, it is not a pool of cash. Recall that the net worth is merely a record of the funds that have been invested in the facility over time and that most of the funds shown here are therefore not available for spending or investing.

The administrator might also check the cash accounts of the Old Well to see if the cash for purchasing the items is available. But this is not suitable either, for if the Old Well owes $367,000 to various creditors, as indicated by the current liabilities section on the balance sheet, any available cash may be needed to meet these obligations.

In order to get an idea of the funds available to purchase the needed equipment, the administrator must look at the amount of available working capital. Current assets remaining after current liabilities have been subtracted yields the amount of money that the administrator has at his discretion.

The administrator finds that there is only $36,898 in working capital available to purchase equipment for the nursing department and that the facility probably should not purchase new equipment at this time. Because current assets include relatively nonliquid accounts, such as inventory and prepaid insurance, the working capital may be calculated by excluding these accounts from the total current assets.

RATIO ANALYSIS

Another common approach to analyzing financial statements is to perform a ratio analysis. Financial managers generally express the information in financial statements as a series of ratios.

There are an infinite number of ratios that may be derived from financial statements, but the discussion here will be confined to several of the more common measures of financial performance. The References section for part 3 includes several excellent texts that explore financial statement analysis in greater detail.

Usefulness of Ratios

Ratios are useful in several ways. First, financial ratios are no more than fractions using the numbers in the financial statement and are therefore fairly simple to calculate quickly and easily.

Ratio analysis allows the administrator to identify trends in many measures of financial performance of the facility by comparing the same ratio for several periods. Ratio analysis of the financial statements can also be used to compare the financial performance of several facilities. It is one of the most useful tools the administrator has.

That the amount of working capital available is calculated by subtracting current liabilities from current assets has already been mentioned. A positive amount of working capital indicates that the facility is able to meet its current obligations with its current assets.

If all resident/patient revenues were collected before or immediately after they were earned, the facility would have no need for excess working capital. But since third-party payers such as Medicare and Medicaid pay nursing facilities for services sometimes well after services were rendered, the facility must maintain a certain level of working capital to meet expenses during the lag time before the payments are received. (If part of a chain or group of facilities, the same problem is faced by the corporate managers who have the same gaps between services rendered and payments received, but on a larger scale). Even nursing facilities that have predominantly privately paying residents/patients must plan for collections of resident/patient bills to extend over a period of weeks or months. How much working capital should the facility maintain to cover its lag time? One way to get an idea of an appropriate amount is to perform a current or acid-test ratio.

$$Current\ Ratio = Current\ Assets\ /\ Current\ Liabilities$$

The Old Well Home has

$$\$403,898\ /\ \$367,000 = 1.1$$

A current ratio greater than 1 shows that the Old Well is able to meet its current obligations, with a surplus of working capital. Does this mean that a current ratio of 2.5 is even better? Not necessarily; a high current ratio may show that the facility has too much money tied up in current assets and that it may make better use of some of these funds by investing them in an interest-bearing bank account or its equivalent.

Interpreting Ratios

Interpretation of an appropriate current ratio exemplifies a point of caution with the use of any ratio. One ratio itself reveals very little about the performance of the facility. Ratios must be compared either over time or with the rest of the industry. A current ratio of 1.1 may be fine if the ratio for the Old Well in the past has been as follows:

Year 1	Year 2	Year 3	Year 4
.80	.85	.90	1.0

A ratio of 1.1 could also indicate a decline in working capital if past ratios have been much higher than 1.1. Industry comparisons are also important. If the average current ratio for the nursing facility industry, preferably in the same region, is 1.0, then the Old Well may be managing their working capital well. If, however, the industry average is .9, then Old Well might rethink the amount of funds it is keeping available. Thus, interpretation of all ratios is relative to both past performance and industry averages. The administrator of the Old Well will find out what the appropriate current ratio is and adjust his/her own working capital to maintain that ratio.

The Quick Ratio

Another commonly used ratio is the quick ratio. Similar to the current ratio, it is a more rigorous and representative measure of current assets, as only cash and accounts receivable, and sometimes marketable securities, are used to cover current liabilities. (The figure for marketable securities in the example is an approximate one.)

Quick Ratio = (Cash + Acc. Rec. + Mkt'ble Sec.) / Current Liabilities

($60,700 + $53,519 + $25,275) / $367,000 = 0.93

The quick ratio reveals that Old Well is not quite able to cover its current obligations with its most available assets but is quite close to the industry average.

Average Collection Period Ratio

The average collection period ratio shows the average lag time of accounts receivable. Although the administrator of the nursing facility will have relatively little influence in expediting the collection of funds paid by third parties she should attempt to collect privately paid monies from resident/patient's as soon as possible in order to decrease working capital needs. This is, therefore, an important ratio.

Because most insurers reimburse the nursing facility sometimes up to 3 to 5 months after billing, an average collection period of 58 days may be appropriate for a facility with a majority of publicly paid-for residents/patients. The length of time between billing Medicaid and receiving payment varies radically among the states, some paying immediately, some deliberately delaying payment for months in order to manage the state's own cash flow. A number of states now require that all Medicaid billing be submitted electronically.

Accounts Payable Average Payment Period Ratio

A related ratio is the accounts payable average payment period, which shows the average number of days used to pay creditors. Too many days in the payable period may develop into a poor credit relationship with suppliers, and too few may indicate that funds should be invested for a longer time before creditors are paid.

For both accounts payable and accounts receivable considerations, the opportunity cost (loss of use that would otherwise be available for these funds) must be considered. In times of low interest rates, when the use of money is low, the opportunity cost is less than in times of high interest rates, that is, when using money is more costly.

Net Operating Margin Ratio

The net operating margin is the proportion of revenues earned to the amount of expenses used to earn those revenues. A low operating margin may indicate that rates for services should be raised or expenses reduced.

$$\text{Net Operating Margin} = \frac{\text{Operating Revenues} - \text{Operating Expenses}}{\text{Operating Revenues}}$$

$$(\$334{,}693 - \$339{,}078) \, / \, \$334{,}693 = -0.013$$

The Old Well's negative operating margin shows that operating revenues do not cover operating expenses and that the administrator should consider increasing charges for services, if the market will allow it, or reducing operating costs, in order to increase the facility's operating margin. Another approach to this ratio is operating income as a percentage of revenues, which is best compared with industry averages for an indication of performance.

Debt-to-Equity Ratio

The debt-to-equity ratio is a measure of the long-run liquidity of the facility, or the ability of the facility to meet its long-term debts. A low proportion of debt to equity indicates that the facility could incur more long-term debt, all other things being equal, if needed; whereas a high debt-to-equity ratio (when compared to the industry) probably shows that the facility may have more debt than may be advisable, all other things being equal. This ratio is of particular interest to would-be creditors.

$$\text{Debt} \, / \, \text{Equity} = \text{Long-Term Debt} \, / \, \text{Total Equity}$$

$$\$4{,}135{,}202 \, / \, \$3{,}529{,}508 = 1.17$$

There are, of course, many other parameters of financial performance that will be of interest to the administrator. The foregoing are some of the more commonly used ratios.

VERTICAL ANALYSIS

A third method of analyzing the financial statements is to perform a vertical analysis. A vertical analysis converts each item on the income statement, balance sheet, or other financial report to a percentage of some total item on the same document.

A vertical analysis of the Old Well income statement, using the year-to-date values, is shown in Table 3-6. Like the preceding ratios, these ratios are useful when compared over time or with other facilities. For example, an unusually high ratio of supplies to total expenses in July may indicate that supplies are being wasted or pilfered, provided there has not been a change in the type of services that would warrant a greater use of supplies. On the other hand, although their percentage for July may be higher than for any month that year, if supplies as a proportion of total expenses are consistently higher in July than any other month, then the administrator knows that this is a pattern that may or may not be a cause for concern.

The administrator can accumulate valuable information from the financial statements by performing both ratio and vertical analyses. By comparing these ratios over time and with other facilities, trends and patterns in the operation of the facility can be identified, which is perhaps one of the most important functions of financial statement analysis. Awareness of such patterns enables the administrator to pinpoint problem areas in the facility and make more knowledgeable financial decisions.

Table 3-6. Old Well Home Income Statement: Vertical Analysis

	July 'X1	Year to date	Vertical analyses	
Revenues				
Operating revenues				
Revenues				
Operating revenues				
Nursing				
Skilled				
Intermediate				
Total nursing	357,603	2,207,814	100%	94%
Ancillary				
Physical therapy	9,974	61,839	45%	
Occupational therapy	9,890	59,340	43%	

Table 3-6. (Continued)

	July 'X1	Year to date	Vertical analyses	
Social services	2,866	16,909	12%	
Total anciHary	22,730	138,088	100%	6%
Gross operating revenues	380,333	2,345,902	100%	
Less deductions	45,640	281,508	12%	
Net operating revenue	334,693	2,064,394	88%	
Non-operating revenue				
MisceDaneous				
Meals	430	2,494	16%	
Concession	1,358	8,691	54%	
Beauty shop	790	4,819	30%	
Total misc.	2,578	16,004	100%	51%
Interest	2,640	15,312	49%	
Non-operating revenue	5,218	31,316	100%	
Total revenues	339,911	2,095,710		
Expenses				
Operating expenses				
Salaries				
Nursing	135,192	833,151	68%	
Dietary	15,582	93,492	8%	
Administration	9,551	54,441	4%	
Laundry	3,409	20,454	2%	
Housekeeping	13,435	81,282	7%	
Maintenance	5,287	32,145	3%	
Physical therapy	9,652	60,808	5%	
Occupational therapy	3,450	20,735	2%	
Social serv	2,146	13,305	1%	
Total salaries	197,705	1,209,812	100%	59.0%
Supplies	31,393	189,928	9.2%	
Activity	2,065	12,390	0.6%	
Capital equipment	200	1,600	0.1%	
Utilities	8,764	52,594	2.6%	
Telephone	163	1,043	0.1%	
Insurance	4,000	24,018	1.2%	
Taxes (real estate)	3,313	19,878	1.0%	
Capital costs				
Interest	27,816	166,896	30%	8.0%
Mortgage payment	24,029	144,174	26%	7.0%
Depreciation	39,627	237,762	43%	11.5%
Total capital costs	91,472	548,832	100%	
Total expenses	339,078	2,060,085	100%	
Net income Qoss)	833	35,625		
Income tax (@ 45%)	375	16031		
Profit after tax	458	19,594		

3.6 Additional Accounting Procedures for Maintaining Control Over the Facility

Although accounting processes are similar in every institution, the procedures for managing finances will vary from facility to facility, and so will the best methods of control.

In financial management, control refers to the development and maintenance of systematic ways to identify problems when they occur to permit the administrator to intervene appropriately. To maintain control, the administrator and the staff normally develop policies for all office procedures. Identifying possible financial problems as soon as they arise enables the staff to deal effectively with them through the use of recognized policies.

There are several tools available to assist the administrator in controlling financial operations. Procedures should be arranged so that no single person has complete responsibility for any area of the facility's finances. A system of checks and balances can be established so that part of one person's task is completed or reviewed by another. Furthermore, each employee can be required to take vacation time so that no one has uninterrupted control of certain office tasks. It is important to have procedures in place that reduce temptation to a minimum. Even the best procedures set up by the most sophisticated corporations have not been able to prevent the occasional embezzlement of funds at facilities. Eternal vigilance is necessary in such money matters.

ACCOUNTS RECEIVABLE: BILLING FOR SERVICES RENDERED BY THE FACILITY

The facility cannot receive monies for services rendered until the resident/patient has been billed for them. Delays in billing create an opportunity cost: the loss of use or availability of funds when cash owed to the facility is not yet in its possession.

Financial Review of Applicants

Some states require that admissions be on a first-come first-served basis for any applicant the facility is capable of providing appropriate care for. Other states allow the facility to make admissions decisions based in part on financial considerations.

The payment source should be established at the time of admission. If the client is not paying with his own funds, written agreement to pay must be obtained from the person who controls the residents/patient's funds. In addition, present and potential Medicare and Medicaid needs should be determined. These agencies will normally pay for care only after an authorization number has been established for a recipient. A significant number who enter the facility as Medicare or private-paying persons quickly exhaust their savings. The social worker must anticipate which persons will become eligible for Medicaid and begin the application process several weeks in advance of actual eligibility in order to achieve a steady payment stream for care rendered.

Just as the facility must remove employee temptation to embezzle facility funds, so also must the facility constantly seek to minimize temptations for resident/patient's money managers to withhold money legitimately due the facility. Experience has taught that Social Security and similar checks that have been pledged to pay for the resident/patient's care are best sent directly to the facility rather than to a family member who may feel more pressing financial needs than payment of the facility charges.

Resident/Patient Ledger Card

When the resident/patient's source of payment has been confirmed, a resident/patient ledger card is made up for each person admitted, listing the name, room number, source of payment, and daily (or routine) service charges. The charges and the billing and collection procedures must be explained to each resident/patient and sponsor.

Preparation of Invoices

In every case, charge slips for each service not bundled into the daily rate must be collected from each service center on a daily or weekly basis. Since these charges are distinct from routine room-related services, a special revenues journal may be created to record them.

Routine Charges

Once the ancillary charges for the billing period have been determined, they are added to the resident/patient's routine charges. The routine charge is the charge for room and board, which usually includes basic nursing care, room, and meals. Facilities will package their charges variously, depending on a number of considerations. Some offer a broad range of services from which resident/patients may choose.

Daily Census Form

The routine charge may be determined on a daily, weekly, or monthly basis and is calculated with the aid of the daily census form. This is a summary of the facility's occupancy that lists, for each day, admissions, discharges, and transfers by level of care, if more than one is offered by the facility. The daily census form is normally prepared by the nursing unit (often called *the midnight census*) and is submitted to the business office.

Resident/Patient Census Report

A resident/patient census report is drawn up by the bookkeeper (usually for the month) by compiling the information from the patient census forms (Figure 3-5).

The patient census report is in turn used to calculate the total routine charge for each resident/patient or service recipient (for example, outpatient physical therapy charges). Routine and ancillary services are finally calculated for each resident/patient and service recipient and entered on each resident/patient's or service recipient's accounts receivable ledger card (Fig. 3-6, Ledger Card) and in the billings journal.

To expedite the billing process, the billings journal should be divided by payer type (private pay, Medicare, Medicaid, Veterans Administration, hospital reserve bed contract, HMO, PPO, IPO, Workers' Compensation Fund, or similar third-party payer). (In addition to building serve new long-term care facilities of its own, the Veterans Administration is subcontracting with private nursing homes for care [usually shorter termed] of the growing number of aging and aged veteran population). The billing process and services covered vary with each payer, but each bill should itemize any ancillary charges (when permitted by the payer) to expedite the processing of invoices by third-party payers. Increasingly, billing may be done by electronic submission using computers and

OLD WELL HOME

MONTH/YEAR 06/x1

ROOM AND BED	ROOM RATE	PATIENT NAME LAST	INITIAL	PATIENT NO.	DAY OF MONTH 1	2	3	4	5	6	7	8	9	10	11	12	13	14	15	16	17	18	19	20	21	22	23	24	25	26	27	28	29	30	31
117	70	Jones			x	x	x	x	x	x	x	x	x	x	x	x	x	x	x	x	x	x	x	x	x	x	x	x	x	x	x	x	x	x	
118	70	Rose			x	x	x	x	x	x	x	x	x	x	x	x	x	x	x	x	x	x														

					TOTALS		
Private	Agency	Medicaid	Medicare	Other	Billings		
240.00		2100.00			2340.00		
100.00		1400.00			1500.00		

FIGURE 3-5. Patient Census report.

ADDITIONAL CURRENT ENTRIES – COMPLETE SECTION A AND B

ACCOUNTS RECEIVABLE
INVOICE SUPPLEMENT

ADJUSTMENTS TO PRIOR MONTHS – COMPLETE SECTION A AND C

S E C	FACILITY NO.	FACILITY NAME				
		OLD WELL HOME				
C A	PATIENT NUMBER	INVOICE NUMBER	YR/MO	NUMBER	INVOICE DATE	PATIENT NAME
		3012-758-01	x10/8	1	8/29/21	Ross, M. L.

TRAN CODE	DATE MO/DAY	OPEN ITEM	DESCRIPTION	PRIVATE	AGENCY	MEDICARE	VETERAN	OTHER
A	/							
V	/							
E								
N	/							
T								
S								

TOTAL

TRAN CODE	DATE MO/DAY	ROOM-BED	NO DAYS	RATE	AREA	LEVEL	PRIVATE	AGENCY	MEDICARE	VETERAN	OTHER
C	8/29	118	30	70.00	S	S	275.00		2100.00		
U	/										
R											
R	/										
E											
N	/										
T											

TOTAL   275.00   2100.00

	STATUS	NON-COLLECT

TRAN CODE	DESCRIPTION	PRIVATE	AGENCY	MEDICARE	VETERAN	OTHER
A	PHYSICAL THERAPY			240.00		
D						
J						

TOTAL   240.00

	STATUS	NON-COLLECT

AREA
C = CERTIFIED
R = RESIDENTIAL

LEVEL
UNCLASSIFIED
SKILLED
7 = RESIDENTIAL
9 = HOLD/OOD

STATUS CODES
1 = PRIVATE
2 = AGENCY
3 = MEDICARE
4 = VETERAN
5 = OTHER

SECTION C

EXPLANATION OF ADJUSTMENTS

ADJUSTMENTS	TRAN CODE	TRAN CODE	OPEN ITEM	NO. OF DAYS	RATE	AREA	LEVEL	PRIVATE	AGENCY	MEDICARE	VETERAN	OTHER	STATUS	NON-COLLECT
	65													
	65													
	65													
	65													
	65													
	65													
	65													
	65													
	65													
	65													
	65													
	65													
	65													
	65													
	65													
	65													
	65													
	65													
							TOTAL							

FIGURE 3-6. Ledger card.

modems. Some state Medicaid programs require electronic submission, which usually means the facility receives payment on a more timely basis.

BILLING MEDICARE, MEDICAID, OTHER THIRD PARTIES, AND PRIVATE PAYERS

Billing is becoming a more complex process because of the increasing variety of payment agreements that nursing facilities are negotiating with third parties. Medicaid patient care costs are normally billed and paid for monthly, usually with one composite bill for all Medicaid residents/patients submitted to the state or its designated payer. Medicare bills, on the other hand, are normally submitted for the individual resident/patient and sent to a fiscal intermediary. Medicare (and Medicaid) payers sometimes pay promptly; other times they request clarification on bills, the purpose of which is to delay final payment in order to ease their own cash flow problems. It is a complicated game in some states.

More and more third-party payers are negotiating contracts with nursing facilities that also vary in method of payment. Often a third-party payer (a health maintenance organization, for example) will negotiate a separate payment schedule for each member they send to a nursing facility. Others may negotiate a flat rate for all members it refers to a particular nursing facility, regardless of acuity level. For some residents/patients the monthly fee negotiated by their third-party payer will be all-inclusive; others will be on an itemized service use basis. In these circumstances both the facility administration and the third-party payer administration are jockeying for a position that, whatever the payment arrangement, covers their actual costs.

Intense pressures on third-party payers to hold down costs are being passed on to the nursing facility.

Accounting for Deductions from Revenue

Besides contractual discounts, charity care and bad debts also reduce revenue. Charity care is provided to a resident/patient when the service is not reimbursable and cannot be paid for privately. Bad debts, on the other hand, are resident/patient accounts that are past due but still subject to collection.

Contractual discounts are often the largest source of deductions from revenue in nursing facilities. Because most deductions cannot be confirmed until payment has been received, they are accounted for in the billings journal when known rather than estimated. The payment from public insurers will be accompanied by a medical assistance remittance and status report. This report lists the resident/patient's name and claim number, the service dates, the description of services rendered, the total amount billed to the program, and the allowed and not allowed charges, with an explanation code stating why the service was not reimbursed. Entries n the *T* account for deductions from revenue would be as follows:

Billings Journal

	Debits	Credits
2/27	Cont. Disc. $450.00	
2/27		Acc. Rec. $450.00

Submitting and Resubmitting Claims

The amount of the deduction is also included on the resident/patient's accounts receivable ledger card. If the deduction is invalid, the fiscal intermediary should be contacted for an explanation of the deduction. The claim can then be resubmitted, accompanied by the information needed to justify the request for payment. Medicare intermediaries are constantly issuing bulletins defining and redefining what covered charges include and exclude. Understanding Medicare billing, especially Medicare Part B, is one of the more complex yet important tasks of the facility staff. In an era of razor-thin net operating margins, appropriate billing can have a significant impact on the result. So can inappropriate billing.

Medicare has many rules, one of which is that facility bills will be paid as expeditiously as possible so long as the amount of "inappropriately" billed services do not exceed 5% of all the facility's Medicare billings. What Medicare deems appropriate and inappropriate is a moving target requiring constant business office attention. Once this 5% threshold is violated, each bill submitted by the facility for a future time period is scrutinized and payment slowed. Some facilities have found that the best way to ensure that Medicare billings are appropriate is to have weekly "Medicare meetings" attended by nursing (usually the director of nurses and other relevant nurses), the business office manager, the director of rehabilitative therapies, the admissions/social worker director, and the administrator. At these meetings each Medicare resident/patient is reviewed for appropriateness of the Medicare-specific care being given and an assessment made of future days of appropriate Medicare coverage that can be anticipated during the 100-day limit for each spell of illness experienced by this person.

Medicare Cost Reconciliation Settlement

When Medicare pays a facility for providing care to patients/resident, the amount of reimbursement is based on the cost of that care. However, instead of calculating the actual cost of providing care for each Medicare beneficiary in each facility, Medicare makes an estimate of how much the care for residents/patients in each facility should have cost and then pays the facility periodically, based on that estimate. If the estimated amount of reimbursement received during the year is less than the cost of providing the care, Medicare will make up the difference at the end of the year by paying the facility a Medicare Cost Reconciliation settlement, or requiring any overpayment be returned. Any funds due from Medicare are recorded in the cash receipts journal as follows:

Cash Receipts Journal

	Debits _____	Credits _____
11/23	Due from Medicare $375.00	
11/23		Cont. Disc. $375.00

Sometimes services that are not allowable by their insurer (e.g., occupational therapy or some types of dental care) will be provided to patients who cannot pay for them. These services are considered charity care and are written off as essentially non-billable. A special account should exist in the chart of accounts for this type of care, separate from other types of uncollectibles. Each facility needs policies to govern the circumstances and extent of charity care that will be given.

COLLECTING MONEY OWED TO THE FACILITY

An appropriate collection policy will depend on the facility's past experience with its payers. For bills delinquent by 1 month, a letter may be sent as a reminder. A telephone call to the payer (logged into a written record) may be made after an appropriate interval. The collection policy must indicate if and under what circumstances a collection agency or other procedure will be used.

Account Write-Off Recommendation

Problem collections are most effectively handled with diplomacy and firmness, and an effort should be made to accommodate the payer if there is a valid reason for delinquent payment. If a patient's accounts are eventually determined to be uncollectible, some type of account write-off recommendation form is filled out (Figure 3-7), with one copy re-

Facility _____ # _____ Date _____

Patient Name _____ # _____ P__ A__ M__ VA__ Other __ Balance $_____

Admission Date _____ Discharge Date _____ Expired: Yes ☐ No ☐

Readmission Date _____ Discharge Date _____

Readmission Date _____ Discharge Date _____

Name and address of responsible party _____

_____

Home phone _____ Business phone _____

Date and amount of last payment _____

Brief History of account: (attach copy of form H-0611) _____

_____

_____

_____

Should account be assigned to a collection agency? Yes ☐ No ☐

Facility opinion by _____ Date _____

*Regional concurrence by _____ Date _____

**Corporate concurrence by _____ Date _____

If Medicare—Include all intermediary correspondence.

Is coinsurance involved& Yes ☐ No ☐ If yes, please provide dates and amounts: _____

_____

_____

_____

_____ /_____
Administrator   Date

_____ /_____
Regional Controller   Date

_____ /_____
District Director/Director of Operations   Date

*For all accounts over $250.00
**For all accounts over $500.00.

FIGURE 3-7. Recommendation for write-off of uncollectible account.

tained in the resident/patient's file and another going to the accountant, so that the total of uncollectible accounts can be recorded in financial statements.

Nursing facilities, like hospitals and other health-care providers, are victims of the cost shifting phenomena in the United States. Because of public relations and other considerations, it is exceedingly difficult for facilities to discharge resident/patients whose bills are uncollectible, but who have no place else to go.

HANDLING CASH

Cash is easily mismanaged. It is easily concealed. The typical facility will keep only a small amount of cash on the premises, often not more than $500, as most transactions will take place through business office accounts.

Procedures

All cash must be handled by at least two employees, both of whom are bonded. One person should be responsible for receiving the cash, for example, opening the mail or taking a check in person. This should not be the same person who is responsible for making bank deposits. Immediately upon receipt checks should be stamped "For Deposit Only" in the name of the facility and a daily remittance list prepared for all cash received. One copy of this list should be retained by this employee, and another should go to the person making the bank deposits.

Cash receipt slips should then be prepared, with one copy going to the payer and another to the accountant or the accountant's file. The bookkeeper should record the cash received in the cash receipts journal and also on the patient's own sheet in the patient accounts receivable ledger (Figure 3-8).

Cash should be deposited in the bank daily to prevent its being mislaid and to earn the maximum amount of interest on available funds. At the end or each month entries in the cash receipts journal are posted into the general ledger and these figures checked against the cash receipts entries in the patient accounts receivable ledger.

ACCOUNTS PAYABLE: THE FACILITY'S BILLS

Accounts payable are monies owed to creditors for purchases made by the facility. A nursing home's creditors usually furnish foodstuffs, linens, medical supplies, pharmaceuticals, laboratory tests, office, housekeeping, and maintenance supplies, for example. A file should be set up for each regular vendor or supplier, as well as a miscellaneous vendor file for all unusual or incidental purchases.

When a purchase order is made out and sent to the supplier, a copy of the purchase order should be placed in the appropriate file. When the order is received, all supplies should be delivered to a storeroom with the exception of foodstuffs. A receiving slip will accompany the shipment; this should be checked against the items as they are received and against the purchase order to make sure all items purchased were delivered (and, incidentally, that supplies that were *not ordered* are not deliv-

FACILITY NO. _____   PAGE _____ or _____

DATE OF DEPOSIT 09/12/19X1   FACILITY NAME Old Well Home

PATIENT'S NAME LAST NAME INITIAL	C A S H	MISCEL- LANEOUS	PRIVATE	AGENCY	MEDICARE	VETERAN	OTHER	POSTED TO INVOICE NO.
Jones, F.A.					2375 00			3012- 756-01
TOTALS FOR EA. COLUMN	Ⓐ							
	ACCOUNT	1211	1212	1213	1210	1217		

MISCELLANEOUS RECEIPTS SUMMARY		
ITEM	ACCOUNT	AMOUNT
EMPLOYEE MEALS - FOOD SALES	4820	
VENDING MACHINE INCOME	4860	
TOTAL A MUST EQUAL TOTAL B		Ⓑ

REDEPOSITED ITEMS RECEIVED FROM	AMOUNT

TOTAL OF
THIS DEPOSIT $_____
                        ACCOUNT 1130

FIGURE 3-8. Accounts receivable record.

ered and signed for). Any back-ordered items on the receiving slip should be noted. The approved receiving slip is then placed with the purchase order in the vendor file.

Invoices from creditors are usually sent to the facility at the beginning of each month. The receiving slip and purchase order should be checked against the invoice to confirm that the unit price is the same as when the shipment was ordered and that all supplies charged in the bill were actually received.

All invoices should be approved by the administrator according to owner policies, but practically speaking the administrator designates appropriate individuals to share in this task. These invoices are then recorded in the accounts payable journal by department. For example, medical supplies and pharmaceuticals may be attributed to nursing, foodstuffs to dietary, linens to housekeeping, and so on. Invoices are placed in an invoice file.

At the end of the month the accounts in the payables journal are added up, and this sum should equal the total of all invoices in the invoice file. Bills are usually payable within 30 days. Creditors should be paid at the latest possible date, unless a discount is offered for early payment. This does not mean that accounts payable should be chronically delinquent while available funds remain in the bank; it is important to maintain a good credit relationship with suppliers. Suppliers, often middlepersons, are dependent on reasonably prompt payment of invoices for their own business operations.

At the beginning of the month the invoices in the invoice file should be used to pay all bills due in that month. Checks should be signed by two designated employees, and all payments should be recorded in the cash disbursements journal at the time checks are written. Invoices should be marked paid and placed in the vendor file, along with the receipt of payment statement when it is received. These source documents are retained until the end of the year for the accountant's records.

INVENTORY: CONTROLLING SUPPLIES AND EQUIPMENT

A system of inventory control is needed to measure the amount and type of supplies used by each department. Under accrual accounting one must be able to measure all expenses incurred in order to match them with the revenues earned in a time period. Consistent records of the cost of supplies enable price and usage comparisons to be made over time between departments or services. These records are also valuable in the budgeting process.

A system of inventory control discourages waste and pilferage of supplies and provides a means of keeping supplies at optimal levels. Overstocking, especially of time-limited supplies, may result in opportunity costs: the cost of monies unnecessarily tied up in inventory and the cost of possible obsolescence. Excess inventory also increases the opportunity for pilferage. On the other hand, frequent shortages of needed supplies can impinge on the quality of care, result in frustration among

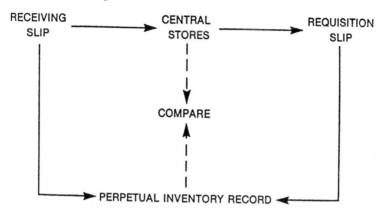

FIGURE 3-9. Perpetual inventory record.

staff, or require costly rush orders to meet supply needs. In the early 1990s a management approach to this continuing problem was initiated, called "just in time" inventory. One well-known example was Harley-Davison Motorcycles, which moved to this type of inventory with notable success. Today, its management views just-in-time inventory as much a liability as an asset. (The real problem at the Harley plants, it turned out, was not the timing of the arrival of inventory, but the quality and appropriateness of the inventory when it arrived.)

Ideally, the focal point of inventory control is a locked central storeroom (Figure 3-9). All supplies should be delivered to a central storeroom as soon as they are received. A limited number of employees should have access to central stores, usually one employee on each shift, though access to supplies must be balanced so that supplies may be obtained when needed but are not subject to unwarranted use. Smaller facilities may find a central storeroom impractical, in which case decentralized storerooms can become the responsibility of personnel in the individual departments.

Perpetual Inventory

A perpetual inventory system is recommended to maintain a precise count of inventory on hand, that is, an accurate count of supplies used and those remaining in the storeroom. At the beginning of each fiscal year (ideally more often), all inventory in the central store (or the decentralized storeroom) should be physically confirmed. This is the *beginning inventory* for the time period.

Additions to inventory are noted form the receiving slips that are included in each shipment of supplies. The beginning inventory and the *inventory received* by the storerooms make up the *total available inven-*

Table 3-7. Old Well Home Perpetual Inventory Record

Item #400 Syringes, disposable	# Units	Cost/unit	Cost
July			
Beginning inventory	4	$7.00	$28.00
Goods received	5	$7.00	$35.00
Total goods available	9	$7.00	$63.00
Ending inventory	3	$7.00	$21.00
Goods used	6	$7.00	$42.00
August			
Beginning inventory	3	$7.00	$21.00
Goods received	6	$7.00	$42.00
Total goods available	9	$7.00	$63.00
Ending inventory	4	$7.00	$28.00
Goods used	5	$7.00	$35.00

tory. When supplies are removed from a storeroom, a requisition slip identifying the supplies and date issued, by department, must be filled out. Supplies issued by storerooms may be taken as the supplies actually used in providing care for all residents. This, of course, does not account for those supplies remaining in each department or sublocation that have not yet been used.

For this reason, department heads should be encouraged to keep initial levels of supplies in their departments. A requisition slip should be initialed by a department head or other designated person, which not only provides a check on the unjustified removal of supplies from the storeroom, but also is the objective measure of the supplies used during a particular period.

The receiving slips and requisition slips are the source documents for keeping the perpetual inventory record (Table 3-7). At the end of each year or other time period, the inventory in the storeroom should be counted and compared with the ending inventory from the perpetual inventory record. If the physical count of the storerooms and the inventory record do not match, this may indicate pilferage, misuse of requisition slips, or inaccuracies in the record-keeping system.

It is advisable for the business office to maintain a list of all inventory items used by the facility, the number of items in one unit, and the current price per unit. This log acts as a reference for determining the cost of the inventory used by each department and for establishing the total volume of supplies remaining in the storeroom.

Table 3-8. Inventory

Item #400 Syringes, disposable	# Units	Cost/unit	Cost			
August						
Beginning inventory	3	$7.00	$21.00			
Goods received	6	$7.00	$42.00			
Total goods available	9	$7.00	$63.00			
Ending inventory	4	$7.00	$28.00			
Goods used	5	$7.00	$35.00			
September		Ust in-first out			First in-first out	
Beginning inventory	4	$7.00	$28.00	4	$7.00	$28.00
Goods received	5	$8.00	$40.00	5	$8.00	$40.00
Total goods available	9	4 @7.00	$68.00	9	4 @7.00	68.00
		5 @8.00		OR	5 @8.00	
Ending inventory	5	4 @7.00	$36.00	5	$8.00	$40.00
		1 @8.00				
Goods used	4	$8.00	$32.00	4	$7.00	$28.00

LIFO OR FIFO

To account for the effects of inflation or deflation on the price of inventory, the GAAP recognizes two methods of inventory costing: last in, first out (LIFO), and first in, first out (FIFO). The LIFO method assumes that inventory added last to stores is used first, thus (in times of inflation) making the value of the goods remaining in inventory lower than that of the goods used to provide services. The FIFO method assumes the opposite: that the older and less expensive supplies (in times of deflation) are used for services, and the higher-priced goods remain in inventory longer. The difference in the effect of these two methods is shown in Table 3-8. Either method of inventory cost may be adopted, but the one selected should be used consistently and should be mentioned in the notes to financial statements.

PAYROLL

Payroll is another source of cash outflow. As mentioned in part 2, it is the largest expense in the nursing facility, accounting for over 50% of total costs in most cases. It also makes up about 85% of the facility's controllable costs. (A controllable cost is one over which the administrator has influence.) Because it is the primary expense of the facility, accurate accounting records are essential.

PAYROLL JOURNAL

The payroll journal lists all paychecks disbursed in the time period, by department. At the end of the pay period the hours worked are entered in the payroll journal, as derived from the time cards or sheets and the salaried employees staffing plan. Overtime hours are compensated at a higher rate, as indicated in part 2, and are listed in a column separate from the regular rate. Gross pay is then calculated by multiplying hours worked by the hourly rate:

(Pay Rate x Reg. Hrs.) + (Overtime Rate x Overtime Hours) = Gross Pay

Payroll Deductions

Payroll deductions must be subtracted from gross pay to arrive at the employee's net pay. They include federal, state, and sometimes municipal taxes, as well as various other deductions that must be made.

The amount of federal, state, and local tax deducted is a percentage based on the employee's income. The percentages are supplied by the various government agencies. The Federal Insurance Contribution Act (FICA) deduction is the employee's contribution to the Social Security fund, described in part 4.

A certain proportion of the employee's paycheck is withheld, matched by the employer, and remitted on a quarterly basis to the Internal Revenue Service, which collects taxes for the federal government. Because this payroll tax is part of the cost of providing services, it must be attributed to the time period in which the employee was earning the wages. The cumulative amount of payroll tax is entered in the accounts payables journal for each month as a credit to the taxes payable and a debit to cash.

Other deductions from the employee's pay may include meals and uniform expense. If the employee health plan requires some contribution by them, this would also be noted in the payroll journal as a deduction. Deductions for each employee are calculated and subtracted from gross pay to arrive at the net pay. A separate column should exist for bonuses or other adjustments to net pay. At the end of each month, salary totals for each department are posted to the general ledger. A page from a typical payroll journal is shown in Figure 3-10.

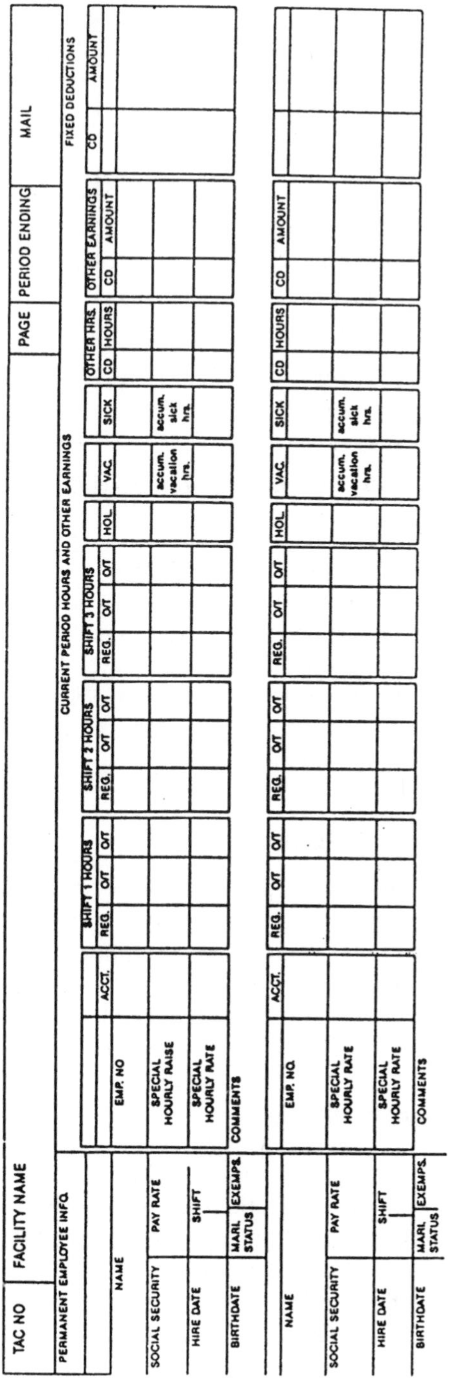

FIGURE 3-10. Page from payroll journal.

| Facility | Old Well Home _____ | # _____ | | Month ending | 06/30/X1 |

Patient Name	Beginning Balance	Deposits	Disbursements	Ending Balance
Jones, F.A.	$210.00	$90.00	$25.00	$275.00

FIGURE 3-11. Patient trust-funds trial balance.

Employees who divide their time between two or more departments should be listed in the department where the majority of hours are spent, with a portion of their earnings and taxes allocated to the second department. Some reimbursement programs, such as Medicare, may require record keeping for the hours each day spent by an employee attributable to each Medicare resident/patient.

Separate Payroll Bank Account

The facility should maintain a separate bank account solely for payroll. The person preparing the payroll does not write his own paycheck. All paychecks should have two signatures or be approved by the administrator before being disbursed. The paycheck number and the date of issue are recorded in the payroll journal to identify checks that are misplaced or to stop payment on checks that are not cashed within a reasonable period of time. Checks are best distributed to each employee in person.

Preparation and maintenance of the payroll is largely a bookkeeping function, although larger facilities may have a separate department devoted to this task. In recent years a number of electronic payroll services have been offered by banks and other financial service groups. A telephone call to the bank or data transmission by computer modem sends information to the financial service or corporate office, which in turn delivers the checks to the facility at a specified time. (The modem is an electronic device that can transmit computer data over telephone lines from the facility computer to the bank computer.)

PROTECTING THE RESIDENTS' FUNDS

Legal Responsibilities

Nursing facilities are frequently asked by residents to safeguard their assets. Any agreement to take responsibility for these assets must be conformed through a legal contract signed by both the facility and the resident/patient or the sponsor. This contract establishes a trust relationship between the resident and the facility, and sound procedures for managing these assets must be adhered to so that the relationship is not violated. Administrators vary in what they will protect on behalf of residents. Some may keep jewelry and similar items in safekeeping. In general, experience suggests that cash be the primary or only resident asset the facility will take responsibility to safeguard. Valuables other than cash are best managed by a legal representative of the resident.

Separate Accounting

A separate book should be kept to record information about any funds held in trust for resident/patients (Figure 3-11). A copy of a receipt signed by the resident/patient or sponsor is kept in an envelope accompanying this book.

Interest Bearing Accounts

Patient funds deposited with the facility are to be managed in accordance with §483.10(c) of the federal requirements. (See Allen [2000], *Nursing Home Federal Requirements and Guidelines to Surveyors,* 4th ed., §483.10(c) Protection of Resident Funds.)

CONCLUSION

Matters such as inventory and payroll should not occupy too much of the administrator's time. However, it is important that all of these details be properly managed by the staff, and experience seems to show that when the administrator understands the fine points of financing and occasionally reviews these matters knowledgeably with them, the staff tend to pay attention to details also. The result is that the administrator is freed to deal with broader policy, while procedures such as payroll and managing resident/patient accounts function smoothly.

3.7 Depreciation

Depreciation has been mentioned to some extent already. Capital assets are those used to provide services during more than one time period; in the course of operations they lose value as a result of use, wear and tear, or obsolescence.

To account for this loss of value to capital assets in the accrual system of accounting, the cost of the asset is spread over the time period that it is used. This must be done because the total cost of acquiring the asset could not properly be attributed to the month in which it was purchased, when it is actually an expense for providing services for several years to come.

IDENTIFYING DEPRECIABLE ASSETS

Assets that can be capitalized or depreciated differ from other assets of the facility in that they are used in operations for more than one time period and will not be converted into cash within the year. Many facilities set a minimum value for depreciable assets, usually somewhere about $500. A calculator, for example, may be used in the business office for many years, but its acquisition cost may be so low that the depreciation expense over its useful life would be negligible. The asset must be tangible and by definition must be owned by the facility. Thus, leased equipment cannot normally be depreciated. (Some leases, in which the lessor agrees not to take depreciation, can be depreciated under some circumstances).

All new assets meeting these criteria are considered depreciable assets. Any alterations of the present fixed asset that affect either its value or its useful life, such as renovation, are depreciable expenses. Repair of damages or regular maintenance of the asset cannot be considered part of the depreciable expense.

DETERMINING DEPRECIATION EXPENSE

There are several methods of calculating depreciation expense, but all methods are based on the historical cost of the asset, its useful life (sometimes preset by tax or other regulations), and its salvage value, if any.

1. *Historical Cost.* The historical cost of the asset is the cost of acquiring the asset that is depreciated over several time periods. In addition to the purchase price, the cost of taxes, shipping delivery, installation, and so forth can be included along with any other one-time costs associated with acquiring the asset.
2. *Useful Life.* The useful life of the asset is the number of years the item can be expected to be used by the facility. This must be an estimation. However, the IRS has useful-life estimates for most assets that are mandated in reporting taxes or, in most instances, in calculating depreciation reports for Medicare, Medicaid, and some other third-party payers.
3. *Salvage Value.* A capital asset may have some value at the end of its useful life. A van, which normally has an IRS-determined useful life of 5 years, might be such an asset.

STRAIGHT-LINE DEPRECIATION

There are several methods for figuring the depreciation expense, once the historical cost, useful life, and salvage value are determined. Straight-line depreciation is a method in which the historical cost of an asset is spread evenly over its useful life so that the depreciation expense is the same in every time period that it functions.

$$\frac{\text{Historical Cost}}{\text{Useful Life}} = \text{Annual Depreciation Expense}$$

If the Old Well purchases new physical therapy equipment worth $20,000 with an estimated useful life of 5 years, the annual depreciation expense for the equipment would be:

$$\frac{\$20,000}{5} = \$4,000 \text{ per year depreciation}$$

After the first year the value of the physical therapy equipment on the books would be:

$20,000 – $4,000 = $16,000

Hence, the $16,000 is called the book value of this asset.
   Straight-line depreciation has the advantage of simplicity.

ACCELERATED DEPRECIATION

This method attributes most of the depreciation expense to the first years of the asset's life, thus enabling the facility to write it off more quickly and thereby gaining a tax advantage through earlier tax recognition of the investment. Among the several types of accelerated depreciation are the sum-of-the-years digits and double declining balance.

PURPOSE OF DEPRECIATION

We have already mentioned that depreciation must be calculated to adhere to the accrual system of accounting. To ignore the very real cost of depreciation is to underestimate the expense of providing services and to overestimate the value of the assets of the facility. For this reason, depreciation is included on the income statement as an operating expense and is subtracted from the historical cost of fixed assets on the balance sheet to reflect its impact on the financial position of the home.
   Probably the most important reason for recognizing depreciation is asset replacement. Because the asset will eventually have to be replaced, the present asset should be expensed over its useful life to accumulate the funds needed for its replacement. Although chances are that an asset purchased 10 years later will be more expensive than the original, this is not always the case. Some assets remain about the same for replacement while others actually may decrease in replacement costs. Computers, for example, have become less expensive yet provide more capabilities because of advances in technology and competition among computer makers (Johns & Saks, 2001).
   Few facilities actually "fund" depreciation, that is, put cash in an interest-bearing account reserved for replacing equipment. Such a fund

would appear as funded depreciation in the capital or new worth section of the balance sheet.

ENTERING DEPRECIATION INTO THE ACCOUNTING RECORDS

A portion of the depreciation expense may easily be attributed to each time period by dividing the annual depreciation expense by the number of accounting periods in the year. Because depreciation is entered in the general journal at the end of each month, Old Well's new physical-therapy equipment depreciation expense after the first month of purchase under straight-line depreciation would be as follows:

General Journal

	Debit _____	Credit _____
1/29 Depreciation expense	$333.33	
1/29 Reserve for depreciation		$333.33

Categorization of Fixed Assets

The chart of accounts should have an account for each type of fixed asset owned by the facility. These assets can be categorized generally as

- land and improvements
- buildings
- fixed equipment
- major movable equipment
- minor movable equipment

or in more specific categories that are more useful to the facility.

In addition, depreciation schedules should be maintained for each category of assets (Table 3-9) and for each type of depreciation, if accelerated and straight-line are both used.

If two different schedules are used to depreciate the same assets—one for reimbursement and one for other purposes—there will be a difference in depreciation expense for each asset every year. Because the total amount of depreciation taken for each asset should be the same (total depreciation will equal the historical cost less salvage value), this difference between the two depreciation expenses is a difference of timing. Depreciation in this case may be regarded as a charge that must be deferred to another time period or as revenue that is accrued if depreciation will be recognized in a later accounting period.

Table 3-9. Old Well Home Depreciation Schedule

Item	Cost	Date Purchased	Life	Method Depreciated	Year	Depreciation, per year	
						Annual	Cumulative
Plant: main	$5,767,004.00	6/19X0	30	Strt. line	X0	$192,233.47	$192,233.47
Hall welsh					X1	192,233.47	384,466.94
Hall & Garage					X2	192,233.47	576,700.41
					X3	192,233.47	768,933.88
					Etc.		
Kitchen	$398,600.00	6/19XO	15	Strt. line	X0	$26,573.33	$26,573.33
Equipment					X1	26,573.33	53,146.66
					X2	26,573.33	79,719.99
					X3	26,573.33	106,293.32
					Etc.		

3.8 Using Costs in Managerial Decisions

EFFICIENCY

Efficiency, discussed in part 1, may be defined as input over output, or the amount of input used for a certain level of output. Costs, as a component of input, are generally easier to control than are revenues or other measures of output. Revenues are subject to limitation by competition from providers of similar services and by government regulation through insurance and medical assistance programs. Knowledge of costs and the ability to control and reduce them permit liquidity of limited funds, making them available for other uses.

3.8.1 Types of Costs: Variable and Fixed

VARIABLE COSTS

All costs can be regarded as variable, fixed, or semi-variable. Variable costs are those that fluctuate directly and proportionately with changes in volume. That is, if volume is increased or decreased by a certain percentage, variable costs will rise or fall, respectively, by the same percentage. The cost of disposable medical supplies in the nursing department will vary directly with the number of similar care type and level patients served. The cost of food in dietary or the cost of postage for resident/patient billing will also vary with resident/patient volume.

FIXED COSTS

Fixed costs, on the other hand, do not relate to changes in volume. The cost of the director of nursing's salary will not change with fluctuations in the number of residents. This does not mean that the director's salary cannot change at all, but it will result from an administrative decision rather than a fluctuation in patient volume because federal regulations require that there be a full-time director of nursing. Clearly, if volume varies enough, many fixed costs will not remain the same. If resident/patient volume increases substantially, a new administrative position in the nursing department may have to be created to accommodate the additional patient load. "Fixed" costs, then, are said to be fixed only over a relevant range of volume.

AN ADDITIONAL TYPE: SEMI-VARIABLE COSTS

Semi-variable costs do not fit neatly into either a variable or fixed category, as they vary disproportionately with volume. Examples of semi-variable costs might be total nurse's aides' salaries, which depend more on resident/patient volume and level of care needs than does the director of nursing's salary, which does not fluctuate directly with these variables.

Utility costs that are based on ranges of usage rather than actual usage may also be considered semi-variable costs. It is helpful to think of semi-variable costs as those having a much narrower relevant range than fixed costs. Semi-variable costs are often broken down into fixed and variable components for use in calculations, and so our discussion here will be limited to fixed and variable costs for the sake of simplicity.

TOTAL VARIABLE COSTS

While total variable costs (TVC) change with volume, variable costs per unit do not. If disposable syringes are $1 each, the cost per syringe per patient will be $1, whether 100 or 150 patients receive injections using

Table 3-10. Behavior of Fixed and Variable Costs

Patients	Director of Nursing		Disposable medical supplies	
	(TFC)	FC/Unit	TVC	VcAjnit
100	$44000.00	440	100	$1.00
125	$44000.00	352	125	$1.00
150	$44000.00	293	150	$1.00
	(No change)	(Change)	(Change)	(No change)

syringes purchased at one cost in one batch. Total fixed costs (TFC), however, do vary per unit with changes in volume. If the director of nursing's salary is $44,000 (exclusive of benefits, etc.) and she oversees the care of 100 residents/patients, the director's salary cost per resident/patient would be $440 (exclusive of benefits, etc.). If that same director of nurses oversees 150 resident/patients, the cost drops to $293 per resident/patient. Familiarity with the costs of the facility maximizes the administrator's ability to control its finances.

The behavior of variable and fixed costs is summarized in Table 3-10. As can be seen, fixed costs decrease with an increase in volume. Because the nursing facility generally has a high proportion of fixed costs, maintaining a high volume of service is of paramount concern to their administrators.

A closer study of the concept of fixed and variable costs reveals how it can be used to aid in decision making. Because all costs (even semi-variable ones) can be considered fixed or variable,

Total Fixed Costs + Total Variable Costs = Total Costs

Because total variable costs are a function of the variable cost per unit and the number of units, the equation can be expanded.

TFC + (Variable Cost Per Unit x Volume Units) = Total Costs

$$\text{TFC} + \left(\frac{\text{Variable Costs}}{\text{Unit}} \times \text{Volume Units}\right) = \text{Total Costs}$$

$$\text{Break-even Volume in Units} = \frac{\text{Fixed Cost}}{\text{Rate}} - \text{Variable Cost}$$

Thus, if three of these values are known, the remaining value can be calculated.

The administrator of Old Well wants to find the average variable cost of medical supplies used per resident/patient during the month. The general ledger shows that the total costs of the nursing department for 1 month are $12,000. The administrator has determined that fixed cost accounts in that department amount to $9,000 and that medical supplies are its only variable cost. The patient census report for the month shows that there have been 3,000 resident/patient days or an average of 100 resident/patients over 30 days. To calculate the variable cost per patient in the nursing department:

$$\frac{(\text{Total Costs} - \text{Total Fixed Costs})}{\text{Volume units}} = \frac{\text{Variable Costs}}{\text{Units}}$$

($12,000 — $9,000) / 100 resident/patients = $30 per resident/patient

Thus, the variable cost of providing nursing services in this particular month was $30 per resident/patient.

VOLUME OF SERVICE UNITS

These equations can be used to determine the volume of service units required to break even. Because total costs (TC) equal total revenues (TR) at the break-even point, total revenue (TR) can be substituted for total costs (TC) in the above equations to give the costs or volume needed to break even.

If the total costs of the physical therapy department are $6,500 per month, and the total fixed costs are $5,200, and the variable cost per patient visit to physical therapy is $8, how many patient visits are needed per month to break even in this department?

$$\text{Total Costs} = \text{Total Revenue}$$
$$= \$6,500 = \$5,200 + (\$8 \times \text{Volume Unit})$$
Volume units ($6,500 − $5,200) / $8 = break-even number
Volume units = 162.5 visits per month

We have assumed that the physical therapists are employees of the facility and that their salaries comprise a significant portion of the fixed costs of the department. If physical therapy is provided on a contractual basis, the therapists' salaries would become a variable cost if they were paid for each visit.

3.8.3 Additional Types of Costs: Indirect and Direct

Costs may also be categorized as direct and indirect. In order to discuss them, however, we must first define revenue centers and cost centers.

REVENUE CENTERS

Revenue centers are units of the facility, usually departments, that generate revenue, usually though resident/patient care. Revenue centers in the nursing facility will normally be nursing, possibly physical therapy, occupational therapy, pharmacy, laboratory, and medical support. It may also be any other department or center that is earning revenue, such as a cafeteria that serves a large number of guest meals or a profitable day-care program. If pharmaceuticals or medical supplies are included as part of the routine care and are not separately charged, they would not be revenue centers.

As facilities add service areas such as assisted-living wings, home health, and hospice care, these become additional revenue centers. If the facility earns a significant amount of revenue from interest on investments, interest may also be considered a revenue center.

COST CENTERS

Cost centers are units of the facility that are identified with certain costs. Revenue centers are almost always cost centers because the revenue-earning departments also have costs directly associated with them. Interest as a revenue center has little or no costs associated with it. All other departments, such as administration, maintenance, housekeeping, and usually dietary and laundry are cost centers. Depreciation, interest, insurance, telephone, utility, and transportation expenses may also be considered cost centers. These are all identifiable costs of the facility, and the concept of cost centers will become clearer as we proceed.

DIRECT COSTS

Direct costs are those directly attributable to a revenue center or directly providing resident/patient care. In the nursing facility direct costs are often called resident/patient care costs. Direct costs of the nursing department would include all nursing salaries, payroll taxes, benefits, medical supplies, expenses associated with capital equipment used only in the department, and any other costs associated directly with this department.

INDIRECT COSTS

Indirect costs are those that cannot be directly associated with a revenue-producing center, yet support the functions of the resident/patient care centers (or other care centers, such as an adult day-care center). Indirect costs of the nursing department would be administration, payroll, utility, housekeeping, maintenance, dietary, laundry, plant depreciation, tax, and interest expenses that keep these departments running. For this reason, indirect costs are also known as support service costs.

Support Service Costs

These indirect costs must be allocated to all the revenue-producing departments that are also cost centers in order to be included in the charge for services in each revenue center and to reflect the total cost of providing that service. To find the total costs of the revenue-producing department, then, the support costs must be spread over all revenue-producing departments in some systematic way. This process is known as cost finding, as it yields the total costs of the resident care centers (and other centers such as adult day care).

The concept of cost finding illustrated is schematically in Figure 3-12, where the total costs of both the support and service (or revenue-earning) centers are shown. To find the total cost of providing resident/patient Service Centers A and B, some portion of the support centers must be allocated to the revenue centers. Support Center No. 1 divides its support equally between Service Centers A and B, so 50% of the costs of support Center No. 1 are attributed to each resident/patient service center.

Support Center No. 2 provides more services to Service Center B, and this is reflected in the proportion of Support Center No. 2's costs that go to Service Center B. When the costs of both support centers are allocated, the total cost of providing services A and B are known.

THE VALUE OF COST FINDING

Cost finding yields a representative picture of the entire expense of providing each service. This information is used in deciding whether a particular service should be discontinued or supported. For example,

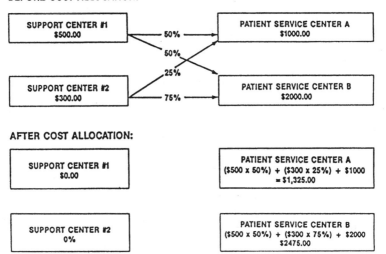

FIGURE 3-12. Cost allocation between two support and two revenue centers.

unless all direct and indirect costs are calculated for providing a service such as adult day care, it is difficult to determine the cost-effectiveness of offering such a service. Cost allocation is a subjective process in that there is an almost infinite number of ways to perform cost allocation properly. Numerous facilities offered adult day care in the early 1980s, but when they stopped to determine the full actual costs of earning the daily charges for day care, they discovered that most of the programs were cost-ineffective (Maddox et al., 2001).

ALLOCATING INDIRECT COSTS

There are several methods for allocating indirect costs, among them the step-down and reciprocal methods. Providers who are reimbursed on a cost basis must usually use the step-down method unless another method is approved. We will discuss that method in some detail here and briefly explain the reciprocal method at the end of this section.

The step-down method derives its name from the shape of the completed worksheet and involves the systematic allocation of all cost centers all other cost centers that use the "services" of the cost-center expenses being allocated. Support costs are spread not only over revenue centers, but also over other support cost centers.

Once a support cost is divided among the other cost centers, no more costs can be allocated to that department. Therefore, the order in which support costs are allocated affects the final cost of the revenue centers. As a rule, cost centers that are used by most of the other cost centers are allocated first.

The basis of allocation also affects the outcome of the cost-finding process. In allocating housekeeping costs to the departments that use housekeeping services, the basis for allocation might be the number of employees in the department, the square footage of the departments, or some other criteria. Likewise, administrative costs might be allocated on the basis of number of employees, total salary of employees, volume of services provided, or total revenues earned in each department. These alternatives are examples only; clearly, the basis for allocation varies.

Third-party reimbursement will indicate the basis for allocation that should be used for residents/patients for whom they reimburse, but in any case the method the facility uses should remain consistent to enable comparison of the resulting costs in different time periods.

The Step-Down Process

Cost allocation is best illustrated through a step-by-step example of the step-down process. The scenario provided in Table 3-11 is necessarily simplified; cost allocations for most health care organizations are usually performed by computer because of the volume and complexities involved in larger, more departmentalized or multiprogram facilities.

Other Methods of Cost Finding

Two other approaches to cost finding are the reciprocal and cost-apportionment methods. The reciprocal is similar to the step-down method, except that it recognizes reciprocal services provided between cost centers, such as administration and maintenance. Because of the calculations involved and the extent of these services in most organizations, reciprocal allocation is performed by computer.

RATE SETTING

One of the primary uses of the cost-finding process is to develop a basis for setting rates for the services provided by the revenue centers. Once the costs of the revenue centers are known, the average cost per unit of service can be calculated by dividing the total cost of the revenue center by the expected service volume.

Table 3-11. Old Well Home Step-Down Worksheets: Preliminary Worksheet

Cost Centers	Capital (sq. ft.) %	Plant (sq. ft.) %	Admin. (1) (-FTE)-(1) %	Main. (1) (sq- ft.) %	Laundry (lbs. dry) %	Housekeep (sq. ft.) %	Dietary (meals) %	Soc. Serv. (visits) %	P.T. (visits) %	O.T. (visits) %	NURSING %	TOTAL %
Support & revenue centers												
Administration												
Maintenance (2)	1.5	1.5	0.5									
Laundry	9.0	9.0	3.0	9.4								
Housekeeping	8.0	8.0	7.4	8.4	5.0							
Dietary	10.0	10.0	7.3	10.5	15.0	12.8						
Social services	0.5	0.5	0.1	0.5	0.6							
Physical therapy	7.0	7.0	2.5	7.3	2.5	8.9						
Occupational therapy	2.0	2.0	0.4	2.1	2.5	2.6						
Nursing	59.0	59.0	78.8	61.7	75.0	75.2	100.0	100.0	100.0	100.0	100.0	100.0
TOTAL	100.0	100.0	100.0	99.8	100.0	100.0	100.0	100.0	100.0	100.0	100.0	100.0

Note: 1. FTE = Full-Time Equivalent Employees
2. Total maintenance costs include all utility costs.

The unit of service must first be determined. In the physical therapy department, a unit of service is normally calculated as a 15-minute segment for which charges are made.

The average cost per unit of service offers a basis for rate setting, because rates should approximate the cost of providing the service. But other factors, such as demand for services, competitive rates, expected inflation rates, contractual discounts, and frequency of uncollectibles must be considered in achieving realistic rates.

3.9 Budgets and Budgeting

CONSIDERATIONS IN BUDGETING

The budgeting process in the nursing facility is a period of planning. The physical budget is more than a record of anticipated expenses for the next fiscal year: It represents a careful examination of internal and external changes that management believes will affect the operation of the facility and the strategy to deal with these changes for some time to come. Thus, the budget is a reflection of the administrator's short- and long-term goals for the facility. Most organizations also have a 3- to 5-year budget plan following the next fiscal year as a guide to long-range planning.

The budget is a tool to be used throughout the year, rather than a document that, once completed, is filed away. It can be changed as conditions change, and it provides a meaningful comparison between actual and projected expenditures and revenues.

Most facility administrators use the budget in a monthly review with department managers on how the year is unfolding and what changes need to be undertaken.

3.9.1 Two Methods of Budget Preparation

Budgeting is done in any number of ways, and the individual facility or multifacility operation will develop its own particular style. In general, two methods of budget preparation are used: the top-down and the participatory method.

THE TOP-DOWN APPROACH TO BUDGETING

With the top-down approach, the administrator alone (or corporate) prepares the annual budget with little or no guidance from department heads. This method is most suitable for smaller facilities with few departments, where the administrator is familiar with all the costs of the facility. Top-down is also often the approach used by chains, in which case the local administrator is given a suggested budget with the corporation's goals already built into it. The top-down method is quick, but has the disadvantages of possibly stifling innovation or imposing an unpopular or unrealistic budget on department heads or chain facility administrators.

THE PARTICIPATORY APPROACH

The participatory method of budgeting requires input from staff members on several levels of the organization. The administrator provides guidelines for the preparation of departmental budgets by the department heads and other key personnel. These budgets are then reviewed by the administrator, adjusted as necessary, and combined into one organizational budget.

Participatory budgeting is more appropriate for larger facilities. Although it is time-consuming, it furnishes an opportunity for communication between the administrator and department heads, and results in input into the budget from those who are most knowledgeable about the daily operation of the individual departments.

Participatory budgeting will be used to describe the budgeting process in this section, as it is considerably more involved than the top-down approach. However, the process described is equally applicable to the latter.

Participatory budgeting augments the role each participant plays in the operations of the facility. Department heads and others become more aware not only of the costs of their areas and the resources available to the facility, but also of the needs of the other departments. Budgeting also brings greater recognition of their own roles to the participating staff, and although the budget process is often time-consuming and frustrating, the staff is rewarded by the knowledge that their experience and ideas are valued.

Finally, the budget communicates information about the facility to external parties who have an interest in its status, such as the board of directors or stockholders, third-party payers, planning agencies, accreditation teams, rate review commissions, and unions. The administrator must often be able to justify proposed expenses and revenues to them.

3.9.2 Five Steps in the Budgeting Process

There are countless ways to prepare the budget, whether by the administrator alone or with the input of key personnel. The optimal method will depend, among other considerations, on the size of the facility, whether it is free-standing or a unit in a small or large chain, and the administrator's time constraints.

In designing the budgeting process the administrator first decides what information is desired and how detailed it must be and the maps out the logistics of the activity. The administrator determines who the participants will be. In the case of top-down budgeting, the administrator and perhaps other administrative personnel, such as the bookkeeper, comptroller, or business manager, will be involved. Participatory budgeting usually includes the administrator, the accountant or the comptroller, bookkeeper, human resources director, and department heads and their assistants. The budget timetable must also be defined. At least 2 to 5 months before the beginning of the next fiscal year should be allowed for the entire process.

STEP 1: ASSESSING THE ENVIRONMENT

The initial step in the budgeting process is the assessment of the external and internal environments (Hitt et al., 2001). The budget cannot be prepared in a vacuum. As mentioned in part 1, the political, economic, and social environments outside the nursing facility walls are not static. Although the administrator does not have control over these aspects of the external environment, ignorance of the trends affecting the nursing facility industry, and failure to anticipate their effects on the operations of the facility, leave the administrator less able to deal effectively with changes (Hitt et al., 2001). Such trends may occur as one or more of the following:

- increased or decreased competition
- new types of competition, for example, a local hospital opening long-term care beds; increased capacity of local home health agencies to treat at home; emergence of additional hospice care agencies
- altered reimbursement policies
- amended licensing laws
- revised quality-review regulations

- swings in the economy (e.g., inflation, deflation, or stagnation
- changes in prevailing wage rates
- reduction or enlargement of the potential service population
- changes in availability of key personnel
- changes in disease patterns among residents/patients
- changing system pressures from hospital discharge patterns due to Diagnostic Related Group (DRG) pressures
- changing third-party payer situation, with new patterns of providing and paying for care emerging
- increasing acuity level among the resident/patient population

Some, if not most, of these fluctuations in the external environment may affect the plans and operations of the facility, and there are others that are not mentioned here.

STEP 2: PROGRAMMING

After the external environments and their anticipated effects on the facility have been evaluated, the facility's objectives for the coming year are determined. This process is sometimes known as *programming*; in effect, it results in a program for the facility to follow. Through this programming the administrator can alter internal operations over which he has control in order to respond to the external (and internal) influences on the facility.

How might an administrator use programming to cope with external events? In periods of rising inflation the cost of living goes up. This usually results in a demand for higher wages. If the administrator is aware of this trend, an objective might be to index the salaries, that is, raise them by a certain percentage to approximate the increased costs of living by a certain time during the following year. An increase in salary expense can then be included in the budget, thereby preventing a situation in which funds are not set aside for this purpose. Such an oversight could result in recruiting problems, high staff turnover, or a strain on operating funds when a salary increase is finally provided.

Similarly, if a competitor is opening a facility nearby, a contingency fund could be set aside in the following year's budget to raise salaries to meet the new competitor's salary scale, should this become necessary (Hitt et al., 2001).

Other considerations for programming are changes in (a) service volume, (b) services offered, (c) payer mix, (d) human resources needs, and (e) capital needs. The cumulative effect of expected external and internal events should determine the objectives of the facility for the next year(s), which in turn form the basis of assumptions made in the budgeting process.

The completed budgeting process should result in four types of budgets: the operating budget, the cash budget, the capital budget, and the pro forma financial statements.

STEP 3: DEVELOPING THE OPERATING BUDGET

The operating budget has two parts: the expense budget and the revenue budget.

The Expense Budget

The expense budget, the type with which we are most familiar, lists the anticipated expenses of the facility for the coming year and is prepared largely by the department heads. The budget timetable should indicate when the final departmental expense budgets are due.

The heads of all service units should indicate the expected resident/patient service volume, while support departments (such as dietary) should be able to estimate the number of meals that will be served. Budgeting offers an opportunity for communication among departments. After all, dietary must know the expected resident/patient volume in the different areas of the facility in order to calculate the number of meals that will be served and types of diets likely to be prescribed.

Additionally, department heads should review staff positions and note any recommended changes in the staffing pattern. In larger facilities, recommendations for salary changes may be the responsibility of the personnel director and may be based on competitive salaries in the community or union agreements if employees are so organized.

Department heads should also check equipment in their departments for repair or replacement needs. Included in this assessment would be estimates of the costs of repair or replacement, supported by professional estimates, manufacturer price sheets, and the like. If equipment needs are extensive, it may be worthwhile for department heads to develop a plant and equipment budget for their departments, which will facilitate preparation of the capital budget.

The cost of supplies and other expenses are often a significant portion of departmental costs. Any change in the volume of supplies needed and the cost per unit should be noted on the budget. Catch-all or miscellaneous categories should be kept to a minimum, as there can be little control over unidentified costs.

Anticipated expenses should be broken down by months or another customary accounting period used in the facility. Monthly expense budgets also facilitate preparation of the cash budget.

Determining Expenses. Several strategies can be used in determining expenses. One tactic is to increase all of the current year's expenses by a certain percentage. Although this method is quick, it defeats the purpose of budgeting and the effort involved in environmental assessment and programming.

It is more productive for the department head to identify monthly and yearly trends in costs and utilization to help reduce expenses. For example, occupancy of the nursing unit might be consistently below average during the winter holidays, but regularly above average in late January and February. Identifying such trends is useful in budgeting for monthly costs on volume levels. It is also often helpful to identify the source of variances in the current year's budget and allow for them in the preparation of the new budget.

In setting up the expense budget a checklist can be used to make sure all expense items in departments are included. A good source for this checklist is the chart of accounts, which should list all expense accounts by department.

All budget participants ought to know how and by whom the final budget levels are decided. Finally, the organizational expense budget is separated by months, and the individual department budgets retained for comparison of actual with budgeted performance in each department throughout the year.

The Revenue Budget

The second section of the operating budget is the revenue budget, which projects the monthly income for the next fiscal year. The revenue budget need not be prepared on a departmental basis; fewer departments are involved in determining revenues than in determining expenses, and nonoperating revenues are generally under the control of the administrator. Also, service revenues are based on the prices charged for services, which are determined by administrative decision. Hence, the revenue budget is usually prepared at the administrative level.

Operating Revenue Estimates. To estimate operating revenue, all revenue centers are listed, with the number of residents/patients appearing by type of payer. Total resident/patient service revenue is calculated by multiplying the expected service volume in each revenue center by the charge per unit of service. As mentioned in the section on cost finding, rates for services may be determined in several ways. For publicly insured persons, the allowable rate per unit of service may be somewhat less than charges; the reimbursable rate should be used in projecting revenues for these persons.

For privately paying residents/patients, charges can be based on the cost plus profit for providing the service, using the results of the cost-finding process and break-even analysis. Rates may also be based on competitive charges for similar services in the community or on the price that the market will bear.

Nonoperating Revenue. Nonoperating revenue, such as interest income, borrowed funds, and charitable donations, is dependent on any number of factors, but is relatively predictable on a monthly basis. This revenue is added to the monthly operating revenue to arrive at the total expected revenue.

Total revenue can then be compared with total budgeted expenses. If revenue seems inadequate to meet expenses, the administrator can check the validity of the predicted service volumes. If service levels seem reasonable, the administrator can seek to increase patient service volume, reduce budget expenses, or raise rates.

Using the Operating Budget: Variance Analysis

As a managerial tool, the operating budget is used throughout the fiscal year to measure performance by a technique called variance analysis, which is a comparison of actual versus budgeted monetary and volume values at the end of each month.

Actual expenses that deviate significantly from the budgeted amounts can be investigated to identify the source of the variance (as mentioned in part 1). Such variances may be anything from an inadvertent miscalculation of costs or patient volume to serious mismanagement by a particular department. Typical sources of overage are items such as using more pool labor than anticipated or a number of employees working unanticipated or unauthorized overtime. Once the source of variances is known, the budget can be adjusted accordingly or the cause of the variance can be dealt with. Budget variance analysis provides the administrator with an important means of control over the finances of the facility.

STEP 4: THE CASH BUDGET

The next step in the budgeting process is preparation of the cash budget. As its name implies, it is prepared on the cash basis of accounting, although it is based on the revenues and expenses from the operating budget. Note that the operating budget is prepared on the accrual basis of accounting: Projected revenues are based on the income earned in the time period, not on the amount of cash received for services during the month.

The cash budget is an estimate of the cash inflows and outflows for the next 12 months, enabling the administrator to identify months with possible cash shortages and overages. This information can be used to defer expenditures that are not urgent to a month with high cash inflows or to retain overages in one month to cover anticipated cash shortages in the next. A cash budget is useful for anticipating the effects of such events as when three pay periods occur in one month or anticipated large Medicare payments at known intervals. Corporate-owned facilities may have little need of a cash budget inasmuch as corporate funds can cover any temporary shortages in the cash flow needs of the facility. Some administrators rely on the cash budget for daily operations and sometimes prepare weekly or even daily cash budgets a month in advance.

Determining Cash Inflows and Outflows

To develop the cash budget, cash inflows and outflows must be determined. Because the facility has less control over cash inflows, especially those received from third-party payers, projecting them is somewhat complicated. First, all payer sources must be identified. These will usually be private payers, Medicare, Medicaid, insurance companies, HMOs or IPOs or similar organizations, the Veterans Administration and all other known or anticipated sources of income for services expected to be rendered. The lag time between the billing of services and receipt of payment is determined. Most private payers do so within 30 days of billing, but time lags for Medicare and Medicaid may vary considerably. This can be used to measure the percentage of revenues that will be received from each payer in each month.

When cash inflows from resident/patient services are known, monthly cash receipts from nonoperating sources are computed to give total cash receipts for each month.

Cash outflows are somewhat easier to estimate, as most cash disbursements, such as salaries and supplies, are made at prespecified intervals. Using the expense budget and the facility 's experience with suppliers and other creditors, the amount of cash disbursements can be determined for each month. An insurance policy that is paid on a triennial basis may be due in February, for example.

As with the operating budget, the cash budget is updated as conditions or needs change throughout the year, whatever the reason. The cash budget can be a useful planning tool.

STEP 5: THE CAPITAL BUDGET

The capital budget is a summarization of all anticipated capital (items with a life of more than 12 months) expenditures in the budget year.

Although many capital purchases and projects may be needed, all might not be readily affordable in the course of a single year. The capital budget is the result of the decision concerning capital projects that will be undertaken, and, most important, how they will be financed. If a competitor is to open a large new facility nearby, for example, a contingency capital item might be funds for renovations of a portion of the facility to compete should census drop precipitously.

Pro Forma Financial Statements

The budget process concludes with the development of the *pro forma* financial statements. The pro forma statements are the preliminary financial statements based on budgeted amounts. The pro forma income statement, for instance, is derived from the operating budget and shows the net income (or loss) expected under the budgeted expenses and revenues.

The budgeting process can be costly in terms of time for the administrator and all other budget participants. However, it involves a thorough investigation of the facility's finances through such tools as cost finding, break-even analysis, rate setting, programming, and cash flow analysis. Through these processes, budgeting familiarizes the administrator with the costs of running the facility and maximizes her ability to manage successfully.

3.10 Business and Financial Management

Thus far in part 3 we have focused on the internal business and financial matters of the nursing facility. We now turn to examine the broader business and financial context within which the nursing facility manages its affairs.

In this section we will

- look briefly at the sources of law and the court systems
- review a number of legal terms
- discuss the issue of risk management for a nursing facility
- examine a number of business and financial concepts and terms, insurance terms, and terms associated with wills and estates

3.10.1 Sources of Law

The daily business of the nursing facility is conducted within the context of the United States legal system.

Constitution. The Constitution is the written agreement establishing the fundamental law of the United States of America, setting forth the conditions, mutual obligations, and rights of the federal and state governments and laying down basic principles of government. The Bill of Rights guarantees specific individual rights.

Statutes. Statutes are the laws under which we live. In the United States they are the acts passed by the federal and state legislatures (Noe et al., 2000). Lesser governmental bodies, such as county commissions, adopt ordinances; administrative agencies function by means of regulations.

Common Law. Common law is the accumulation of opinion handed down by judges. It is an outgrowth of court decisions over hundreds of years. Our common law originated in England, where judges followed unwritten principles of common sense in addition to statutory laws. Common law principles change over time with the changing values and needs of society.

Regulations. To implement statutes (laws) passed by legislative bodies, the executive branch of government (the president and the various federal agencies) writes regulations (Noe et al., 2000). These regulations are the official interpretations of the intent of each statute. As a consequence, regulations become, in effect, part of the law. One may challenge a regulation on the grounds that the "official interpretation" is unconstitutional or inconsistent with the legislative intent of the statute.

The federal requirements for nursing facilities are an example of regulations. These were written by the executive branch of the federal government during the process of spelling out the details of how the legislation would be interpreted and implemented. The federal requirements for nursing facilities (see Allen, 2000, pp. 1–67) were written by the employees of the Health Care Finance Administration, which administers Medicare and Medicaid. The federal requirements published in the *Federal Register* as, for example, the Omnibus Budget Reconciliation Act (OBRA) regulations (the Nursing Home Reform Amendments of 1987) have the effect of law when federal inspectors visit a nursing facility and issue deficiencies based on both the written regulations (i.e., Allen, 2000, pp. 1–67) and a set of "interpretive guidelines" published in 1999. These interpretive guidelines, although not law or regulation per se, are very real; they are the guidelines used by federal certification inspectors to record deficiencies and levy fines.

These requirements (not the interpretive guidelines) along with other federal administrative agency regulations, are published in the *Code of Federal Regulations* (often refereed to as CFR).

The president of the United States has the prerogative of issuing executive orders under various statutes. Executive orders also have the effect of law. President Lyndon B. Johnson, for example, issued Executive Order 11246, requiring all federal contractors to use affirmative action guidelines designed to hire and promote women and minorities within their organizations (Noe et al., 2000).

Code. A code is a compilation of statutes and regulations. The statutes, together with the regulations written by the administrative assigned to implement each statute, are systematically collected and placed into codes of law. The United States Code, often referred to as USC is an example.

3.10.2 The Court Systems

Federal Courts. The United States Constitution authorizes the creation of the Supreme Court and any additional courts Congress chooses to establish. Currently, entry into the federal court system is at the level of federal district courts (general courts of original jurisdiction). *Jurisdiction* is the power to hear and decide a case. Between these and the federal Supreme Court are 12 courts of appeal, which together cover the 50 states and hear cases in the event a party is dissatisfied with the judgment of the federal district court based on what the dissatisfied party views as an error (Noe et al., 2000).

The federal government also operates other courts, such as a Court of Claims, the Court of Customs and Patent Appeals, the Tax Court, and federal bankruptcy courts.

State Courts. The court systems vary from state to state. The lowest level of the state system is the magistrate court, which deals with misdemeanor cases, traffic violations, and small claims. Above the magistrate courts are the state circuit courts, or district courts, where more serious cases are tried.

Circuit or district courts have original jurisdiction over both civil and criminal cases. Most states have courts of appeal, which normally do not have original jurisdiction and therefore limit themselves to appeals from lower courts in the state. Finally, each state has a supreme court. This is the court of final appeal in all matters except those involving a federal issue that is appealable to the United States Supreme Court.

3.10.3 Terms Relation to Legal Matters

Accuse—to directly charge a person with committing an offense that is recognized as being against a law. The accused person becomes the defendant and must answer the complaint or accusation through the legal process.

Acquit—to set a person or corporation free of accusation(s). Acquittal is a decision (verdict) of not guilty and is rendered either by a jury or a judge (in nonjury trials). Under the principle of double jeopardy, a person or corporation cannot be tried again for the same accusation after a verdict of not guilty.

Actionable—conduct giving rise to a cause for legal action. For example, actionable negligence occurs only when a person unreasonably fails to perform a legal duty, resulting in damage or injury to another person. If there is no resulting damage, there may not be actionable negligence even though the person made a mistake.

Adjudication—decision or disposition of a case by the announcement of a judgement or decision by the court or other body.

Admission—the acknowledgement of certain facts by a party in a civil or criminal case. An admission does not necessarily constitute a confession of guilt. For example, the defendant may admit that he was driving the automobile but deny running the red light. The term "confession" is generally restricted to an acknowledgment of guilt.

Affidavit—A written statement given under oath before an officer having authority to administer oaths. A notary public is such a public officer and is authorized to signify by her signature that she witnessed the execution (signing) of certain documents, such as affidavits, deeds, and wills.

Aggrieved party—one whose legal rights have been invaded or who has suffered a loss or injury. The term is frequently used in connection with proceedings by administrative agencies. For example, a person contesting the revocation of her professional license in an administrative proceeding is an aggrieved party.

Amicus curiae—literally, a friend (amicus) of the court (curiae). An amicus brief is a written document that provides the court with information that might otherwise escape attention. A long-term care ombudsman might, for example, appear in a court case on behalf of a resident/patient. The "friend of the court" has no absolute right to appear in the proceeding, so must obtain the court's permission prior to intervening.

Appeal—the request by a party for a lawsuit to a higher court to review a lower court's decision when the party believes the lower court committed an error.

Appearance—the coming into court of a person on being summoned to do so. Appearance without receiving a summons is a voluntary appearance. Appearance in court after papers have been served is an involuntary appearance.

Arbitrator—an impartial person chosen by the parties to an argument to decide the issue between them. Arbitration is used to avoid unnecessary and costly court actions.

Arraignment—an early step in a criminal proceeding at which the defendant is formally charged with an offense.

Assault—see Torts.

Battery—see Torts.

Burden of proof, or burden of persuasion—the obligation of the person bringing an action to prove facts in dispute. In criminal cases, the state must prove its case beyond a reasonable doubt. In civil cases the burden of proof is met by a "preponderance" of the evidence, that is, evidence of superior weight, importance, or strength.

Civil law—pertains to a crime, that is, any act the government has deemed to be injurious to the public and actionable in a criminal proceeding. The criminal acts may be felonies (serious crimes such as murder, arson, rape, armed robbery) or misdemeanors (less serious crimes such as minor traffic violations). A criminal violation may result in either a jail sentence, a fine, or both.

To picture the interaction of civil and criminal law, assume an employee intentionally runs over a resident/patient in the facility parking lot. The employee may be sued by the resident/patient for money damages in a civil action and may also be brought to trial on criminal charges by the district attorney for the same act. (The nursing facility probably will be sued civilly too, particularly if the employee has very little money).

Consent, informed—consent given after full information regarding the matter has been provided to the person consenting. In the nursing facility context, residents/patients must understand the nature and risks of certain treatments before the facility can claim exemption from responsibility for resulting complications

A diabetic resident/patient, for example, may volunteer to participate in an experimental diet program. Unless the resident/patient fully understands the risks involved, the facility may be held liable for subsequent complications. The facility should require the resident/patient to sign a properly prepared consent form.

Consent to one treatment or procedure is not necessarily consent to another treatment or procedure, even if such treatment or procedure is beneficial. If a patient resident consented to a tonsillectomy but the surgeon also removed the appendix, the surgeon may have committed a battery.

Counterclaim—a counterdemand by a defendant against a plaintiff (accuser), not merely responding to the accuser, but asserting an independent cause of action against the accuser. For example, if the resident/patient in the knitting needle illustration (see Torts) sued the orderly for damages for assault or battery, the orderly might counterclaim with a demand for damages for assault or battery.

Damages—money awarded by a court (or jury) to a person who has been wronged by the action of another. The meaning of the terms used to describe the various types of damages available differs from state to state and depends on the type of case. Generally, actual damages, consequential damages, and incidental damages are designed to compensate the person wronged.

Nominal damages are an award of a small sum of money in recognition of the invasion of some legal right of the plaintiff that has resulted in no actual injury or pecuniary loss to the plaintiff. *Punitive damages* are designed to punish the defendant for particularly bad conduct and to deter the defendant from such conduct in the future. (Punitive damages are also sometimes called exemplary damages.) Double and treble damages are types of punitive damages sometimes provided for by particular statutes.

Defendant—in criminal cases, the accused; in civil cases, the one who is sued and who must defend against a claim of wrongdoing brought by another.

Defamation—the communication to a third person of that which is injurious to the reputation or good name of the victim. Oral defamation is slander. Written defamation is libel.

Libel is written publication that exposes someone to public scorn, hatred, contempt, or ridicule, especially if related to an individual's profession or livelihood.

Slander, because it is spoken, is more difficult to establish. The action for slander has been restricted because of the right of free speech and to avoid overloading the courts with trivial cases. Only if slanderous statements lead to actual damages (e.g., loss of employment) can they be actionable, unless the words imply crime, unchastity, or relate to a person's profession or business.

In the cases of both libel and slander, there must be communication to a third party, for example, showing a third party written words or speaking slanderous words in the presence of a third party.

Deposition—a statement given under oath, reduced to writing and authenticated by a notary public. A deposition gives the attorneys for both sides an opportunity to find out what the person deposed (deponent) knows about the relevant event.

Directed verdict—a verdict given by a jury at the direction of a judge. If, for example, a plaintiff fails to make a reasonable case or a defendant fails to make a necessary defense, the judge may direct the jury to render a specified verdict.

Discovery—pretrial devices used by the parties' lawyers to gather information or knowledge about the case. Discovery devices include depositions, interrogatories to parties, and requests for documents and articles. The purpose of discovery devices is to facilitate pretrial settlements and to reduce surprises at trials in order that cases might be decided on their merit (rather than by ambush).

False imprisonment—see Torts.

Fraud—intentional deception that results in injury to another.

Indictment—a formal, written accusation by a public prosecutor, submitted to a grand jury and charging a crime. The grand jury is a body authorized to investigate crimes and accuse (indict) persons within its jurisdiction when it decides a trial is called for.

Injunction—a judicial direction to a party to do or to refrain from doing something. Injunctions guard against future acts, but do not remedy past acts. When the court issues an injunction, the party to whom it is issued is said to be *enjoined.*

Litigants-the parties to a lawsuit, that is, the plaintiff and defendant.

Malice—the intention to commit a wrongful act without just cause or excuse, with the intent to inflict injury. Under some circumstances the law will imply evil intent. Therefore, malice (in law) does not necessarily mean personal hate or ill will. The law will imply malice to an act committed with reckless disregard for another's safety, even though the perpetrator did not dislike the party she injured. For example, the law may imply malice to the act of one who shoots a rifle into a crowd of strangers.

Motion—an application to the court requesting an action favorable to one's side.

Negligence—the failure to exercise the degree of care a reasonable person would exercise under the same circumstances that results in injury to another. Negligent conduct falls below the standard established by society (a jury) for the protection of others from an unreasonable risk of harm. Negligence may arise from either an overt act or from a failure to act.

The term *negligence* is used in several different ways:

1. *Comparative negligence.* In some states one can recover damages even though he was negligent himself. For example, a resident/patient slips and suffers injury partly as a result of the unreasonably slippery floors in the facility and partly because the resident/patient wore slippery shoes. The facility is negligent because it failed to warn the resident/ patient that the floors were unusually slippery. But the resident/patient was also negligent because she wore shoes with slippery soles. In states that recognize comparative negligence, the jury determines how much of the injury should be blamed on the facility's negligence and how much the resident/patient is to blame. The jury then apportions the damages (money) accordingly.

2. *Contributory negligence.* Contributory negligence is similar to comparative negligence in that the victim is partly responsible for the injury. However, in states where the doctrine of contributory negligence applies, all recovery by the victim is barred. Contributory negligence is a favorite of defendants because they can win the case by convincing the jury that the victim was just the least bit to blame for the injury.

3. *Negligence per se* (conduct treated as negligence without proof). It is usually necessary to show failure to exercise a reasonable degree of care.

Negligence per se is found where the act complained of is in violation of a safety statute. Negligence per se also includes acts that are so clearly harmful to others that it is plain to any reasonable person that negligence must have occurred.

4. *Criminal negligence.* Recklessness or carelessness resulting in injury or death punishable as a crime. Criminal negligence implies reckless disregard or indifference to the safety or rights of others.

Prosecutor—a public official, either elected or appointed, who conducts cases on behalf of the government against persons accused of crimes.

Risk, assumption of—the principle that a person may not recover for an injury received through voluntary exposure to a known danger.

Res ipsa loquitur—a Latin phrase that literally means "the thing speaks for itself." The defendant's negligence is inferred from the mere fact that the event happened and that the instrumentality causing the injury was under the exclusive control of the defendant. *Res ipsa loquitur* could apply to an otherwise unexplained gas furnace explosion in a nursing facility.

Res judicata—Latin for "a thing decided." Once a court of competent jurisdiction has decided a matter, that decision continues to bind those parties in any future litigation on the same issue.

Retainer—a fee paid an attorney in advance for services on a case. In exchange, the attorney must refuse employment as the client's adversary in the case.

Search warrant—a written order from a judge permitting certain law enforcement officers to conduct a search and seize specified things or persons. Warrants are issued on sworn testimony or affidavits supporting probable cause. Law enforcement officers may not search or seize items or persons not within the scope of the search warrant.

Stare decisis—a Latin phrase meaning "to stand by that which was decided earlier." The doctrine of *stare decisis* means that once a court has laid down a principle of law as applicable to a certain set of facts, it will adhere to that principle in all future cases in which the facts are substantially the same. *Stare decisis* gives the law a measure of predictability. However, a court will reverse itself occasionally where considerations of public policy demand it. For example, nonprofit health care institutions were once immune from lawsuits. Public policy has demanded that such immunity no longer apply.

Subpoena—a written order issued by a court to require the appearance of a person in court. A person failing to appear may be held in contempt of court.

Subpoena duces tecum—a written court order for a person to bring certain objects or documents in his or her possession to a judicial proceeding. The court, for example, may require a nursing facility administrator to bring resident/patient records to a court proceeding.

Summons—a written instrument notifying a defendant that a lawsuit has commenced against her. Failure to appear may result in a default judgment, wherein the defendant has a judgment entered against her for failure to appear.

Tort-a wrong; literally, "twisted." A tort exists when (a) a legal duty is owed by a defendant to a plaintiff, (b) that duty is breached, and (c) the plaintiff is harmed as a direct result of the breach of duty.

For example, the duty to provide care to residents/patients is imposed on the nursing facility by virtue of its holding itself out as a health care provider. If the facility breaches its duty to provide care for a resident/patient and that person is harmed as a direct result of the breach of duty, a tort has occurred. The general term includes several specific types of bad or wrongful conduct. Assault, battery, false imprisonment, and negligence are among the types of conduct labeled by the law as torts.

An *assault* is an attempt to inflict bodily harm on another person that creates well-founded fear of imminent peril; it does not require actual physical touching. An assault can be the basis for a civil action (actions outside criminal practice) and/or a criminal action (violation of criminal laws). In the civil action, the person assaulted brings the action seeking to be awarded money. In the criminal action, the district attorney brings assault charges of the purpose of punishment.

The tort of assault is closely linked to, and often confused with, the tort of battery. *Battery* is the unlawful touching or application of force to another human being without his consent. For battery to occur there must be an intent to touch, actual touching, and a lack of consent. If the touching is knowingly consented to, it is not battery.

Assault has been defined as a "failed battery," because an assault must cause apprehension of immediate harmful contact, without actual contact. For example, if the doctor ordered pills, and the nurse approaches the resident/patient with a 4-inch long needle, causing apprehension of immediate contact in the resident/patient, it is an assault. When the nurse actually use the needle (touching), it becomes a battery (unless the resident/patient has consented).

To illustrate the differences between assault and battery consider the following. An orderly bumps into a female resident/patient's breast. If it is purely accidental, no battery has occurred. If the orderly intended to bump into the resident/patient's breast, it may be battery. The angry patient retaliates by throwing a knitting needle at the orderly. If it misses but the orderly is apprehensive about immediate harmful contact, the resident/patient has committed an assault. If the knitting needle hits the orderly, it is battery (even if the orderly was not apprehensive of the contact). The orderly then throws a towel at the resident/patient. If it hits the resident/patient, it is a battery. If it misses the resident/patient but the resident/patient fears immediate harmful contact, it is an assault.

False imprisonment is another tort occasionally related to assault and battery; it is the confinement of another human being within fixed boundaries against his or her will. Numerous circumstances within the nursing facility can give rise to false imprisonment. If a competent resident/patient refuses bed rails and the nurse raises the bed rails anyway, false imprisonment has occurred.

If a physician leaves orders to restrain a competent resident/patient in a wheelchair and that resident/patient refuses, tying the resident/patient in the wheelchair will constitute false imprisonment. It may also be a battery). Another common example of false imprisonment occurs when the competent resident/patient demands to be released from the facility and the facility will not allow the resident/patient to leave.

Tort-feasor—the person who commits a tort.

Warrant, arrest—a written order from a judge having authority in that jurisdiction for the arrest of a person.

Witness—a person who gives sworn testimony in a court proceeding.

3.10.4 Risks Assumed by the Operation of a Long-Term Care Facility

The act of obtaining a license to operate and operating a long-term care facility automatically brings a set of risks to the facility. Some of these are defined below.

EMPLOYER'S LIABILITY ACTS

Various states have statutes that set forth the extent to which employers are liable to their employees for injuries to them. Generally, the employer is held responsible only for injuries to employees that occur in the course of their work. Workers' compensation acts and the federal Employer's Liability Act are examples. Employer's liability acts usually pay for physician and hospital costs. These statutes eliminated the earlier claims by employers that the employee knew the hazards of a job and accepted them when agreeing to work for the facility.

Often these statutes also hold the employer responsible for negligent acts of fellow employees within the zone of employment. The zone of employment is the physical area within which employers are liable (legally responsible) under workers' compensation acts. This usually includes the parking areas, entryways, and other areas under the control of the employer.

STRICT LIABILITY

An employer held strictly liable is subject to liability without fault, that is, without the employee's having to show employer fault.

Vicarious or Imputed Liability

The employer is held responsible for the acts of employees within the scope of their employment. For example, if a nurse's aide carelessly drops a resident/patient from a wheelchair, causing injuries, the employer is normally held liable for the injuries. *Respondeat superior* is a Latin term meaning "let the master answer for the acts of [his] servants," or "let the employer answer for the acts of [his] employees."

Scope of Employment

The range of employee activities held by the courts to be the legal responsibility of the employer is called the scope of employment. Basically, it includes any acts performed in the process of carrying out one's duties. Ascertaining the scope of employment is important when determining the employer's liability for the acts of employees.

The nurse's aide who is hurrying down the hall to aid one resident/patient and knocks down and injures another who is on crutches is likely to be found acting as a servant within the scope of employment, resulting in employer liability for the accident. An employee may be found acting within the scope of employment even if the employee is doing her job contrary to the instructions of the employer.

Borrowed Servant

A borrowed servant is a person under the temporary employ of another person. In a nursing facility, a nurse employed by the local community college as a nursing instructor, who is temporarily working under the direction of the nursing facility's director of nurses might be found to be a borrowed servant. Under the concept of *respondeat superior,* the nursing facility might be found liable for the wrongful acts of the "borrowed" nurse.

Independent Contractor

An independent contractor is one who agrees to perform a certain job and remains in control of the means and methods of performing the job. Because an independent contractor is not an employee, the doctrine of *respondeat superior* is not applicable to the independent contractors. Therefore, the nursing facility would not be liable ordinarily for the negligence of an independent contractor.

Determining whether a person is acting as an employee, with the facility liable for the employee's negligence, or as an independent contractor, without this liability, depends on a number of factors:

* the extent to which the facility controls the details of the work
* whether the person is engaged in a distinct occupation or profession
* whether the work is usually done under the direction of the employer or by a specialist without supervision
* the skill required
* the portion of time the person is employed
* who supplies the equipment used
* whether the work is part of the regular business of the facility
* whether the facility and worker believe they have formed an employer-employee relationship
* whether or not the person is in business

Depending on the circumstances, physical therapists under contract to the nursing facility and private duty nurses may (or may not) be considered independent contractors. Because facilities would naturally prefer to have a number of its employees viewed as independent contractors in order to reduce liability, courts do give great weight to the label the facility places on the worker. Liability for injuries sustained by a resident/patient under treatment by a physical therapist on contract to the facility might more nearly be ascribed to the facility than an injury to a resident that is caused by an outside painting contractor employee.

MANAGING RISKS

How Much Risk?

How much risk is faced in an average 100-bed nursing facility over a year? Assuming that each nursing facility resident will have at least 20 contacts with staff members each day, more than 2,000 contacts occur daily between staff and resident/patients in this typical nursing facility. Over the course of a month, 60,000 contacts occur; in a year nearly three quarters of a million contacts occur. Within the nursing home industry, based on the nearly 17,000 nursing facilities certified by Medicare and Medicaid, approximately 12 billion such contacts occur each year. Each of these 12 billion annual contacts potentially incurs risks to the facility. Consider the following.

Care Decisions of a Nurse Aide. Not too long ago, an Alabama jury awarded $2.5 million in punitive damages to the family of an 86-year-old nursing home resident/patient who strangled to death while restrained in a Posey vest. Not realizing that vests are color coded, the nurse's aide chose a vest to match the resident's gown rather than body size. She then put the vest on the resident backwards, causing the resident to choke to death. The J. T. Posey Company, a codefendant, was found not guilty of negligence because it had warned the nursing home that the vests' V-neck should be placed in front (*Quality Care Advocate*, 1989, p. 6). Nurse aides provide the preponderance of hands-on care in nursing facilities.

Registered Nurse and Allied Health Professional Performance. In a Pennsylvania nursing facility, a night shift registered nurse, annoyed by the "disturbing" noise produced by a resident/patient's respirator, turned the respirator off while she and a respiratory therapist cleared a 65-year-old man's breathing passages. Then they left the room without turning the respirator back on. Twenty minutes later, an alarm on the respirator sounded in the resident/patient's room. The registered nurse returned to the room and found the patient dead in what the coroner called a "therapeutic misadventure."

Staff Performance Under Stress. At a nursing facility in a southern state with more than 150 beds, 9 people died, 141 were hospitalized, and 98 received significant injuries and treatment for smoke inhalation from a fire started by smoking materials at the foot of a resident/patient's bed. State and local officials said the nursing facility had undergone recent inspections and was in compliance with state fire codes. An administrator for the group of facilities said the nursing facility was fully up to code, was well equipped to deal with fires, prohibited smoking in bedrooms, and had fire alarms, smoke and heat detectors, and fire-resistant doors. Fire and effective or ineffective staff responses can occur at any time (Johns & Saks, 2001).

Uncontrolled Resident/patient Behavior. At a Dade City, Florida, facility an 89-year-old resident beat his roommate and another sleeping resident to death with his cane, then injured four others in a room-to-room rampage sparked by squabbles with roommates.

Uncontrolled Behavior of the Director of Nurses. A jury award $15 million to the estate of a resident whose family claimed was given Darvocet (a mild painkiller) in place of morphine (a more powerful painkiller) for a period of one month, under the instructions of the director of nurses. Facility owners could show that the resident's physician had written prescriptions for both morphine and Darvocet to be administered as judged medically needed. The jury debated less than 2 hours and found for the plaintiff's family.

What Is a Risk?

A risk can be defined as any event or process that can lead to actions which result, directly or indirectly, in economic losses or damage to the facility or its reputation.

Each of the foregoing events are risks to be managed. One writer in this field (Kapp, 1987) has cited several definitions of risk management that appear in the literature. "A program that attempts to provide positive avoidance of negative results. Liability control; loss prevention" (Showalter, 1984). "Prediction of patient injury, avoidance of exposure to predicted and other risks, and minimization of malpractice claims loss (Orlikoff, Fifer, and Greeley, 1981).

Troyer and Salman define risk as "exposure to the chance of injury or loss; a hazard or dangerous chance." They note that there are "many considerations other than professional liability," and define loss control broadly as an attempt to prevent "financial, human or intangible harm." They include personnel and intangible resources such as position in the community as risks to be managed (Troyer & Salman, 1986).

Essentially, risk management is identifying and solving problems before they get out of hand, thus preventing being sued.

For a definitive discussion of the legal aspects of risk management in long-term care see *Preventing Malpractice in Long-term care: Strategies for Risk Management* (1987) by Marshall B. Kapp. Troyer and Salman's *Handbook of Health Care Risk Management* (1986) provides a broad statistics-oriented treatment of risk management.

Facilities must ensure that the environment is as free of hazards as possible to prevent unexpected and unintended injury. On average, during the years 1993 to 1999, surveyors judged about 80% of facilities to be adequately ensuring the risk of unintended or unexpected injury (see Figure 3-13). But study Table 3-12 and a very mixed pattern emerges. In 1999 some states' surveyors found that more than 40% of facilities risk injury-management programs that are deficient (Michigan and Mississippi) while in one state (Arkansas), surveyors found 0% programs deficient. Risk management appears to be highly subjective, but nevertheless highly important to the administrator of a facility.

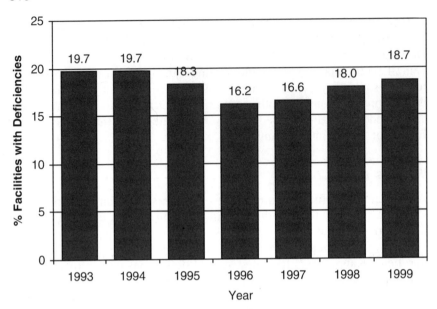

FIGURE 3-13. Accident hazards in the environment, U.S. nursing homes, 1993–1999.
Nursing Facilities, Staffing, Residents and Facility Deficiencies, 1993–1999, Department of Social & Behavioral Sciences, University of California San Francisco.

TERMS RELATING TO RISK MANAGEMENT

Civil liability. The three primary sources in health care malpractice suits are (a) failure to obtain effective consent before intervening in the life of the resident/patient; (b) breach or violation of a contract or promise, (c) rendering substandard, poor-quality care (Kapp, 1987).

Claims-made policy. The insurance company pays for the claims made only during the term of the policy and only for events occurring during the term of the policy (Kapp, 1987). (See occurrence policy.)

Durable power of attorney. Appointment of an agent who is empowered to act on behalf of the person creating the power in case of future incompetence (Maddox et al., 2001). (Ordinary power of attorney ends when the person creating the power becomes incompetent.)

Empty shell doctrine. The view that the facility merely provides a workplace for health professionals and has no corporate liability for their actions. Abandoned after Darling v. Charleston Community Memorial Hospital (1965), in Illinois, in which the facility was held liable for acts of staff.

Table 3-12. Percentage of U.S. Nursing Facilities with Accident Environment Deficiencies, 1993–1999

State	1993	1994	1995	1996	1997	1998	1999
AK	0.0	0.0	23.1	0.0	14.3	7.1	0.0
AL	14.9	24.6	19.2	15.9	13.8	11.6	22.2
AR	23.8	26.0	30.0	35.9	24.7	23.3	24.4
AZ	8.5	18.5	24.1	44.4	43.2	36.4	25.3
CA	32.5	35.9	26.0	27.8	28.8	31.7	33.0
CO	32.5	26.9	17.7	17.9	18.3	17.0	16.0
CT	11.5	7.1	6.0	2.6	1.2	4.4	3.8
DC	13.3	0.0	23.1	11.1	4.5	14.3	21.4
DE	18.9	20.9	27.3	45.9	31.0	22.2	14.7
FL	5.8	7.1	8.8	8.4	9.5	10.8	10.2
GA	18.9	18.3	19.3	13.0	10.4	17.4	19.6
HI	4.0	3.8	4.8	0.0	7.1	9.1	7.7
IA	10.6	10.9	6.8	11.0	17.4	20.8	21.1
ID	16.9	9.0	6.3	25.7	16.9	24.1	14.1
IL	39.0	40.5	36.9	30.1	33.9	30.2	34.8
IN	13.5	18.8	24.1	29.6	37.6	35.6	34A
KS	29.7	17.7	21.5	27.7	23.9	24.3	30.3
KY	5.0	1.5	4.3	2.5	7.7	16.4	21.6
LA	13.9	11.5	9.5	4.8	5.9	6.5	6.8
MA	13.9	9.6	8.1	2.9	2.5	2.3	3.9
MD	8.5	10.5	9.7	4.8	5.1	8.8	6.0
ME	20.0	19.8	15.7	8.8	17.6	15.3	21.1
MI	17.4	20.1	34.7	30.9	33.7	35.8	40.3
MN	17.6	15.0	15.0	5.3	3.9	12.7	6.6
MO	15.5	8.2	8.3	8.7	7.3	8A	8.7
MS	31.1	34.6	34.2	26.3	24.4	32.5	46.2
MT	20.0	26.0	10.0	18.3	5.3	8.7	4.1
NC	4.6	6.2	6.0	8.5	8.7	9.9	12.9
ND	6.3	0.0	2.4	1.1	2.7	6.8	2.3
NE	8.7	11.3	8.4	7.0	8.2	10.4	9.6
NH	12.1	10.4	5.6	8.6	2.7	5.3	4.5
NJ	1.9	5.8	4.0	3.0	2.1	4.2	1.0
NM	2T.5	31.2	11.7	6.3	1.6	13.6	2?.1
NV	9.7	22.5	19.4	25.6	7.9	22.0	25.0
NY	10.3	8.7	11.9	10.0	6.6	5.9	11.8
OH	30.9	31.0	32.9	25.8	22.7	21.5	22.3
OK	3.9	9.1	10.7	5.8	6.5	6.4	10.7
OR	19.9	12.0	14.0	8.4	14.5	8.4	7.7
PA	15.0	18.0	12.7	12.3	12.3	14.4	14.0
RI	18.2	6.5	6.1	9.3	12.0	15.7	8.7

Table 3-12. (Continued)

State	1993	1994	1995	1996	1997	1998	1999
SC	28.1	23.1	13.6	21.2	23.4	23.9	23.8
SD	25.9	29.2	26.1	15.0	30.7	34.9	30.6
TN	21.5	15.8	20.7	12.0	11.1	17.5	21.9
TX	24.5	25.4	20.4	13.3	13.3	14.0	13Z
UT	35.2	36.7	26.3	30.4	30.8	28.1	13.5
VA	3.7	10.3	'11.8	10.7	8.0	22	4.6
VT	22.0	5.6	12.5	5.4	2.7	29	9.5
WA	41.8	32.0	27.9	27.0	27.9	33.6	30.9
WI	15.2	18.3	16.5	9.8	16.3	21.5	13.9
WV	67.5	48.4	31.3	4.5	9.0	2.9	6.7
WY	32.1	26.5	15.8	13.5	22.2	37.5	36.1
US	19.7	19.7	18.3	16.2	16.6	18.0	18.7

Nursing Facilities, Staffing, Residents and Facility Deficiencies, 1993–1999
Department of Social & Behavioral Sciences
University of California San Francisco

Euthanasia. A "good" or "easy" death. Active euthanasia in the nursing facility setting is involvement of facility care givers in nonaccidental termination of a resident/patient's life (Evans et al., 2000).
Guardianship. Appointment by a probate court of a substitute decision-maker for an incompetent person.
Malpractice system. The purposes of this system are (a) the just financial compensation of innocent, injured residents/patients and (b) the maintenance of a high level of care by deterring undesirable provider practices (Kapp, 1987).
Occurrence policy. The insurance company pays for claims for events occurring during term or policy regardless of when claims are filed (Kapp, 1987).
Palliative care. Alleviating suffering even where "cure" of underlying disease is no longer possible (Maddox et al., 2001).
Resident/patient's rights. Sources—common law (judges' opinions) based on society's values; and specific statutes (legislative law resulting in rules and regulations defining resident/patient rights).
Standard of care. The duty to have and to use the degree of knowledge and skill that is usually possessed and used by competent, prudent, similar health-care providers in like or similar circumstances (Kapp, 1987).
Substandard care. Four elements are required for a civil lawsuit: (a) duty owed, (b) breach or violation of that duty, (c) damage or injury, and (d) causation (Kapp, 1987, p. 4).

3.10.5 Business-Related Concepts and Terms

In the health care field, the nursing home industry is second in size only to the hospital industry in total dollars received and spent each year. The gross income of the larger nursing home chains is in the billions. The following is an introduction to some of the vocabulary of the business of running what is a $100 billion-plus industry.

ADDITIONAL ACCOUNTING CONCEPTS

Activity-based costing. An accounting method that assigns identifiable costs and allocates common costs to specific activity areas in the facility, sometimes known as departmental area costing. This allows the facility to identify the profit contribution of each activity or departmental area (Argenti, 1994). Similar to or the same as the step-down accounting method described earlier.

ARR Accounting Rate of Return. A method of measuring the potential profitability of an investment. ARR is calculated by dividing the net income by the amount (or average amount) of the investment (Argenti, 1994):

$$\frac{\text{Net income}}{\text{Investment}} = \text{ARR}$$

American Institute of Certified Public Accountants (AICPA). This national organization of certified public accountants develops standards for its members and offers advice to such governmental agencies as the Securities and Exchange Commission (SEC) (Argenti, 1994). The decisions of this group usually become the standard of practice.

Allowance for bad debts. A provision a facility makes for uncollectible accounts receivable. On the balance sheet, net receivables—the amount the facility realistically expects to collects from resident/patient billings—is calculated by reducing the accounts receivable by the allowance for bad debt (Argenti, 1994).

Annual report. A detailed statement of the facility's financial position at the end of its reporting year, either fiscal or calendar. Annual reports, as described before, contain the facility's income statement, balance sheet, statement of cash flows, statement of owners or shareholder's equity, management's discussion and analysis of operations, notes to the financial statements, audit opinion, and other selected data. The Financial Accounting Standards Board (FASB) also requires reporting on all other financial activities, for example pharmacy holdings or any other business activities that affect the facility's financial status. (Argenti, 1994).

Audit. An examination of a facility's compliance with accounting standards and policies. There are four types of audit: financial, internal, management, and compliance. In the financial audit an independent certified public accountant examines the facility's financial records and gives an audit opinion. In the internal audit the internal financial officer studies the financial records to ensure they meet facility policies. The management audit examines management's efficiency, and the compliance audit determines whether the facility is meeting specific rules and regulations (Argenti, 1994).

Audit opinion. A report by an independent certified public accountant that gives the auditor's opinion as to the reasonableness of the facility's financial statement (Argenti, 1994).

Big Six. A term given to the six largest CPA firms in the United States. The rankings change over time, depending on the criteria used, such as billings and number of staff. In alphabetical order, the most recent listing is the former Arthur Andersen and Co., Coopers and Lybrand, Deloitte and Touche, Ernst and Young, Peat Marwick Main and Co., and Price Waterhouse (Argenti, 1994).

Certified Public Accountant (CPA). A title given to accountants who pass the Uniform CPA examination administered by the American Institute of Certified Public Accountants and who satisfy the experience requirements of each given state (not unlike the licensing of nursing home administrators through the NAB exam). CPAs are licensed to issue an audit opinion on a facility's financial statements (Argenti, 1994).

Change in accounting estimate. A revision of an accounting forecast or assumption about the facility's expected or experienced performance (Argenti, 1994).

Cumulative effect of a change in accounting principle. In accounting, the income statement account showing the effect of switching from one accounting principle to another. Cumulative effect shows the difference between the retained earnings reported at the beginning of the year under the old method and the retained earnings that would have been reported at the beginning of the year had the method never been changed (Argenti, 1994).

Extraordinary item. In accounting, an economic item that is both unusual and infrequent, such as the replacement of the emergency power generator, which might occur once every 15 years (Argenti, 1994).

Financial Accounting Standards Board (FASB). The independent institution that establishes and disseminates the generally accepted accounting principles (GAAPs) and recording practices. The American Institute of Certified Public Accountants (AICPA) and the Securities and Exchange Commission (SEC) both recognize the statements of the FASB. All practicing CPAs are required to adhere to FASB guidelines (Argenti, 1994).

Generally Accepted Accounting Principles (GAAP). The policies, standards, and rules followed by accountants in the preparation of financial statements and in recording and summarizing transactions (Argenti, 1994).

Materiality. In accounting, the relative importance of an accounting error or omission in a facility's financial statements. A $200 error in an earnings statement of $2 million income would be immaterial, while a $500,000 error would clearly be material (Argenti, 1994).

Qualified opinion. An auditor's report of a facility's financial statement pointing to some particular limitation, for instance, the inability of the CPA to obtain objective evidence of a certain transaction that might directly or inversely affect the facility's financial standing (Argenti, 1994).

Unqualified opinion. Sometimes known as a clean opinion, that is, the report meets all the GAAP requirements (Argenti, 1994).

Agency. A relationship in which one person acts on behalf of and under the control of another. The acts of the agent are binding on the person or business the agent represents. The nursing home administrator is the agent of the facility, thus the facility is bound by the agreements the administrator makes on behalf of the facility.

TERMS RELATING TO ASSETS

Attachment. A legal procedure in which a defendant's property is seized by court order pending the outcome of a claim against the defendant. The purpose is to gain control over property that may be used to satisfy payment of a judgement if the plaintiff's suit is successful.

Bad faith. Generally implies a design to mislead or deceive another. Good faith means being truthful and faithful to one's obligations in business dealings.

Brand mark. The portion of a brand in the form of a symbol, design, or distinctive coloring or lettering; also called a logo (Argenti, 1994).

Life Care Centers of America, for example, has a caregiver standing over a person in a wheelchair; Hillhaven (Vencor) has a rose or flower symbol above their logo.

Intangible asset. An item or right that has no physical substance and provides an economic benefit. The reputation of a nursing facility as the best caregiver in the community is a valuable intangible asset, for example.

Liquidity. The ability of current assets to meet the financial obligation of current liabilities. Having high liquidity enables a facility to take advantage of investment opportunities and to borrow capital or receive a line of credit at a more favorable rate.

Long term asset. An asset with future economic benefits that are expected for a number of years. Long-term assets are reported on the balance sheet as noncurrent assets and include buildings and equipment. A new central building for a life-care community may have a long-term expected asset value of perhaps 40 or more years to come.

Net Present Value. In corporate finance, the present value (i.e., the value of cash to be received in the future expressed in current dollars) of an investment in excess of the initial amount invested (Argenti, 1994). When a proposed project such as building a new wing has a positive net present value, it should perhaps proceed; when a proposed wing shows a negative net present value, it should perhaps be delayed or abandoned.

Note receivable. A contract to receive money at a future date. Notes receivable are reported on the balance sheet as either current assets (less than one year) or noncurrent assets (more than one year).

Off-Balance sheet. An item not reported in financial statements that nevertheless has an impact on the operations of a facility. An example might be an estimate of the monetary value of a strong reputation for quality that a recently purchased facility enjoys.

Present value. The current value of a future payment or stream of payments (Argenti, 1994). Present value is calculated by applying a discount (capitalization) rate to future payment(s). This is sometimes referred to as the "discounted cash flow method" or the "discounted earnings method" (Argenti, 1994). Its purpose is to estimate the fair market value of a potential investment.

TERMS RELATING TO COMPETITION AND RISK

Bankruptcy. Inability to pay one's debts, insolvency. Also refers to the legal process of Chapters 7 and 11 of the federal bankruptcy code, under which the assets of the business or individual(s) are liquidated, creditors paid, and the debtor given a fresh start. In a Chapter 11 reorganization, which is the dominant form (Argenti, 1994) under the bankruptcy code, the debtor's assets are not liquidated. Instead, the debt structure and business are rearranged, creditors are paid some or all of what they are owed under a restructuring plan, and the business continues to function without serious interruption. Under Chapter 7, the conventional form under the 1978 Bankruptcy Reform Act, all the assets must be auctioned or sold in order to pay creditors. A court-appointed trustee gathers and liquidates all assets, then distributes the proceeds to the creditors. In most cases, debts remaining after liquidation distribution are discharged. Generally, debtors at the bottom of the creditor ranking receive little or nothing. Attorneys usually refer to a Chapter 7 bankruptcy as a *straight* bankruptcy.

Better-Off Test. A method of evaluating the strategic impact of an acquisition or business venture on the facility's financial standing. The better-off test stipulates that the new venture must either gain a significant competitive advantage through its functioning or offer a significant competitive advantage to the facility (Argenti, 1994).

Cannibalization. The reduction of income in the sales of a product caused by the introduction of another similar product by the same facility or company (Argenti, 1994). A facility may decide to offer newer forms of physical therapy that reduce the use of current physical therapy methods. If the total combined income is higher using the new method and reducing usage of the old method, cannibalization is justified.

Caveat emptor. "Let the buyer beware." The purchaser buys at his own risk. In recent years, consumer protection laws and the Uniform Commercial Code have implied certain warranties in most purchases, unless the goods are bought "as is."

Competitive advantage. The elements within a facility's operations that give it an edge over its competitors. Building a new enlarged outpatient physical-therapy wing might give facility A competitive advantage over its competitors. If a competing facility B counters by building an even larger and more attractive state-of-the-art outpatient physical therapy wing, facility A is placed at a competitive disadvantage. These are calculations used in developing the corporate strategy to be followed by facility A.

Competitor analysis. The evaluation of the intent and actions of one's competitors (Argenti, 1994). This is part of corporate strategy. The information gained in competitor analysis is used to estimate the probable future actions of competitors, such as their future goals and assumptions about the marketplace.

Cost of entry test. A method of evaluating the strategic impact of the acquisition or start-up of a new business venture for the facility

(Argenti, 1994). This test specifies that the cost of entering the new venture must not exceed the future profits generated by that venture.

Debt-to-assets ratio. A measure of the relative obligations of a facility (Argenti, 1994). Generally, the lower the debt ratio, the more financially sound the facility is believed to be. The ratio is calculated by dividing total liabilities (current and noncurrent) by total assets.

Differentiation. The emphasis a facility places on some important product benefit or set of benefits that is valued by the entire market, but not offered by the competition (Argenti, 1994). Numerous facilities sought to differentiate themselves by being the only one to offer, say, subacute care or an Alzheimer's unit. These competitive advantages through differentiation (Johns & Saks, 2001) are usually short lived as competitors emulate and begin to offer the same services (Hitt et al., 2001).

Externality. Any incidental by-product (positive and negative) associated with a particular course of action chosen by a facility (Argenti, 1994). A positive externality for a facility that chooses to admit subacute patients from local hospitals might be an increased census. A negative externality associated with this course of action would be the necessity to hire additional staff and provide additional training for present staff.

Inflation. An increase in the general price level (Argenti, 1994). Inflation can be viewed as an increase in the cost of doing business or an erosion of the value of the facility's income. Inflation rates usually force facilities to offer higher salary increases in years of higher inflation.

Management's discussion and analysis of operations. A section in the facility's annual report required by the Securities and Exchange Commission that summarizes the reasons for changes in operations, liquidity, capital resources, and working capital available to the facility. The purpose is to assist readers of the financial statements in understanding the effects of changes in activities and accounting procedures (Argenti, 1994).

Perfect competition. A market so competitive that all its participants have virtually no control over the price (Argenti, 1994). Characteristics of a perfect market are thought to be (a) a large number of relatively small buyers and sellers, (b) easy entry and exit from the market, (c) a standardized product, and (d) complete information about market price. Few, if any health care markets meet these requirements.

Price elasticity of demand. The effect price change has on income (Argenti, 1994). This is calculated by dividing the percentage change in quantity demanded (sales) by the percentage change in price. In setting its rates for private paying residents/patients, for example, each facility must calculate the impact on census of any rate increases. Potential private paying persons might go to a competitor if rates at facility A are raised significantly above rates at facility B, all other things being equal.

Return on investment (ROI). A measure of the earning power of a facility's assets (Argenti, 1994). A high return on investments is desirable whether it is a for-profit or a not-for-profit operation. Return on investment is broadly thought of as net income divided by investments, but may be calculated using three different figures: return on assets, return on owner's equity, and return on invested capital.

Return on assets (ROA). Calculated by dividing the net income after any taxes by the average total assets, where average total assets are calculated by adding the ending balance of total assets of the previous year and the ending balance of total assets for the current year and dividing by 2.

Return on owners' equity (ROE). Measures the return that a facility has earned on the funds invested in it. These funds may be invested by shareholders (public or private) or may be, for example, the funds invested by a church in its own facilities. The ratio is calculated by dividing net income after any taxes by investor's equity.

Return on invested capital (ROIC). Tells how well a facility has used the funds given to it for a long time period. Invested capital equals noncurrent liabilities plus owners' equity, and ROIC is determined by dividing the net income after any taxes by the invested capital.

TERMS RELATING TO BENEFITS AND PENSIONS

Accumulated benefit obligation (ABO). The present value of the amount a facility would owe to its pension plan if its eligible employees retired during that accounting period (Argenti, 1994).

Charter. A document issued by a state or other sovereign government establishing a corporate entity (same as an article of incorporation).

Contract. An agreement between two or more persons that creates legally enforceable rights and remedies. Contracts must have the following elements:

- *competent parties* (of majority age and of sound mind)—in the case of some nursing home residents/patients, the courts decide on their competence to enter into a contract.
- *consideration*—something of value given in return for performance of an act or the promise to perform an act. A promise to refrain from an act (that is, giving up a legal right) may qualify as consideration.
- *mutuality of agreement*—the parties must agree willingly; often stated as a "meeting of the minds."

- *mutuality of obligation*—all parties must be bound to some reciprocal performance. A promise by one person to do something at the will of another person without any consideration (benefit) to the first person is not a contract.

An oral contract is an enforceable agreement that is not in writing or signed by the parties. Oral contracts are enforceable, but are subject to limitations. Various state statutes impose monetary limits on oral contracts for the purchase of goods, and almost every agreement dealing with real estate must be in writing to be enforceable.

Normally, no punitive damages are available for breach of contract. A person or facility suing for breach of contract can recover only what would have been received had the contract been fulfilled. Generally, the nonbreaching party can recover money damages, but cannot command performance of actual work. Ordinarily, attorney's fees cannot be recovered by the successful party.

Contractor. One who agrees to do work for another and retains control over the means, method, and manner in which the work is done. A subcontractor is one who deals only with the contractor for performance of some portion of the work to be accomplished by the contractor.

Defined benefit pension plan. A program of pension benefits that employees will receive when they retire. Normally benefits are based on a formula involving years of service and compensation levels as employees near retirement (Argenti, 1994). Whenever a facility establishes a defined benefit pension plan it must ensure that its pension fund has enough assets to pay the promised benefits. Delivering promised health benefits has become a major liability to pension plans in recent years because of the escalation of health care costs.

Defined contribution pension plan. A program designating the annual dollar amount an employer contributes to a pension plan. Under a defined benefit pension plan, specific benefits such as dollar amounts and other benefits are promised. Under a defined contribution pension plan, in contrast, the employer makes no guarantee of future benefits beyond the value of the dollar amount of the funds set aside in the pension fund each year (Argenti, 1994; Noe et al., 2000).

Employee stock ownership plan (ESOP). An employee benefit plan that gives employees shares in the facility. These may be voting shares, but more often are a special class of nonvoting common stock. ESOP rules change with revisions to the IRS code. Employers are allowed a tax deduction for part or all of their donations to ESOPs. Sometimes ESOPs are used as the acquiring mechanism, via bank loans to the ESOP, to achieve management buyout of part or all of a company (Argenti, 1994). ESOPs may borrow from banks and acquire additional shares in the company.

401(k). An employee retirement plan, sometimes called a salary reduction plan (Argenti, 1994). This plan allows employees to set aside a government- and company-specified percentage of their salary in a special retirement investment account. The IRS does not count contributions to a 401(k) plan as income. Contributions and earnings accumulate tax-free until they are withdrawn. Early withdrawals (before age 59½) are subject to full taxation plus a 10% withdrawal penalty. Companies sometimes match contributions. Some long-term care chains use 401(k) plans as a cost-saving device in lieu of a defined pension plan. One drawback to the 401(k) approach is that workers, especially when changing companies, often cash in their 401(k) plans for present needs.

Minimum pension liability. In accounting terms, an obligation recognized when the accumulated benefit obligation of a pension plan is greater than the fair market value of plan assets (Argenti, 1994), which must be shown on the balance sheet as a pension liability. This became so prevalent among American corporations in recent years that the Financial Accounting Standards Board instituted a new rule for accounting for pensions that resulted in companies taking up to billions of dollars of "losses" on their balance sheets to show this obligation.

Pension funds. The money set aside by an employer to meet the obligations under the pension plan. A pension fund is administered by trustees who actually pay the retirement benefits (Argenti, 1994; Noe et al., 2000).

TERMS RELATING TO COST

Acceptable quality level (AQL). The actual percentage, specified by administration, of goods in a lot of incoming materials that a facility will allow to be defective yet still accept the lot as "good" (Argenti, 1994). This applies to such areas like dietary where large deliveries of items such as baked goods or canned goods are received.

Alternative work schedules. A method of increasing worker flexibility by offering a number of different scheduling options. Job sharing by two or more employees is such an option (Johns & Saks, 2001). Nurses have for some years been offered plans like the Baylor plan under which a nurse may work long hours over a full weekend and receive a regular week's pay.

Cost-benefit analysis. A method of determining whether the results of a particular proposed course of action are sufficient to justify the cost of undertaking it (Argenti, 1994). If a facility wished to purchase a similar facility 50 miles away a cost-benefit analysis would assist in deciding whether the purchase should be undertaken.

Default. A failure to perform an act or obligation. A common example is failing to make a mortgage payment.

Deferred expense. An expense incurred in one accounting period that will benefit future accounting periods, also called a deferred charge. Prepaid insurance, as mentioned earlier, is a good example.

Economic order quantity (EOQ). A method of determining the optimum amount of materials that needs to be ordered on a regular basis (Argenti, 1994). The costs of possession (storing, pilferage, obsolescence, spoilage) are compared with the cost of acquisition.

Just-in-time (JIT). An approach to dealing with materials inventories that emphasizes the elimination of all waste and the continual improvement of the production process. This concept was developed in the 1970s by Toyota Motor Company in Japan (Argenti, 1994) to ensure that materials are replenished exactly when they are needed and no sooner or later. JIT is so widespread that traditional materials and supplies inventory is sometimes referred to as "just in case." In the nursing facility, however, nursing supplies for wound care, IVs, oxygen tanks, and the like are of critical importance and must be available when needed.

Marginal costs. The increase or decrease in the total costs that results from the output of one more unit or one less unit; also called the incremental cost (Argenti, 1994). In a nursing facility, for example, adding one more bed might trigger a state requirement for an additional RN on a shift, dramatically increasing the marginal cost of adding one more bed to a wing.

Materials requirements planning. A system of materials or supplies management designed to reduce or eliminate the need for excessive inventories of supplies by analysis of product needs and lead times.

Methods-time measurement (MTM). A system for measuring individual motions called micro-motions, such as reach, grab, and position (Argenti, 1994). One method of changing a resident's bed may take significantly less time than a second method, for example, or designing a facility so that no bed is farther than a certain number of feet from a nursing station might produce more care time.

Price controls. The use of government powers to keep a price either above or below its equilibrium point. Keeping the price of a product above the equilibrium is establishing a "price floor," such as setting the price for a bushel of wheat to ensure that farmers continue to raise wheat. In the nursing facility situation, however, the government has sought to keep the price of a product below its equilibrium level, called a "price ceiling." By paying only the lesser of usual, customary, or actual health care charges in Medicare, the government establishes a price ceiling. This normally results in cost shifting from Medicare or Medicaid residents' costs to charges made to private paying residents/patients.

Queue time. The time that a job or activity takes before a particular facility is available. The amount of time needed for housekeeping and nursing to "turn a room" to make it available for the next resident/patient is queue time that affects the occupancy rate a facility can achieve.

FORMS AND TERMS RELATING TO FINANCING

Additional paid-in capital. An accounting concept of the excess amount over par value that shareholders pay for a company's stock; usually treated as a donation (Argenti, 1994, p. 27).

Arm's length transaction. A business transaction at market-established prices between two unrelated parties (Argenti, 1994, p. 43). For example, a chain establishes and operates its own pharmacy to provide drugs to its own facilities. To be reimbursable as an arm's length transaction that chain must sell drugs to other nursing facility chains and other disinterested purchasers at the same price it "sells" drugs to itself.

Bonds. A debt obligation of a facility or corporation or other body to pay a specific amount on a stated date (Argenti, 1994, p. 66). Facilities usually issue bonds to raise capital for building or renovation projects. Not-for-profit facilities may often be allowed to issue tax-free bonds. Issuing bonds usually involves a very detailed and expensive prospectus that conforms with SEC-required information. Junk bonds are debt securities rated below investment grade by credit-rating agencies (Argenti, 1994, p. 242). Long bonds are 30-year United States treasury bonds or other bonds that mature beyond 10 years. Interest charges used to measure the market in corporate bonds are reflected in basis points: 100 basis points equal one percentage point of interest (Argenti, 1994, p. 59).

Borrowing base. The facility assets used as collateral to secure short-term working capital loans from banks and other lenders (Argenti, 1994, p. 70).

Capital. The amount on the balance sheet that represents ownership in a business; also called equity or net worth (Argenti, 1994, p. 83).

Capital asset. An asset purchased for use rather than resale, including land, buildings, equipment, goodwill, trademarks (Argenti, 1994, p. 84).

Capitalize. To classify an expense as an asset because it benefits the facility for more than 1 year (Argenti, 1994, p. 87).

Capital market theory. A set of complex mathematical formulas that strive to identify how investors should choose common stocks for their portfolios under a given set of assumptions (Argenti, 1994, p. 85).

Commercial paper. Short-term securities (2 days to 270 days) issued by corporations, banks, and other borrowing institutions to raise short-term working capital. Investors buy commercial paper as a very short term investment (Argenti, 1994, p. 99). Commercial paper is unsecured debt that can be sold at a discount or bear interest.

Cost of capital. The rate of return available in the marketplace on investments that are comparable both in terms of risk and other characteristics such as liquidity and other qualitative factors (Argenti, 1994, p. 120).

Disclosure. A necessary explanation of a company's financial position and operating results (Argenti, 1994, p. 151). Impending lawsuits and other liabilities must be part of disclosure.

Federal Trade Commission Act of 1914. The act that established the Federal Trade Commission (FTC) and gave it responsibility for promoting "free and fair competition in interstate commerce in the interest of the public through the prevention of price-fixing agreements, boycotts, combinations in restraint of trade, unfair acts of competition, and unfair and deceptive acts and practices" (Argenti, 1994, p. 183).

Leases.
- *capital lease*—a lease in which the lessee acquires substantial property rights (Argenti, 1994, p. 85).
- *finance lease*—a long-term rental commitment by both lessor and lessee that usually runs for the entire useful life of the asset (Argenti, 1994, p. 184). Usually the total of the payments approximates the purchase price plus finance charges. Most leases are net leases, under which the lessee is responsible for the maintenance of the property, taxes, insurance, and the like. In the nursing home industry most leases are known as net net net, or triple net leases under which the lessor's role is strictly that of a financier whose responsibility extends solely to financing the facility, assuming no liability from the operating of the facility.
- *leasehold improvement*—any refurbishment made to leased property, such as painting, reroofing, redoing the interior (Argenti, 1994, p. 255). Leasehold improvements (if a for-profit facility) must be amortized over the life of the improvement.
- *sale/leaseback*—a transaction in which a facility sells some or all of its hard assets to a leasing company for cash and then leases them back over a period of time (Argenti, 1994, p. 345). This allows for raising immediate capital while retaining control over the assets. A

cash-poor small chain might use this mechanism to obtain money to purchase additional facilities.

Letter of Credit. A bank instrument stating that a bank has granted the holder the amount of credit equal to the face amount of the letter of credit (L/C). This transfers collection risk from the seller to the bank. A "standby L/C" cannot be drawn unless the payee fails to perform or pay as agreed upon by the contract.

Leverage. In accounting and finance, the amount of long-term debt that a company has in relation to its equity (Argenti, 1994, p. 256).

Leveraged buyout (LBO). Purchase of controlling interest in a company using debt collateralized by the target company's assets to fund most or all of the purchase price (Argenti, 1994, p. 256). This has allowed small nursing facility chains to purchase much larger nursing facility chains.

Leveraging. the advantage gained by using debt financing to create asset appreciation (Argenti, 1994, p. 257). This is used by most purchasers or builders of nursing facilities which, in today's market, cost upwards of $4 million for a 120-bed facility. Buying a condominium with a small down payment and a large mortgage is leveraging, as is buying a nursing facility with a small amount of cash and a large loan.

Mortgage. A use of the value of a purchase to borrow money for the purchase of that property by promising to repay the debt on a scheduled basis. The interest rate on most mortgages is set relative to the prime rate (the interest rate established by money center banks as a base against which to calculate customer interest charges). Banks define prime rate as the rate of interest charged to their best commercial customers (Argenti, 1994, p. 313).

Notes. Borrowing money for an agreed upon purpose between a lender and borrower. A *demand note* is a promissory note with no set maturity date; the holder may require payment at any time. Notes spell out the principal amount of the loan and the interest rate and may identify a final date for liquidation of the note (Argenti, 1994). Promissory notes with a term of 5 to 6 years are regarded as medium-term notes (Argenti, 1994, p. 280).

Recapitalization. A revision to a company's capital structure (Argenti, 1994, p. 329), which may involve exchange of debt obligations for equity interests or exchange of one type of debt for another. Some reasons to recapitalize are to reduce debt service that will allow additional borrowing, to clean up a balance sheet prior to a sale or merger, and to increase tax deductions (by for-profit facilities) by substituting interest payments for dividends.

Securities and Exchange Commission (SEC). The federal agency responsible for regulating financial reporting (Argenti, 1994, p. 350) and for monitoring the use of accounting principles, trading activities, and auditing practices of publicly held companies. SEC requirements are issued as Accounting Series releases and Staff Accounting Bulletins.

Stocks.

- *Arbitrage*—the process of simultaneously buying a stock, currency, or commodity on one market and selling it in another (Argenti, 1994, p. 41). The price difference between the two markets gives the arbitrageur his profit.
- *Blue chip*—a common stock with a long history of dividend payments and earnings (Argenti, 1994, p. 65).
- *Book value per share*—the assets of a company available to common shareholders, that is, what each share is worth based on the historical stockholders' equity costs maintained in a company's accounting books (Argenti, 1994, p. 68).
- *Capital stock*—the shares representing ownership of a company—At mid-1990s Beverly (the largest nursing home chain in the United States) had 85 million shares outstanding and the nursing home chain Manor Care had 62 million shares.
- *Common stock*—certificates that represent ownership in a corporation. A variety of types of stock exist and are used by most nursing facility chains such as common stock, preferred stock (see below).
- *Common stock equivalent*—a security that is not currently in common stock form but can be converted to common stock—Executives, for example, are often given stock options, the right to purchase stock at a stated price over a specific time period, as a benefit.
- *Convertible security*—stocks and bonds that can be converted into capital stock at some future date (Argenti, 1994, p. 113).
- *Debenture*—an unsecured bond, normally in a subordinated position (Argenti, 1994, p. 133). Debentures often have convertible features or warrants attached that permit the holders to exchange their debenture or the warrants for common stock on a stated date or when specified events occur (Argenti, 1994, p. 133).
- *Garnishment*—a legal process through which a plaintiff can obtain goods or money belonging to a defendant, held by a third party, that are due or will become due to the plaintiff. Garnishment is similar to attachment.

A person who receives notice to retain assets belonging to a defendant is the garnishee. Thus, the nursing home may be the garnishee when a court directs the nursing home to pay over a portion of an employee's salary to a plaintiff to repay a portion of an employee's debt.

- *Grandfather clause*—provision whereby persons already engaged in a business or profession receive a license or entitlement without meeting all the conditions new entrants would have to meet.

- *Option*—a right that is granted in exchange for an agreed-upon sum to buy or sell property, for example a set amount of stock during some specified time period.
- *Penny stocks*—stocks of young public companies that are not listed on any stock exchange (see below) and typically sell at a very low price ranging from pennies to $10 per share (Argenti, 1994, p. 303). One major nursing facility chain did a reverse split in the mid-1990s (see below) to avoid being viewed as a penny stock.
- *Preferred stock*—a type of capital stock giving its holder preference over common stock in the distribution of earnings or rights to the assets of the company (Argenti, 1994, p. 311).
- *Price/earnings (P/E) ratio*—a measure of the company's investment potential, literally how much a share is worth per dollar of earnings arrived at by dividing the market price per common share by the primary earnings per common share.
- *Reverse split*—a procedure whereby a company buys back a portion of its outstanding stock (Argenti, 1994). One major nursing home chain, in the mid-1990s, reduced the number of outstanding shares dramatically by giving one new share for each four old shares held, thereby increasing the value of each remaining share.
- *Stock dividend*—a dividend paid to shareholders consisting of stock rather than of cash (Argenti, 1994, p. 365).
- *Stock exchange*—a place where securities trading is conducted. There are three major United States stock exchanges: the New York Stock Exchange (NYSE), the American Stock Exchange (ASE), and the National Association of Securities Dealers Automated Quotation System (NASDAQ). The minimum listing requirements for the NYSE are (a) publicly held shares of $1 million, (b) market value of $16 million for those shares, (c) annual pretax net income of $2.5 million, (d) at least 2,000 shareholders, (e) net assets of $18 million. In addition the company must engage a registrar and a transfer agent in New York City.

The American Stock exchange requires (a) 300,000 publicly held shares, (b) market value of $2.5 million for those shares, (c) annual pre-tax net income of $750,000, (d) 900 shareholders of which 600 must own 100 shares or more, (e) net assets of $4 million.

The minimum listing requirements for the NASDAQ are (a) 100,000 publicly held shares, (b) minimum of 300 shareholders, (c) net assets of $2 million, (d) net worth of $1 million, (e) two or more market makers, (f) annual fee of $2,500 or $.0005 per share.

These stock listing requirements are given because most nursing facility chains strive to move up the ladder to the NYSE. One midsize nursing facility chain, for example, was forced to list initially on the ASE, but worked diligently to become listed on the NYSE, which afforded it more status and net worth growth potential.

- *Treasury stock*—shares of common stock that have been issued to the general public, but are repurchased by the issuing company (Argenti, 1994, p. 382). A nursing home chain might choose to repurchase some of its stock in order to increase the value of its remaining shares.
- *Value Line Investment Survey*—an investment advisory service that tracks more than 1,700 stocks in 91 industries (Argenti, 1994, p. 387). There are a number of such investment services available, most of them at public libraries. If you are considering going to work as an administrator for a particular chain, visit the library and learn all you can about their financial position. This information can help you decide whether to interview with the company, and if so will enable you to appear well informed during the interview.

TERMS RELATED TO INCOME

Annual percentage rate (APR). A measure of the true cost of credit (Argenti, 1994, p. 39). APR yields the ratio of the finance charge to average amount of credit used during the term of a loan, or during the time money is owed to the facility in accounts receivable on which interest is charged by the facility after a specified due date.

Cash Cow. A facility or product that generates cash (Argenti, 1994, p. 88). The term, according to Argenti, was coined by the Boston Consulting Group as an element of its growth/market share matrix. The outpatient physical therapy department may be a cash cow for the facility if a large volume of private paying patients use the facility.

Cash Equivalent. Any asset, such as a bond or easily sold stock, held as an investment that can easily and quickly be converted to cash (Argenti, 1994, p. 89).

Cash Flow. The cash receipts less the cash disbursements from a given operation or set of operations for a specific time period. If a facility has $300,000 cash income from accounts receivable for a month and operating costs of $275,000, there is a $25,000 cash flow for that month.

Contribution Margin. The amount by which sales exceed the variable costs (such as supplies and labor costs) of a service. The money left over is available to cover fixed costs such as mortgages, insurance, and the like. A contribution margin can be calculated for each income-producing area of the facility.

Lien. A claim on the property of another person(s) as security for a debt owed. A lien does not give any title (ownership) to the property; it is a right of the person holding the lien to have a debt satisfied out of the property to which the lien applies. If a general contractor building a nursing home is not paid money due under the terms of the contract, he/she may seek to have a lien placed on the facility until the indebtedness is satisfied. Similarly, regular creditors of the nursing facility, if not paid within a specified period of time, might seek to have a lien placed against the facility.

Perceived Value Pricing. A pricing approach based on the buyer's perception of value rather than the seller's cost (Argenti, 1994, p. 304). A facility with a strong reputation for quality care may choose to price daily room rates above the prevailing market rate in its community.

Profit Margin. The ratio of income to sales (Argenti, 1994, p. 321). There are two types of profit margin: gross profit margin and net profit margin. *Gross profit margin* shows the percentage return that the facility is earning over the cost of providing services. It is calculated as gross profit divided by sales.

Net profit margin (also known as return on services rendered) shows the percentage of net income generated by each service-billed dollar in for-profit facilities. It is calculated by dividing the net income after tax by sales.

Rate of Return. The annual percentage of income earned on an investment (Argenti, 1994, p. 328). There are a number of ways to calculate rate of return. These are variously termed return on investment, return on equity, return on total assets or return on sales. Rate of return on fixed-income securities is usually calculated as the current yield, that is, the annual interest or dividend payments divided by the price of the security. Some bonds, for example, may have been purchased above or below face value and may or may not have an additional payout at maturity or when called before maturity. In such cases a *yield to maturity* rate of return is calculated, which assumes the asset is held until maturity.

TERMS RELATED TO OWNERSHIP

Article of incorporation. The instrument that creates a corporation under the laws of a state.

Business Combination. The process of associating two or more different companies (Argenti, 1994, p. 77). According to Argent, there are three forms of business combination: statutory merger, statutory consolidation, and acquisition. A *statutory merger* occurs when two separate companies combine in such a way that one of the companies will no longer exist: X + Y = X. A *statutory consolidation* occurs when two or more separate companies combine and both companies no longer exist and a new company is formed: $X + Y = XY$. A number of hospital mergers are of this nature, for example, the Columbia-Hospital Corporation of America combination of two hospital companies. An *acquisition* occurs when two separate companies combine in such a way that both keep their separate identities: $X + Y = X + Y$.

Core competence. The particular capabilities of a company that separate it from competitors and serve as the basis for growth or diversification into new lines of business. One nursing home chain, Manor Care, has been particularly successful in attracting and maintaining a large share of the private-paying-patient market in the communities they serve, possibly being that company's core competence (Hitt et al., 2001, pp. 113–114).

Corporation. An association of shareholders (or even one shareholder) created by statute and treated by the law as a person. In effect, it is an artificial person with a legal existence entirely separate from the individuals who compose it. A corporation may have perpetual existence: may buy, own, and dispose of property, sue and be sued, and exercise any other powers conferred on it by statute.

Normally, a stockholder's liability is limited to the assets of the corporation; thus, stockholders avoid personal liability for their corporation's acts. Corporations are taxed at special rates, but usually stockholders must pay an additional tax on any profits received from the corporation (dividends).

A small corporation earning a modest profit may elect to be taxed as a partnership (see Partnership below). Stockholders, in this case, avoid personal liability for the acts of the corporation and avoid double taxation. A corporation choosing to pay federal taxes as a partnership is called an *"S" corporation.* For tax purposes all income and losses of a corporation pass through to its shareholders.

To qualify for "S" status, a corporation and its shareholders must meet the following criteria: (a) it must be a domestic corporation and not part of an affiliated group of corporations; (b) it must not own 80% or more of the stock of another corporation, (c) not have more than 35 shareholders, and (d) not have any nonresident aliens as shareholders; (e) shareholders must be individuals, estates, or some trusts, not corporations or partnerships; (f) it must issue only one class of stock. Voting and nonvoting shares of stock are permitted (Argenti, 1994, p. 343).

Each state enacts its own corporation laws. Some states, like Delaware, give the officers and board of directors more freedom from minority shareholder controls and thereby attract unusually large numbers of groups who incorporate under their state's laws. Some types of corporations are:

- *De facto* corporations are those that exist in fact without actual authorization by the law. Three conditions must be met: (a) that a statute exists under which it could be incorporated; (b) that it behaves in such a way as to appear to be functioning as a corporation; and (c) that it assumes some corporate privileges.
- *Public corporations* are created by authorization of the federal government and the states to accomplish certain purposes. They include town, counties, water and sewage districts, and radio and television stations. The United States Postal Service and the Corporation for Public Broadcasting are two such entities.
- *Private corporations* are corporations created by private individuals for nongovernmental purposes.
- *Professional corporations* are associations of one or more professionals, such as physicians, dentists, or physical therapists, nurses, who become a corporation.

Courts may choose to ignore the protection provided to stockholders from personal liability, typically when it can be shown that the purported corporation is found to be the "alter ego" of a principal (person). When, for example, it can be shown that the purported corporation does not hold stockholder meetings, generally ignores the duties and activities associated with operating a corporation, and neglects other corporate formalities, the courts may ignore the stockholders' usual immunity from personal liability and assign personal liability to the stockholders for acts of the corporation. If the incorporation itself was undertaken to defraud, the courts may hold the stockholders and officers personally liable for acts of the corporation.

Decentralization. The diffusion of authority, responsibility, and decision-making power throughout different levels of a company (Argenti, 1994, p. 137). Beverly Enterprises, long the largest publicly owned nursing home chain, chose, a few years ago, to move its national offices from the West Coast to a central United States location and to give each region decision making power formerly reserved to the national office.

Horizontal integration. A growth strategy in which a company buys a competitor at the same level of services (Argenti, 1994, p. 215; Hitt et al., 2001, p. 535). Several nursing chains have purchased others in recent years, thus increasing the amount of horizontal integration of the industry.

Joint venture. A legal form of business organization between companies whereby there is cooperation toward the achievement of common goals between entities that were, prior to the joint venture, separate. A *contractual joint venture* is joint venture not created as a separate legal corporate entity. It is an unincorporated association set up to attain specific goals over a specified time period. An *equity joint venture* has two or more partners based on the formation of a legal corporation with limited liability and the joint management of it by the partners. Profits and losses are shared on the basis of their equity in the joint venture. In addition, there are *hybrid joint ventures* which take a variety of shapes.

Limited liability company or limited liability corporation. Companies or corporations that provide the flexibility of a partnership with the same kind of financial protection offered by a "C" (incorporated) corporate structure. Wyoming passed the first state law allowing this form in 1977, and over 40 states are now following suit. In 1988 the IRS ruled that it would treat limited liability companies as partnerships for tax purposes. The limited liability company provides liability protection for its owners similar to that of a corporation, but allows the limited liability corporation or company to be taxed as a partnership.

Limited liability partnership. A new form of partnership used by professional groups such as physicians, nurses, or physical therapists to limit a partner's liability to the partnership's general contractual debts, the partner's individual malpractice, and the wrongful acts of persons acting under the partners' direct supervision. Unlike the standard partnership, there is no individual liability for the malpractice of the other partners. About half the states have adopted this type of business formation. In some states, protection extends even to the partnership's contractual debts that exceed the value of the partner's interest (Lasser, 1995, p. 6).

Merger. A combination of two or more companies (Argenti, 1994, p. 281). The combination may be accomplished by the exchange of stock, by forming a new company to acquire the assets of the combining companies, or by a purchase.

Minority interest. An ownership interest of less than 50%. In consolidated financial statements, minority interests are shown as a line item in the noncurrent liability section of the balance sheet (Argenti, 1994, p. 281).

Partnership. A contract between two or more persons to pool resources and efforts for the purposes of conducting a business operation. Normally, partnership status requires an agreement to divide profits and assume indebtedness in some proportionate share. Unlike stockholders in a corporation, the partners do not have limited liability, unless it is a limited partnership—an entity in which one or more persons are designated general partners (who assume unlimited personal liability for the acts of the partnership) and one or more persons are designated limited partners (whose liability is limited to their investment). Limited partners do not share in the management of the partnership (Argenti, 1994, p. 258).

Privately held company. A company whose ownership shares, unlike publicly held companies, are not publicly traded (Argenti, 1994, p. 315). A privately held company may be of many forms including corporations, partnerships, proprietorships, limited partners, joint ventures, and limited liability corporations. The same accounting principles apply to privately held companies as to publicly held companies. However, reporting requirements from regulatory agencies such as the Securities and Exchange Commission and public stock exchanges do not apply to them. Hence, in most reports on nursing home chains and ownership, privately held companies' financial statements are usually not shown because they choose not to make them available to the public at large. Privately held companies do make their financial statements available to lenders, private investors, and, as required, some state agencies.

Product liability. The liability of manufacturers and sellers for products they place on the market that cause harm to a person because of defects.

Sole proprietorship. Ownership of a business by one individual. Before incorporation became popular among physicians, most of them were the sole proprietors of their office practices.

Vertical integration. Expansion by moving forward or backward within an industry (Argenti, 1994, p. 390). For example, nursing home chains frequently integrate backwards by owning and operating their own pharmacies. Some chains are integrating forward by owning and operating home health agencies.

3.10.6 Insurance Terms

Actuary. A person who computes insurance costs, usually for the purpose of determining rates to be charged—an especially important

function for the continuing care retirement communities that take
lifetime responsibility for their residents.

Annuity. A fixed amount of money payable periodically by an insurer
under the terms of an insurance contract. Normally, the annuitant
(the person receiving the payments) has no rights other than entitlement to payments for a fixed period of time. Often, nursing facility
residents/patients have insurance annuities that can be applied to
their costs of care.

Beneficiary. The person named in an insurance policy to receive the
proceeds or benefits under the policy.

Binder. A contract for temporary insurance until a permanent policy can
be issued.

Coinsurance. A division of responsibility for losses or risks between the
insurer and the insured. The insured individual might agree to pay,
for example, the first $50 of any claim.

Life insurance. Insurance that may be one of several types. Whole life
insurance policies can build cash value (i.e., can be turned in by the
insured for cash) and normally pay dividends (interest on the cash
value). Term insurance, on the other hand, has no cash value; hence,
no dividends. When term insurance expires, no value is left. Whole
life insurance costs more than term insurance. With computers, an
almost infinite variety of types of policies can now be offered as
variations on these two basic forms of life insurance.

TYPES OF INSURANCE

- fidelity or bond coverage of key employees
- pharmacy
- vehicle and driver
- workers' compensation
- property damage—coverage against fire, flood, earthquake damage
  to buildings, furniture and fixtures, building contents
- furnace and machinery
- business interruption
- accounts receivable—protection against loss of income from destruction of financial records
- comprehensive general liability or casualty against losses sustained
  by residents, visitors, or others, resulting from negligence not related to rendering professional services
- directors' and officers' coverage for acts done in their official capacities
- malpractice or professional liability coverage protecting against losses
  sustained by others, resulting from negligence related to the rendering of professional services (Kapp, 1987, p. 37–38)

3.10.7 Terms Associated with Wills and Estates

Administrator. A person appointed to transfer the property of one who dies *intestate* (without leaving a will) to those who succeed in ownership. The estate (or property) of persons who die *testate* (with a will) is administered by an *executor* of the estate, who is usually named in the will.

Codicil. See Will.

Decedent. The person who has died.

Competence. The capability of a person to make a will. A person is judged capable or competent if he understands the nature and extent of his property, the identity of the property owned, and the consequences of the act of making a will.

Estate. A term that originally referred to ownership of land, but now refers broadly to all real and personal property a person owns or leaves at death.

Incompetence. Inability to function within limits judged normal by a court of law. A *guardian* must be appointed if a person is found to be incompetent. The guardian must handle the incompetent person's affairs until the court determines that competency has returned, in which case the guardian is discharged.

Living will. Some nursing facility residents/patients make a "living will," which governs the type(s) of treatment to be given the resident/patient in the event the resident/patient becomes comatose or in a similar condition. Several states have passed laws establishing living wills as valid legal instruments. A living will has noting to do with disposition of property (Maddox et al., 2001, p. 611).

Probate. The process of proving that an instrument presented as a will is in fact the valid and duly executed will of the deceased person. Some states have probate courts to conduct theses procedures.

Will. A person's declaration as to how she wishes her real and personal property to be disposed of after death. A will may call for actions desired by the decedent (testator), but must dispose of some property, real or personal, to be valid. Originally "will" referred to real estate and "testament" to personal property. *Last will and testament* refers to the most recent valid will left by the decedent.

A *holographic will* is an entirely handwritten will. In some states a will may be handwritten and need not be witnessed to be valid. A *codicil* is a supplement or amendment to a will. Codicil literally means "to say along with." A codicil must meet the same formal requirements as the will.

REFERENCES: PART THREE

Allen, J. E. (2000). *Key federal requirements for nursing facilities* (4th ed.). New York: Springer.

Argenti, P. A. (1994). *The portable MBA desk reference.* New York: Wiley.

Evans, J. G., Williams, T. F., Beattie, B. L., Michel, J-P., & Wilcock, G. K. (2000). *Oxford textbook of geriatric medicine* (2nd ed.). New York: Oxford University Press.

Harrington, C.H., Carrillo, M.S., Thollaug, S.C., Summers, P. R., & Wellin, V. (2000). *Nursing facilities, staffing, residents, and facility deficiencies, 1993 through 1999.* University of California at San Francisco, Department of Social and Behavioral Sciences.

Hitt, M. A., Ireland, R. D., Hoskisson, R. E. (2001). *Strategic Management: Competitiveness and globalization* (4th ed.). Cincinnati, OH: South-Western College.

Johns, G., & Saks, A. (2001). *Organizational behavior* (5th ed.). Toronto, Canada: Addison Wesley Longman.

Kapp, M. B. (1987). *Preventing malpractice in long-term care* (p. 480). New York: Springer.

Lasser, J. K. (1995, July). *Monthly tax letter. J. K. Lasser's Tax Letter*, p. 4.

Maddox, G. L., et al. (2001). *The encyclopedia of aging* (3rd ed.). New York: Springer.

Orlikoff, J., Fifer, W., & Greeley, H. (1981). *Malpractice prevention and liability control for hospitals.* Chicago: American Medical Association.

Showalter, J. S. C. (1984). Quality assurance and risk management. *Journal of Legal Medicine, 5,* 497.

Troyer, G. T., & Salman, S. L. (1986). *Handbook of health care risk management.* Rockville, MD: Aspen.

PART FOUR

Environment: The Industry, Its Laws and Regulations

4.1 Origins, Overview, and Current Profile of the Nursing Home Industry

4.1.1 Origins: Long-term Care— A 400-Year Tradition

Long-term care administration is not a new phenomenon. It did not, as is sometimes perceived, spring suddenly into existence after the 1965–1966 passage of Titles 18 and 19, which amended the Social Security Act of 1937.

Every nation has its own tradition of providing care for the aged, chronically ill, and disabled that reflects the demands of the particular culture. Like other American institutions, the United States health care system was modeled on the English one, just as our legal system has its foundation in English common law.

EARLY NURSING HOME ADMINISTRATION

Throughout most of English and American history, until about 1850, little distinction was made between the long-term care facility and the hospital. The long-term care facilities in England were called hospitals, but their functions were more similar to what we know of as a nursing home. From the twelfth through the fifteenth centuries, nearly 700 shelters for the aged, the destitute, and pilgrims were built in England (Dainton, 1961). These institutions housed populations similar to those deemed long-term (or custodial) residents in today's nursing homes: the aged, those without means of support in their own homes, and persons with disabilities.

State Medicaid officials are concerned about inappropriate or unnecessary placement of persons in nursing homes. This has probably been the complaint of many a community that has found it necessary to look after those who cannot do so themselves. Before 1453, all of these facilities were associated with monasteries, in theory, but were administered by men appointed by the king and the local bishop (Freymann, 1980). Did administrators receive training for their jobs in those days? Probably so, in an apprenticeship system not unlike our administrator-in-training programs of today.

In 1536, King Henry VIII, in a dispute with the Catholic Church, closed all the monasteries and their health care facilities simultaneously. One of the most famous, St. Bartholomew's "hospital" (St. Bart's as it was called) in London, had been operating since A.D. 1123. There are no records, however, that St. Bart's had any medical staff during those first 400 years. Pressure to provide care for poor people forced the king to reopen St. Bart's in 1546. He took away responsibility for managing the facility from the bishops and appointed local citizens to direct such facilities throughout England. In this process of removing health care from the Church's charge, the king appointed what is believed to be the first recorded board of citizen directors of a public hospital, consisting of 30 leading citizens. This board decided that the reopened St. Bart's could accommodate 400 of the aged, 650 "decayed" householders, 200 idle vagabonds, 350 poor men overburdened with children (no mention of overburdened women), and 20 sore and sick persons (Freymann, p. 1980, pp. 21–22).

In sum, the board viewed the hospital as providing 99% long-term care and 1% acute care. The shift from chronic to acute care slowly evolved over the next 400 years.

During those years, physicians had little or no contact with what were being called hospitals. Medical care, such as it was, was provided on a sole practitioner basis to those who could afford to pay. In essence, physicians served primarily the upper classes in the patients' homes or in private clinics. Times have not changed much. The majority of nursing home patients today are recipients of Medicaid assistance; they are aged, chronically ill, and poor; and they have lost the ability to earn an income to support themselves or have not saved enough during their lifetimes to sustain them in their later years. The well-to-do usually remain in their homes or move to a continuing care retirement community that admits only those who have ample means to pay.

Nursing homes, like the hospitals, acquired the ability to "cure" or offer effective restorative care to patients in the same way as hospitals did during the late nineteenth and early twentieth centuries.

HOME HEALTH CARE VERSUS INSTITUTIONAL CARE: A 400-YEAR DEBATE

For the average person in most societies, to be very old or chronically ill is to be eventually without means of a steady income. These conditions are becoming ever more closely linked, and it is as much an economic condition as one of health.

An issue hotly debated in the United States Congress and the state legislatures is nursing home versus home health care. Which is better, less expensive for the state? Is health care provided to older and chronically ill persons in their own homes better and less costly? Or is it more frugal and at least as desirable to institutionalize them in a long-term facility and pay for their care where economies of scale prevail?

This controversy has its roots in the Elizabethan Poor Law of 1601. Queen Elizabeth I required each local community to care for its poor by providing cash and in-kind help to enable them to remain in their own homes. In the century that followed, in England and in its colonies in the New World the major mode of assistance to older person, the chronically ill, and disabled person was a program to allow them to stay in their own homes as long as possible.

Our present-day state legislatures and the Congress are now warning that projected increases in the number of older and chronically ill Americans in the early part of this century may bankrupt federally funded programs and state treasuries. When faced with the same issue early in the eighteenth century, the English government and our colonial predecessors decided to provide public welfare and health assistance only in institutional settings. In 1722, England enacted a new Poor Law that established almshouses, or workhouses, where it was hoped the aged, chronically ill, those with disabilities, and other persons receiving assistance could be cared for less expensively (Hunter, 1955). This was emulated in Philadelphia (1722), New York City (1734), and Charleston, South Carolina (1735).

1830 TO 1930: NURSING HOME CARE IS OUT—HOME HEALTH CARE IS IN

During the early nineteenth century the pendulum swung back toward providing in-home assistance to the aged, the chronically ill, and poor people. In England this was known as the Speenhamland System (Frey-mann, 1980), in which a minimum annual income was guaranteed to everyone—what Democrats have called the "minimum annual income" and Republicans have called the "safety net" through which no one should be allowed to fall. But these programs are expensive and suspected by many to be abused by persons who are not truly needy. As a result, the pendulum swung back toward a requirement that persons needing assistance move into institutional settings, where care was believed to be less expensive and less subject to abuse.

Between 1830 and 1930, when America was a land of great economic opportunity for all, the predominant mood was to insist that aid to the aged, chronically ill, and persons with disabilities be available only in what were called public workhouses.

These institutions fostered two trends that are important in the history of long-term care in the United States. First, they had infirmaries for the ill among their population that were the origins of the early public hospitals in this country. Second, as care for subpopulations in the work-houses moved steadily toward specialization, the basis for the current long-term nursing home population was established.

SEPARATING LONG-TERM CARE FROM ACUTE CARE: PRECURSORS OF THE NURSING HOME

To understand the process by which long-term care facilities and acute care hospitals evolved from the same institution, let us consider the Philadelphia Almshouse in 1734. Its operations included an infirmary from the inception. It was not until 19 years later that the first American private or voluntary hospital, the Pennsylvania Hospital, was opened in the same city. By 1795, 114 of the 301 residents/patients of the Philadelphia Almshouse were classified as sick (Freymann, 1980). Its medical functions were finally recognized in 1935. At that time a reorganization was undertaken and the name changed to Philadelphia Hospital and Almshouse (read: "long-term care facility" for Almshouse). In 1903 the hospital section became the Philadelphia General Hospital.

By 1920 the Philadelphia Almshouse and the Philadelphia General Hospital were officially separated (Freymann, 1980). From the original combined facility, two separate institutions had emerged: an acute care hospital and a long-term care organization.

Emergence of Specialization

The Publick Workhouse of New York City illustrates the slow emergence of health-care-services specialization from an early nonspecialized long-term care facility. It had been established in 1734, predating the New York Hospital, which opened in 1769. By 1825 the medical functions of the workhouse infirmary, which until then had operated without medical personnel, had been given administrative recognition when the first resident physician was appointed to its staff. At the same time, the name was changed to Bellevue Hospital (Freymann, 1980). Then began a process of specialization of care that led to the current structuring of our nursing home long-term population. In 1831 people who were blind were removed to specialized care; in 1848 the hospital assumed care of the acutely ill in addition to responsibility for children, those with mental retardation, epilepsy, and other infirmities; and those who were insane, aged, or chronically ill.

Subsequent removal of certain categories of patients to facilities that delivered specialized care occurred in the second half of the century, so that by 1900 the Bellevue Hospital had evolved into an institution providing care to older persons and those with infectious diseases, chronic illnesses, and infirmities (disabilities).

THE TWENTIETH CENTURY

Short-term acute care and long-term care for the aged and those with chronic illnesses had evolved as the primary functions remaining from what had begun nearly two centuries earlier as the public almshouse. This process laid the groundwork for the development of short-term acute care hospitals and long-term care institutions in the twentieth century. This was a response to the great strides in clinical medicine in the early years of the twentieth century. When physicians were actually able to cure their patients of many diseases, separation of short term acute car and long-term care into distinct facilities seemed indicated.

The first specific remedy in the pharmacopoeia of modern twentieth-century medications—Salversan, for syphilis—was discovered by Paul Ehrlich in 1907. In 1912 L. J. Henderson observed that "a random patient, encountering a random physician with a random disease has, for the first time, a better than even chance of profiting from the encounter" (Blake, 1959, p. 13). Astonishing progress was to be made through the rest of the century.

SEPARATING LONG-TERM CARE FROM SHORT-TERM CARE—TWENTIETH CENTURY

From 1900 to 1954, the age-adjusted death rate in the United States fell by 57%. This occurred in three identifiable stages: From 1900 to 1919, engineering and preventive measures accounted for a 1% drop per year; from 1920 to 1935 mortality decreased 0.7% per year; and between 1936 and 1954, with the introduction of sulfonamides and antibiotics, the decline in the death rate was 1.5% per year.

With the ability to cure many common diseases, the typical hospital rapidly evolved into an institution that focused primarily, if not exclusively, on short-term acute care. Some specialized in long-term care and some assigned a wing to long-term care, but the time had come for a more complete separation of the long-term care functions.

During these years, deaths due to infection were reduced from 33% to 4% (Freymann, 1980), with dramatic implications for channels of health care delivery. Until the appearance of AIDS, the health community thought infectious diseases, in the United States at least, had been conquered.

GENESIS OF THE CURRENT NURSING HOME INDUSTRY

Federal Government Reimbursement

With hospitals focusing more and more exclusively on short term acute care, pressure mounted for long-term support to older persons, those with chronic illnesses, and disabilities. In response, the United States once more tried giving financial support to persons in their home instead of having them occupy a nursing home or other institutional bed. It began when the New York Old Age Security Act of 1930 was enacted under the leadership of Franklin D. Roosevelt, who was then governor.

Like its federal successor, which would not appear until 1935, the New York Act provided cash income to persons in need of economic support in their old age. But it excluded those who were in public and private institutions. Similarly, its health care provisions emphasized short-term acute episodic care to the exclusion of direct payments for long-term care in institutions. Those needing such care were expected to pay for it out of direct cash assistance made to them through the Act. This was a step in the right direction, but these cash payments were usually not large enough to support the resident/patient in a full-time institutional setting. In any case, few institutions at the time were able to deal with this population.

Short-term hospital beds were far more available than long-term ones. More and more acute care beds were being built to match the ever increasing capacity of the medical profession to effect cures. Not much thought was given to the needs of patients with chronic diseases. Their care had traditionally been the responsibility of the states and of the cities and counties within those states. As life expectancy increased, so did pressures to develop a care system for this burgeoning sector of the population (Maddox et al., 2001).

The states, cities, and counties were unwilling to assume the economic burden generated by the development and searched for resources other than their own tax bases to meet the cost of this care. A partial solution was to come through judicial interpretations of a seemingly minor provision of the federal Social Security Act.

The Social Security Act of 1935. As a response to the growing numbers of aged persons who could not afford to pay the costs of living from their savings, Congress passed the Social Security Act of 1935. It amounted to an old-age insurance policy. Older people then were able, if they chose, to use the cash to pay for the first small nursing homes that sprang up. Today this legislation, primarily through the Title 19 and Title 19 amendments of 1965, provides a substantial proportion of the cash flow that supports the modern nursing home industry (Maddox et al., 2001).

Like the New York Old Age Security Act on which it was in part patterned, the Social Security Act sought to enable older persons, and subsequently those with chronic illnesses and disabilities, to stay in their homes by funding to support them. It also enabled them to choose to enter the small mom-and-pop nursing homes that became available. In its earliest form the act was almost entirely a cash assistance program, and the monthly Social Security check was to be the extent of federal governmental participation. This explains why the federal act, like the New York legislation, excluded payments to persons who were institutionalized. Similarly, no home health program, such as exists currently, was set up or envisioned.

Legislative and Judicial Origins of Today's Nursing Home Industry

By limiting Social Security payments to noninstitutionalized persons, the federal Social Security Act left to the states, counties, and cities the onus of paying for long-term institutional care for the aged, chronically ill and disabled. This seems to have been the intention of the Congress. However, the act did make federal dollars available for up to half the costs for noninstitutionalized care for the long-term care population. Under pressure to provide assistance for institutional care, local officials sought ways of making this sector of the community eligible for federal dollars, despite the original intent of the federal lawmakers.

BACKING INTO THE CURRENT SOLUTION

The solution (for the state and local officials) came in a series of court cases concerning persons in need of long-term institutionalization who had been placed by local officials in private homes for care. Often these were the homes of retired nurses or other persons seeking supplemental income. The courts ruled that these private homes or boarding houses were "nonpublic" institutions and therefore eligible for federal dollar reimbursement. In this way, state and local officials were successful in shifting a significant portion of the costs of long-term care from the local and state governments to the federal government. Once the federal government began systematically paying for long-term institutionalized care through the Social Security Act, the nursing home industry began an expansion phase that appears likely to last through the aging of the baby boomers—some time past the period 2010 to 2025 A.D.

4.1.2 Overview and Context of the Nursing Home Industry

PROFILE OF THE CURRENT NURSING HOME INDUSTRY

Every day more than 5,000 Americans celebrate their 65th birthday and enter the "elderly" sector of the population. In 1900, 4% of the population were aged 65 or older; in 1980, 11% were in that group. By 2030, 18% are expected to be 65 years or older (see Table 4-1).

Table 4-1. U. S. Population 65 Years of Age and Older and Percentage of Total Population: Selected Years and Projections, 1950–2030

Year	No. 65 or over in thousands	Percentage of U.S. population
1950	12,397	8.1
1970	20,087	9.9
1980	24,927	11.2
2000	.31,822	12.2
2010	34,837	12.7
2020	45,102	15.5
2030	55,024	18.3

Source: U.S. Bureau of the Census from "An Overview of Long Term Care," P. Doty, L. Korbin and J. Wiener, *Health Care Financing Review,* Spring 985, Vol. 6, No. 3, p. 69.

Table 4-2. U. S. Percentage Increases in U.S. Population for 10-Year Intervals, by Age Groups: Selected Years and Projections, 1950–2010

Year	All ages	65–74 years	75–84 years	85 years or over
1950-1960	18.7	30.1	41.2	59.3
1960-1970	13.4	13.0	31.7	52.3
1970-1980	8.7	23.4	14.2	44.6
1980-1990	10.0	13.8	26.6	20.1
1990-2000	7.1	–2.6	15.6	29.4
2000-2010	6.2	13.3	–2.4	19.4

Source: U.S. Bureau of the Census from "An Overview of Long Term Care," P. Doty, L. Korbin and J. Wiener, *Health Care Financing Review,* Spring 985, Vol. 6, No. 3, p. 69.

INCREASED LIFE EXPECTANCY

Increased life expectancy accounts for much of the change in the older population that is of the most direct concern to the nursing facility administrator and staff. Since 1900, life expectancy has increased from 46 years to 75 or more years. A greater number of people are reaching age 65.

Increased Proportions of the "Old-Old"

As a group, older Americans are growing older all the time. The 64–74 cohort, now referred to more and more often as "young-old," increased at approximately the rate of the general population during the 1980s and 1990s. Those 74 to 84 and 85 and older are increasing at twice the rate of the general population (Liu, Manton, & Allston, 1982). Thus, by the year 2000, a full quarter of older persons would fall into the old-old category (see Table 4-2 and Figure 4-1). The striking increase in health care needs of the age group 85 and older is dramatically changing the face of the nursing home facility population. Active life expectancy continues to rise (Evans et al., 2000)

Fewer Men, More Women

As the older population grows even older, their age group becomes more and more dominated by women. In 1900, men in all age groups outnumbered women 102 to 100, but by 1975 the ratio had reversed, with 69 men for every 100 women. In the 1990s this was reduced even further to 66 men for every 100 women. The preponderance of women is even more pronounced in the 75+ age group: The ratio of men to women in

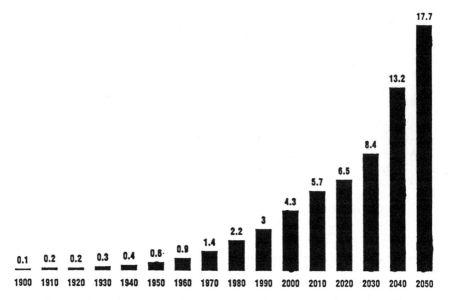

FIGURE 4-1. U.S. population group aged 85 and over from 1900 to 2050.
Source: United States Department of Commerce, Bureau of the Census.

1900 for this age group was 96 men for every 100 women; in 1975 it had decreased to 58 men per 100 women; and today, even fewer—54 men— are expected to be alive for every 100 women. It is no wonder that most of the residents in nursing facilities are women (Evans et al., 2000).

THE NEED FOR INSTITUTIONAL CARE

Most older persons live outside institutions. About 1 out of 20 persons aged 65 and over reside in nursing homes at any one time. For those over 75, however, the proportion increases to 1 in 10 (Vladeck, 1980). One of every five persons aged 65 and older will eventually spend time in a nursing home (Pegels, 1981; Evans et al., 2000).

A total of 1,640,000 older Americans are estimated to need institutional care, as were 710,000 working-age adults and 90,000 children (see Table 4-3). When community-based long-term care is added to institutional care needs, 57% of older persons, 40% of working-age adults, and 3% of children were calculated to be in need of such care in 1995 (see Figure 4-2).

Table 4-3. Number of Persons Needing Long-Term Care in Institutions and in Community Settings (in 1995)

Age -group	Numbers in thousands		
	In institutions	At home or in community settings	Total population
Children	90	330	420
Working-age adults	710	4,380	5,090
Elderly	1,640	5,690	7,330
Total	2,440	10,400	12,840

Note: Based on our analysis of information from HHS and the Institute for Health Policy Studies at the University of California, San Francisco.

Source: J. L. Ross (April, 1995), Long-Term Care: Current Issues and Future Directions United States General Accounting Office: Report to the Chairman, Special Committee on Aging, U.S. Senate. GAO/HEHS-95-109, *Long Term Care Issues,* p.8.

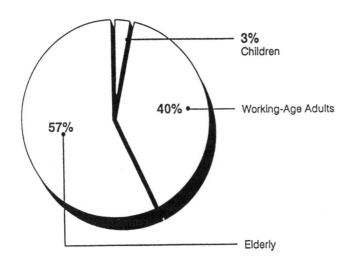

FIGURE 4-2. Need for institutional and community based long-term care, 1995.

Note: Includes people needing long-term care in institutions or in the community. Children are those under 18 years old, working-age adults are those 18 to 64 years old, and the elderly are those 65 years old and older.

Source: Based on our analysis of information from HHS and the Institute for Health Policy Studies at the University of California, San Francisco. From: Ross, J. L. (April, 1995). LongTerm Care: Current Issues and Future Directions. United States General Accounting Office: Report to the Chairman, Special Committee on Aging, U.S. Senate. GAO/HEHS-95–109, Long-Term Care Issues, p. 7.

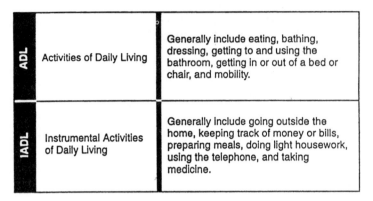

FIGURE 4-3. Definitions of activities of daily living (ADL) and Instrumental Activities of Daily Living (IADL), 1995.
Source: Ross, J. L. (April, 1995) Long-Term Care: Current Issues and Future Directions. United States General Accounting Office: Report to the Chairman, Special Committee on Aging, U.S. Senate. GAO/HEHS-95–109, Long Term Care Issues, p. 5.

INCREASING DEPENDENCY LEVELS AMONG OLDER PERSONS

As individuals age, they become susceptible to chronic conditions (explored in depth in part 5). Therefore, it is no surprise that older Americans also dominate the dependent population. Of people relying on others for eating, bathing, dressing, getting to and using the bathroom, getting in or out of a bed or chair, and mobility in general, approximately 7 in every 10 are older persons (Weissert, 1989). These are called the activities of daily living (ADL). Persons more able to care for themselves are described in the concept of instrumental activities of daily living (see Figure 4-3).

Older persons have higher dependency rates than the non-aged population, and aged women are much more likely to have dependency in mobility and personal care than aged men. Old-old nonwhite females are especially hard hit. Their dependency rates are double those for white males and triple those of nonwhite males. The population at risk for institutionalization is most probably those who need personal care assistance. Studies have shown that nearly 20 times as many nursing home residents need this type of assistance compared to those needing mobility assistance (Weissert, 1989). The extent of future need is illustrated in Table 4-4.

Table 4-4. Projections of Daily Volume of Long-Term Assistance by Source of Assistance, 1980–2040

	Source of assistance				
Year	Institution[a]	Spouse[b]	Offspring[b]	Other relative[b]	Nonrelative[b]
	Number in thousands				
1980	1,187	1,442	1,438	1,213	655
1990	1,623	1,801	1,950	1,610	880
1985	1,411	1,612	1,701	1,414	771
1995	1,861	1,953	2,232	1,814	1,003
2000	2,081	2,049	2,484	1,989	1,110
2020	2,805	2,976	3,392	2,728	1,530
2040	4,354	3,900	5,172	4,028	2,298

[a]These projections refer to a full day of care in an institution.
[b]These projections refer to the number of episodes of caregiving on a given day.

Source: Preliminary data from the DHHS, 1982 National Long-Term Care Survey; 1977 National Nursing Home Survey, National Center for Health Statistics, and Social Security Administration projections as referenced in P. Doty, L. Korbin, and J. Wiener, "An Overview of Long Term Care," *Health Care Financing Review,* Spring 1985, Vol. 6, No. 3, p. 71. .

4.1.3 Nursing Homes

FACILITY CHARACTERISTICS: DO SIZE AND OWNERSHIP MATTER?

In a word: no. Researchers have been unable to establish whether size or ownership affects process and outcomes in terms of quality of care (Harrington et al., 2000). Many researchers have unsuccessfully attempted to demonstrate that not-for-profits deliver consistently better care: Koetting (1980), O'Brien et al. (1983), Greene and Monahan (1981), Hawes and Phillips (1986), Ullman (1987), Nyman et al. (1990), Davis (1991), and Aaronson et al. (1994).

FACILITY TRENDS

Two trends continued over the period 1993–1999. Figure 4-4 demonstrates a slow trend toward increasing chain ownership and increasing hospital ownership. Chain ownership rose from 48% in 1993 to 56% in

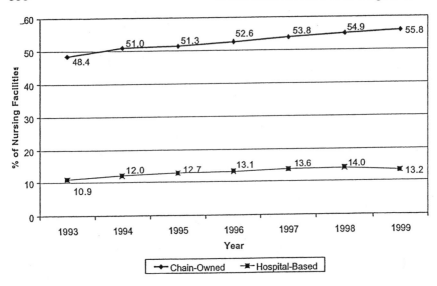

FIGURE 4-4. Percentage of chain-owned and hospital-based nursing facilities, U.s., 1993–1999.

Nursing Facilities, Staffing, Residents and Facility Deficiencies, 1993–1999, Department of Social & Behavioral Sciences, University of California San Francisco.

1999, whereas hospitals increased their share of ownership slightly, from 10% to 13%. Hospitals in some unknown proportion of cases built new stand-alone facilities and sometimes converted acute care beds. Major city and regional hospitals tended to build new competing stand-alone facilities while rural hospitals most often converted acute beds to nursing home beds or into "swing" beds that could be used for either acute or nursing care depending on need.

Number of Facilities: Slightly Down

The total number of Medicare and/or Medicaid certified nursing facilities declined very slightly over the years 1994—1999: from 15,288 in 1994 to 15,086 in 1999. There are an unknown number of noncertified nursing facilities. Some of these are fully private pay stand-alone facilities while some are in, for example, continuing-care retirement communities, but the number, though unknown, is small and may range possibly from 100 to 300.

Number of Beds: Mostly Steady

The number of certified beds in the U.S. varied slightly around the figure of 1,570,000 (Harrington et al., 2000).

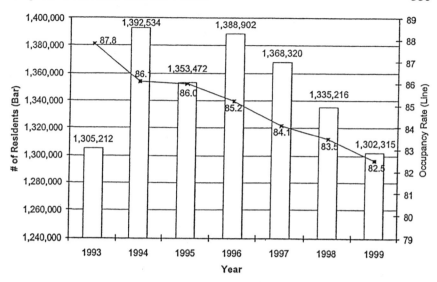

FIGURE 4-5. Percentage of residents and facility occupancy rates, U.s., 1993–1999.
Nursing Facilities, Staffing, Residents and Facility Deficiencies, 1993–1999, Department of Social & Behavioral Sciences, University of California San Francisco.

Average Size of Nursing Facilities

With some slight variations upward and downward in the interval, facilities averaged 104 beds in 1994 and 104 beds in 1999 (Harrington et al., 2000).

Average Occupancy Rates: Declining

Figure 4-5 shows an alarming decline from 88% in 1993 to 82% in 1999. According to Table 4-5 most states experienced a decline. This trend is alarming because, as we have seen in part 3, only with high occupancy (nearly 90%) can the average facility enjoy a positive cash flow.

OVERVIEW OF THE LONG-TERM CARE CONTINUUM

The American long-term care system, insofar as it can be called a system, is loosely interconnected. Each agency and program is separately authorized by various pieces of legislation. No single agency or program is authorized, or indeed able, to coordinate the various efforts on behalf of older persons. Although the act calls for and authorizes coordination,

Table 4-5. Total Number of Residents and Facility Occupancy Rates for Certified U.S. Nursing Facilities, 1993–1999

State	Number of residents							Facility occupancy						
	1993	1994	1995	1996	1997	1998	1999	1993	1994	1995	1996	1997	1998	1999
AK	496	601	526	626	535	601	597	71.7	89.6	90.4	85.4	84.5	89.0	83.8
AL	19,450	19,700	19,750	20,614	19,947	22,330	20,365	95.4	92.4	9Z8	91.5	93.4	9Z8	92.4
AR	19,802	19,990	20,888	20,104	19,919	18,061	16,058	84.5	83.8	82.6	81.3	80.1	77.4	76.2
AZ	10,522	11,554	9,281	12,339	9,758	10,983	7,046	80.9	76.9	76.7	81.8	75.3	77.9	74.9
CA	9P.445	103,000	97.828	99,989	98,412	89,825	87,165	86.2	85.2	86.0	84.1	817	82.7	81.9
CO	16,143	15,681	15,964	15,235	15,349	15,647	16,159	84.4	86.1	86.4	87.9	83.3	83.4	83.4
CT	25,813	27,879	28,248	27,352	29,435	25,683	27,210	91.9	90.1	93.0	93.9	9Z9	91.8	91.6
DC	2,668	2,357	1,918	2,137	2,964	2,089	1,801	92.9	76.0	97.1	86.8	95.1	96.0	90.4
DE	2,989	3,895	3,044	3,274	3,723	2,430	2,973	79.8	80.0	82.4	84.6	78.0	76.7	M6
FL	59,048	61,334	55,486	55,109	57,677	59,754	64,700	$9.6	85.1	86.1	84.5	84.4	82.3	83.0
GA	34,668	34,681	35,709	35,552	30,709	34,960	33,796	95.0	93.5	93.9	93.6	92-2	922	91.7
HI	1,470	2,059	3,215	3,204	3,395	3,651	3,224	92-2	96.0	91.1	93.9	91.9	920	91.2
IA	29,302	28,491	26,966	27,781	26,459	26,227	25,526	87.9	83.7	83.5	82-8	81.6	8ZO	80.0
ID	4,233	4,897	4,870	4,462	4,340	4,533	4,459	82.7	84.6	83.8	83.5	76.2	77A	74.8
IL	77,837	78,032	82,876	83,230	81,724	80,504	81,459	83.8	81.6	80.7	79.1	78.6	77.6	76.0
IN	28,471	40,144	41,217	42,178	42,461	41,169	38,949	77.1	73.7	73.9	73.3	72.0	70.5	70.1
KS	25,496	21,503	23,178	20,503	20,820	22,765	21,777	86.6	83.6	93.8	81.3	80.8	82.2	81.7
KY	19,383	18,216	16,828	20,531	19,074	22,181	20,658	89.3	87.1	88.1	89.1	88.9	89.3	90.0
LA	28,947	29,500	31,763	30,791	30,799	30,922	31,678	85.0	85.4	85.3	82.9	81.4	79-6	78.1
MA	44,411	45,529	43,254	44,076	48,493	44,232	42,803	915	90.4	89.8	90.3	89.4	89.1	88.7
MD	21,943	22,884	20,923	22,491	21,832	16,441	13,790	89.2	86.6	88-2	86.3	83.1	81.9	826
ME	8,034	8,909	7,135	7,812	7,645	6,897	6,676	95.2	93.4	90.8	87.7	87.8	87A	89.5
MI	38,689	41,622	36,582	40,959	40,357	38,032	39,226	90-4	87.6	88.0	86.1	86.9	64.6	84.4
MN	41,489	33,714	36,166	33,651	36,159	36,196	35,526	94.1	93.2	93.7	91.6	92-5	91.0	89.7
MO	33,492	38,583	35,841	36,303	39,236	34,801	35,330	78.8	76.6	74.4	74.5	73.5	72-6	71.0
MS	14,617	14,059	16,089	15,012	15,397	15,717	14,573	96.2	94.8	94.7	94.9	93.5	93.3	94.4
MT	6,030	6,311	6,377	5,628	5,694	5,508	5,609	90.7	89.4	88.2	86.5	83.2	81.7	79.0
NC	31.605	32,557	35,423	33,911	34,770	34,882	33,625	91.5	89.2	93.5	94.3	93.8	91.8	89.8

Table 4-5. (Continued)

State	Number of residents							Facility occupancy						
	1993	1994	1995	1996	1997	1998	1999	1993	1994	1995	1996	1997	1998	1999
ND	6.671	6,450	6.372	6,782	5,649	6,569	6,241	95.3	95.9	96.1	95.3	93.7	93.1	91.4
NE	15.240	15,725	15.517	15,583	15,297	15,057	14,491	89.7	90.2	88.5	88.0	85.9	85.2	83.6
NH	5,659	5,938	6,520	6,532	6,889	6,702	5,631	90.8	90.8	93.1	93.9	93.1	92.5	91.0
NJ	36.283	39.894	40,718	41.529	39,516	39,089	25,453	93.2	91.8	92.6	92-8	91.8	90.7	88.5
NM	5,652	5,425	5,5a8	5,808	4,522	4,989	6,258	88.9	85.1	85.9	84.0	83.7	86.3	88.4
NV	2,668	3.592	3,213	3,208	2,743	3,128	3,100	88.6	90.2	88.8	89.5	89.0	84A	65.1
NY	84.499	101,421	88,160	93,688	87,959	91,264	90,930	96.7	95.0	95.1	95.7	95.6	95.7	94.9
OH	70,611	73,767	72,540	80,378	75,505	75,303	66,696	85.9	83.1	82.8	80.7	80.6	80.0	78.4
OK	21,939	2Z,129	24,999	24,403	22,930	17,656	17,335	79.7	78.1	77.8	76.0	72-9	7Z4	71.2
OR	11,260	11,062	10,807	10,T79	10,491	10,497	9,382	85.0	84.6	83.2	81.2	79.8	78.5	75.2
PA	75,706	83,131	73,849	81,770	84,504	82,239	81,108	90.2	90.9	91.1	90.7	902	89.7	882
RI	7,200	9,102	7,792	8.330	8,617	8,293	8,326	93.9	95.3	91.8	93-2	91.7	89.2	87.7
SC	12.389	11,723	13,625	14,648	15,172	14,017	12,673	86.8	86.4	87.2	88.1	86.8	86.0	87.2
SD	7,583	7,377	7,658	6.795	6,641	5,778	5,103	95.9	96.0	94.6	94.7	94.1	923	91.5
TN	31,820	31,315	30,889	33,533	33,864	34,887	34,666	92.7	90.7	90.4	90.9	90.4	89.8	89.6
TX	63,745	84,795	81,822	82,556	79,603	76,125	79,898	76.4	73.2	722	71.0	70.2	68.2	68.2
UT	5,544	5,809	4,588	5,507	5,746	5,436	4,300	81.0	8ZI	81.8	81.9	79.1	77.4	77.8
VA	25,357	27,236	25,088	2S,965	23,861	22,705	24,934	92.6	93.6	94.1	91A	90.9	90.3	89.2
VT	3,274	1,276	3,280	2,899	2,939	2,486	3,091	92.8	95.7	97.0	94.2	9&9	89.2	90.1
WA	23,568	23,650	22,596	21,935	21,329	20,652	19,978	89.7	89.2	86.7	84.8	82.0	81.9	81.1
WI	43.060	41,406	42,466	40,606	39,627	37,873	37,778	91.7	91.7	91.0	89.9	88.4	86.9	84.4
WV	6,257	10,139	5,312	8,230	5,419	4,917	9,880	94.5	93.4	94.9	93.0	69.8	90.4	91.1
WY	1.734	2,490	2,731	2,584	2,414	2,633	2,303	82.9	88.8	87.4	83.8	83.5	83.4	81.6
US	1,305,212	1,392,534	1,353,472	1,388,902	1,368,320	1,335,216	1,302,315	87.8	86.1	86.0	85.2	84.1	83.5	82.5

Nursing Facilities, Staffing, Residents and Facility Deficiencies, 1993-1999
Department of Social & Behavioral Sciences
University of California San Francisco

in reality officials of the Older Americans Act have not been empowered to bring this about (Maddox et al., 2001).

One result has been that older Americans must largely fend for themselves in seeking services in most communities. One proposed remedy for this situation is called "case management," which is the assignment of each older person in need of an assistance program to a specific caseworker, who will help that individual plan and carry out a care program composed of services from a number of different agencies (Maddox et al., 2001; Steinberg & Carter, 1983). This is, in fact, what employees in departments of social services and the Area Agencies on Aging attempt to do. However, funds are insufficient to employ enough staff to assist all older Americans who need this type of assistance, and most of them are left to fend for themselves. In any event, case management can occur primarily if the clients can reach or come under the guidance of an agency in the first place.

Figure 4-6 describes the major sources of services available to older Americans moving from the least restrictive to the most restrictive.

The nursing facility plays at least two major roles in this continuum. First, it may be simultaneously providing rehabilitative services to almost anyone receiving a combination of long-term services. It is estimated that 25% of all older persons use the services of a nursing facility at some point. Second, the nursing facility is the major provider of intensive services for persons no longer able to care for themselves and in need of nursing care on a 24-hour basis. It is estimated that at any one point in time, 5% of all older persons are residents/patients in nursing facilities.

An overview of the major federal programs supporting long-term care services for older persons and persons with disabilities, fiscal year 1993, is presented in Table 4-6, which gives the programs, their objectives, fiscal year 1993 funding levels, administrators of the programs, and the services offered.

HOME- AND COMMUNITY-BASED LONG-TERM CARE OPTIONS

Table 4-7 provides an overview of various types of services offered under home- and community-based services in 1995. Dramatic growth in the number of home health care agencies during the years 1990—1997 increased competition for the typical nursing home patient. However, the number of home health care agencies declined after the Balanced Budget Act of 1997 required prospective payments for care given, thereby drastically reducing cash flow to home health agencies.

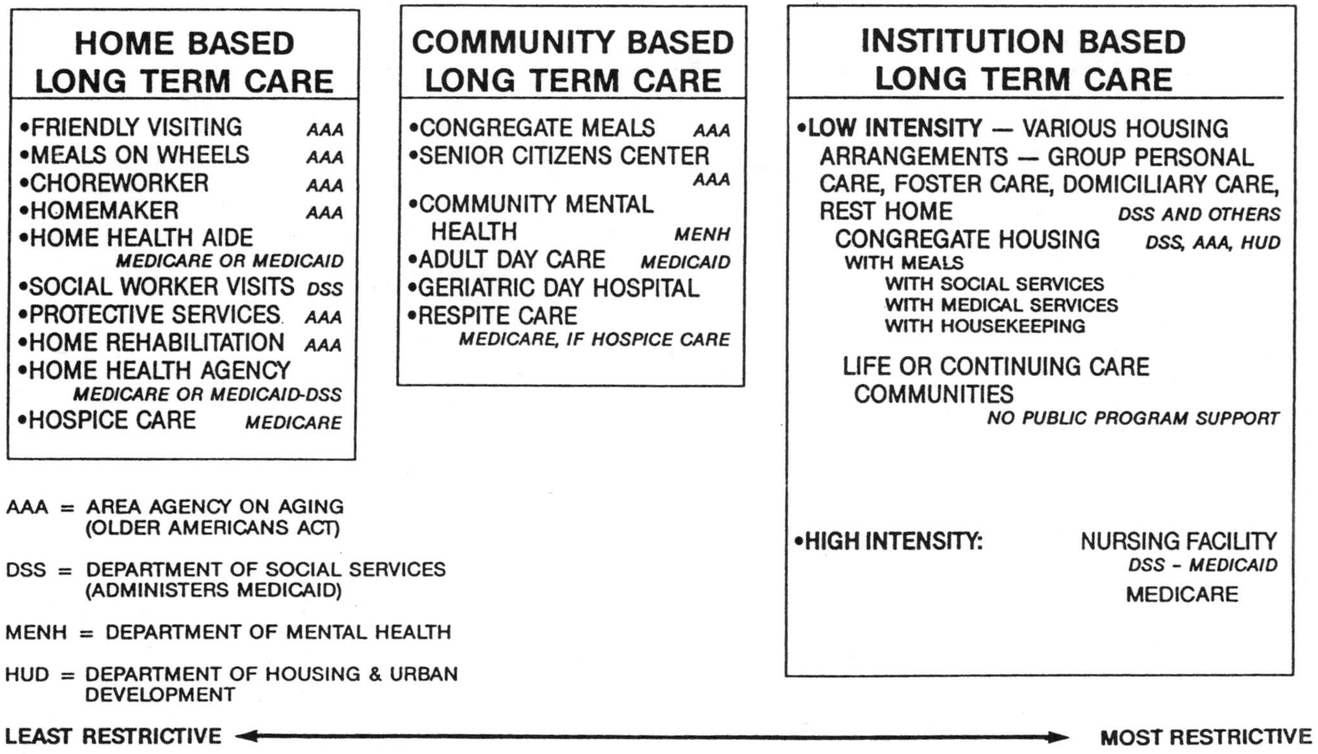

HOME BASED LONG TERM CARE

- FRIENDLY VISITING   *AAA*
- MEALS ON WHEELS   *AAA*
- CHOREWORKER   *AAA*
- HOMEMAKER   *AAA*
- HOME HEALTH AIDE
          MEDICARE OR MEDICAID
- SOCIAL WORKER VISITS   *DSS*
- PROTECTIVE SERVICES   *AAA*
- HOME REHABILITATION   *AAA*
- HOME HEALTH AGENCY
       MEDICARE OR MEDICAID-DSS
- HOSPICE CARE   *MEDICARE*

COMMUNITY BASED LONG TERM CARE

- CONGREGATE MEALS   *AAA*
- SENIOR CITIZENS CENTER
            AAA
- COMMUNITY MENTAL
     HEALTH   *MENH*
- ADULT DAY CARE   *MEDICAID*
- GERIATRIC DAY HOSPITAL
- RESPITE CARE
      MEDICARE, IF HOSPICE CARE

INSTITUTION BASED LONG TERM CARE

- LOW INTENSITY — VARIOUS HOUSING
  ARRANGEMENTS — GROUP PERSONAL
  CARE, FOSTER CARE, DOMICILIARY CARE,
  REST HOME   *DSS AND OTHERS*
     CONGREGATE HOUSING   *DSS, AAA, HUD*
       WITH MEALS
         WITH SOCIAL SERVICES
         WITH MEDICAL SERVICES
         WITH HOUSEKEEPING
     LIFE OR CONTINUING CARE
     COMMUNITIES
        NO PUBLIC PROGRAM SUPPORT

- HIGH INTENSITY: NURSING FACILITY
                DSS - MEDICAID
                MEDICARE

AAA = AREA AGENCY ON AGING
       (OLDER AMERICANS ACT)

DSS = DEPARTMENT OF SOCIAL SERVICES
       (ADMINISTERS MEDICAID)

MENH = DEPARTMENT OF MENTAL HEALTH

HUD = DEPARTMENT OF HOUSING & URBAN
       DEVELOPMENT

LEAST RESTRICTIVE →   ← MOST RESTRICTIVE

FIGURE 4-6. Overview of the long-term-care continuum.

Table 4-6. Major Federal Program Supporting Long-Term-Care Services for Older Individuals

Program	Objectives	Fiscal year 1993 federal spending (billions)*	Administration	Long-term-care services
Medicaid/Title XIX of the Social Security Act	To pay for medical assistance for certain low-income persons	Total: $77.4 Long-term care: $24.7 (estimated)	Federal: HCFA/HHS State: State Medicaid Agency	Nursing home care, home, and community-based health and social services, facilities for persons with mental retardation, chronic-care hospitals
Medicare/Title XVIII of the Social Security Act	To pay for acute medical cut for the aged and selected disabled	Total: $138.8 Long-term care: $15.8 (Estimated)	Federal: HCFA/HHS State: none	Home health visits, limited skilled nursing facility care
Older Americans Act	To foster development of a comprehensive and coordinated service system to serve older individuals	Total: $1.4 Long-term care: $.8	Federal: Administration on Aging/Office of Human Development, HHS State: State Agency on Aging	Nutrition services, home- and community-based social services, protective services, and long-term care ombudsman
Rehabilitation Act	To promote and support vocational rehabilitation and independent living services for those with disabilities	Total: $2.2 Long-term care: $1	Federal: Office of Special Education and Rehabilitative Services/Mepartment of Education State: State Vocational Rehabilitation Agencies	Rehabilitation services, attendant and personal care, centers for independent living
Social Services Block Grant/Title XX of the Social Security Act	To assist families and individuals in maintaining self-sufficiency and independence	Total: $2.8 Long-term care: (not available)	Federal: Office of Human Development Services, HHS State: State Social Services or Human Resources Agency; other state agencies may administer part of Title XX funds for certain groups; for example, State Agency on Aging	Services provided at the states' discretion, may include long-term care

*Data represent total fiscal year 1993 obligations as reported in the _Budget of United States Government, Appendix Fiscal Year 1995,_ except for estimates of Medicare and Medicaid long-term-care spending. These figures are estimates for 1993 from the Assistant Secretary for Planning and Evaluation, HHS. Under the Medicaid program, states contributed an estimated $19 billion in support of long-term care in addition to the federal share of $24.7 billion.

Table 4-7. Examples of Home- and Community-Based Services

Service	Description
Case management	Assists beneficiaries in getting medical, social, educational, and other services.
Personal care	Includes bathing, dressing. ambulation, feeding, grooming,and some household services such as meal preparation and shopping.
Adult day care	Includes personal care and supervision and may include physical, occupational, and speech therapies. Also provides socialization and recreational activities adapted to compensate for any physical or mental impairments.
Respite care	Provides relief to the primary caregiver of a chronically ill or disabled beneficiary. By providing services in the beneficiary's or provider's home or in other settings, respite care allows the primary caregiver to be absent for a time.
Homemaker	Assists beneficiaries with general household activities and may include cleaning, laundry, meal planning, grocery shopping, meal preparation, transportation to medical services, and bill paying.

Source: J. L. Ross (April, 1995), Long-Term Care: Current Issues and Future Directions. United States General Accounting Office: Report to the Chairman, Special Committee on Aging, U.S. Senate. GAO/HES-95-109, *Long Term Care Issues,* p. 4.

HOME-BASED OPTIONS

Friendly Visiting

Both the Area Agency on Aging and local volunteer groups arrange for regular visits to older persons living alone. This offers both needed social contact and continuous monitoring of these individuals.

Meals on Wheels

Title 3c of the Older Americans Act pays for home-delivered meals. To qualify, an organization must deliver meals (usually only the noon meal) on each of 5 days or more per week and meet certain standards, including providing one-third of daily nutritional requirements. As a rule, the Area Agency on Aging contracts with groups to provide these meals. Nursing facilities frequently offer Meals on Wheels, both as a public service and as a contact mechanism with potential applicants. The dietary department of the nursing facility automatically meets the various requirements of the program through preparing food for its residents.

Chore Workers and Homemakers

Area Agency on Aging subcontractors offer the services of persons who will come into older persons' homes to perform specific tasks. Chore workers usually do window washing or other less routine tasks. The homemaker visits on a more regular basis and performs housekeeping tasks such as dusting, dishwashing, and laundry.

Home Health Aide

The home health aide, in contrast to the homemaker and chore worker, is expected to perform only health-specific tasks, such as administering medicines, changing bandages, and the like. The home health aide is paid from Medicaid or Medicare funds, not by the Area Agency on Aging. A home health agency can send such an aide if the older person is receiving Medicare services in the home for a specific illness or injury. Over the past few years local Medicaid offices increasingly have been permitted to use Medicaid funds to pay for services (DHHS) designed to prevent or postpone institutionalizing older persons. Originally, these were called Title 19 waivers, for which states had to apply.

In 1984 the Department of Health and Human Services authorized all Medicaid programs to offer a variety of services similar to those available under the Older Americans Act if they were conducive to postponement or prevention of institutionalization. Usually, these services will be funded for up to three quarters of the costs of institutionalizing the client.

Social Worker Visits

The local department of social services, under Title 20 or other authorizations, is permitted to pay for social worker visits to the homes of older persons. This is similar to a social worker or case worker visiting any other client.

Protective Services and Home Rehabilitation Services

The Area Agency on Aging or its subcontractor is authorized to assist older persons to bring their homes up to minimum standards and to provide added security measures to reduce the possibility of break-ins.

Home health Care

Home health care agencies are creating increased competition to free-standing nursing facilities. In the mid-1960s, the federal government fueled an exponential growth in nursing facilities through its funding legislation. Currently, federal (and state) support is resulting in increasing numbers of home health care agencies on the assumption, probably erroneous, that they can provide care more inexpensively than the nursing facility.

An older person is entitled to receive home health care through any one of three programs, all under the Social Security Act: Medicare Part A, Medicare Part B and Medicaid.

Services Under Medicare Part A. Unlimited home health visits at no cost are available to any Medicare recipient hospitalized under Part A and evaluated to need posthospital home health care for the final DRG diagnosis.

Services under Medicare Part B. Unlimited visits, at 80% of cost, are available to persons covered by Medicare Part B who are found to need part-time health care in their home for the treatment of an illness or injury. No prior hospitalization is required, but four conditions must be met: (a) the care must include part-time nursing care, physical therapy, or speech therapy; (b) the client must be confined to his or her home; (c) a doctor must diagnose the need and design the plan; and (d) the agency must participate in Medicare.

Medicare does not cover general household services, meal preparation, shopping, assistance in bathing or dressing, or other home assistance to meet personal, family, or domestic needs (DHHS, 1985). Thus, to keep an ailing older adult who requires various types of home assistance functioning, several agencies, with separate priorities and interests, must be coordinated by the client or by a friend or a caseworker acting in his or her behalf. During the period from 1966 (the year Congress authorized Medicare to pay for home care) to 1988, the number of home health care agencies rose from 1,000 in 1966 to 10,850 in 1988. Home health care agencies are increasingly able to care for persons needing services similar to the skilled nursing facility (Simon-Rusinowitz & Hofland, 1993). A cost-effectiveness study by Greene, Lively and Ondrich (1993) found that 41% of persons studied could be effectively cared for outside the nursing facility (p. 179). There has been a steady movement toward increasing utilization of home health care (Manton, Stallard, & Woodbury, 1994). In 1995 the American Academy of Medical Administrators formed a division for home health care executives, further recognition of the maturing of this field (Shriver, 1995).

In 1982, 1.1 million Americans were receiving home health care; by 1988 the number had risen to 4 million. By 1993 there were 7,400 home health care agencies of which 37% were proprietary, 43% nonprofit, and 20% government and other. A high percentage were certified by Medicare (84%) and Medicaid (83%) (Strahan, 1994). Of all patients receiving home health care, the proportion publicly paid for is even higher: 89% on Medicare, 91% on Medicaid. In short, when compared to nursing-home-care payment sources, a dramatically higher percentage of costs of home health care patients are paid by Medicare and Medicaid. The same is equally true of hospice patients, 90% of whom are both Medicare and Medicaid eligible (Strahan, 1994). It has been estimated that between 5% and 10% of physician time is spent in home health care, some of whom are full-time (Council on Scientific Affairs, 1990). By 1998 some 20,000 providers were delivering home care with annual expenditures of over $40 billion (Maddox et al., 2001).

Medicaid Services. If a Medicaid recipient is found apt to need full-time institutional care, Medicaid can pay for nearly any of the types of in-home services available through either Medicare or the Area Agency on Aging.

The economic rationale of this program is to reduce public expenditures by offering services that allow people to function in their own home where they, or often their family, will be sharing the financial burden, thus reducing public costs. The care rationale to encourage them to remain at home is based on the positive psychological and emotional benefits.

HOSPICE CARE

Hospice care is usually given to persons who are believed to be at the end of their lives, with perhaps 6 months or less to live, who mainly seek alleviation from pain rather than intensive technological medical treatment. Hospice care is usually provided at home. There is a trend for hospice agencies to attend such patients in nursing facilities. Hospice is also offered in freestanding hospice centers for inpatients and in patient wards in hospitals designated as hospice units, as well as to individual patients on other wards.

Medicare Part A pays for hospice care if three conditions are met: (a) there is medical certification that the patient is terminally ill; (b) it is the patient's choice to receive care from a hospice instead of the standard Medicare benefits; (c) the program is provided by a Medicare-certified hospice. People who choose hospice can be given Medicare Part A hospitalization care for events unrelated to their terminal illness, for example, a bone broken during an accidental fall (Maddox et al., 2001).

The Centers for Medicare and Medicaid Services, which administers Medicare and Medicaid, defines hospice as a public agency or private organization that is primarily engaged in providing pain relief, symptom management, and supportive services to terminally ill people and their families (DHHS, 1985). Medicare pays 100% of all hospice services except for 5% of outpatient drugs and respite care.

By 1998, 540,000 terminally ill persons were receiving hospice care through 2,287 agencies. About 68% of hospice patients were 65 and older, and 71% listed cancer as the major disease. About 90% of hospices are not-for-profit. In 1998, 39% were independent agencies, 25% were hospital programs, 35% were part of a home health agency, and 1% were managed by nursing facilities (Maddox et al., 2001).

Conventional wisdom suggests that Medicare is wasteful, spending about 30% of its total on people in the last year of their lives, most of it during their last month (Burke). However, a Medicare program self-study of those expenditures when compared with costs for survivors differed little during 1976, 1980, 1985 and 1988. Payments during the last month do not differ as dramatically as believed. Burke concluded that any evidence that people in the last year of life account for a larger share of expenditures than beneficiaries who are younger is inconclusive. One study suggests that when all medical services are included, the costs for the "older old" might be somewhat less during their last year of life.

A report of a costly investigation by the Robert Wood Johnson Foundation involving 9,000 patients in five large hospitals revealed that an aggressive effort to improve counseling and communications between doctors and terminally ill patients and their families had no impact on the cost and intensity of their end-of-life experience. In short, managing the costs of dying patients is proving to be a complex social phenomenon with which nursing home personnel and the medical care community will be wrestling for some time to come.

COMMUNITY-BASED LONG-TERM CARE

Congregate Meals at Nutrition Sites and Senior Citizens Centers

Under Title 3c of the Older Americans Act, an effort has been made to make congregate meal sites available to as many older persons as possible in both urban and rural areas.

To accomplish this, the Area Agencies on Aging contract with many thousands of groups who serve such meals 5 or more days a week. Often these nutrition sites, as they are called, are rural schools or churches that are usually centrally located. Transportation is usually provided as well as counseling, nutrition education, recreation, and referral services at the same site and time. The Area Agencies on Aging offer a variety of activities and services at these centers and usually congregate meals as well.

Community Mental Health Centers

Mental health legislation over the past two decades has resulted in the establishment of an extensive network of community mental health centers to which older persons may refer themselves or be referred. However, the utilization rate of these centers has tended to be disproportionately low among older persons.

Adult Day Care

An adult day-care program is a community organization providing daytime health or recreational services to groups of impaired older adults in a centralized protective environment, often for long periods of time. Nursing facilities are uniquely positioned to offer adult day-care programs, and some do. Payments for adult day care can come from various sources, including federal revenue-sharing programs, Title 4 of the Older Americans Act, Title 6 of the Social Security Act, and Medicaid (see Trans Century Corporation, Table 1-1).

People enter an adult day care program for a variety of reasons, such as when the caregiver has to be at work during the day. Its primary function is to allow older persons with various kinds of disabilities to remain in the home setting longer.

Often the adult day-care participant in a nursing facility eventually becomes a resident/patient there. This earlier exposure to the environment serves to reduce the trauma usually involved in the transition to institutional care, which is discussed in part 5.

Adult day care began in the mid-1970s. The National Institute of Adult Day Care was established in 1979. The average day-care program cares for about 22 persons, between 9:00 a.m. and 3:00 p.m., at an average cost of $43 per day in 1997 (Maddox et al., 2001). Day care programs normally offer a structured day, including social interaction, exercise, and a hot noontime meal. Some offer case management, health assessment, nutrition education, and therapeutic diets (Weissert, et al., pp. 640–646).

A majority of adult day-care centers are located in nursing homes. The majority of such participants are functionally dependent older white women. Most are unmarried and about a third are mentally impaired. Compared to the nursing home resident, they tend to be younger, less dependent, and have less mental impairment. Few, if any, adult day care programs are physically located in a hospital (Weissert, 1989).

Geriatric day-rehabilitation hospitals are a medical model of the adult day-care program. Adult day-care programs range from offering recreation with no health care to nearly full health services similar in intensity to those of the nursing facility. Several studies have concluded that stand-alone adult day-care centers and day care hospitals achieve the same outcomes (Maddox et al., 2001).

Adult Foster Care

This form of care is typically defined as care for no more than six unrelated persons in a community-based residence (Maddox et al., 2001). Twenty-four hour supervision and care are offered, and sponsorship can be by individuals or public or similar agencies. There are no accurate estimates of how many such facilities exist (Maddox et al., 2001).

Respite Care

Respite care is a relatively new program under Medicare Part A, where it is defined as a short-term inpatient stay that provides temporary relief to the person who regularly assists with home care (DHHS, 1975; Maddox et al., 2001).

Under Medicare, respite care is available only to caregivers of hospice patients. Medicare will pay 95% of the costs and 100% of the costs after the patient has paid a specified amount of coinsurance. Medicare limits inpatient respite care to stays of no more than 5 consecutive days.

Depending on occupancy level, nursing facilities have offered respite care over the years. Some organizational obstacles to their ability to do so are (a) costs involved in the extensive paperwork required at each admission and discharge, regardless of whether the patient is a regular or hospice resident/patient, and (b) costs associated with keeping beds empty for hospice-type admissions, which by definition are of short duration and therefore incur higher administrative costs to the facility.

Informal Caregiving

Estimates are that 2.6 million to 22 million active caregivers are assisting noninstitutionalized older persons in the U.S. An estimated additional 1.69 million persons are informal caregivers in the nursing homes and similar settings (Maddox et al., 2001).

INSTITUTION-BASED CARE

Low-Intensity Institutional Based Arrangements: Housing

An almost infinite range of housing options faces those who are attempting to decide where and how to live their final years. Numerous group-housing arrangements exist. These are variously called group homes, family homes, personal care homes, foster care homes, domiciliary care homes or, often, rest homes. The number of older adults involved varies from three or four in a group or foster home to as many as several hundred in "rest" homes. The major source of public support for these housing arrangements is the local department of social services that administers the Medicaid program. A new variety of caregiving for older persons is emerging, which is called by different names, but is most often referred to as assisted living. Definitions vary confusingly from state to state.

Congregate-care housing arrangements exist in many forms. These usually are publicly supported housing sites for older persons and those with disabilities. Support can come from numerous public sources, including local taxes.

These housing arrangements range from no services to a progressive array that includes meals, social services, housekeeping, and medical care. Often they are high-rise buildings or small complexes that offer the person on low income an approximate equivalent to the services offered to middle-and upper-income Americans in what are called life care or continuing-care communities.

Life-care or continuing-care retirement communities (CCRCs) are a relatively new phenomenon, at least on the scale they are now being offered. This type of setting can be a microcosm of the community at large with its diverse services.

CONTINUING-CARE RETIREMENT COMMUNITIES

This text focuses on the nursing facility. However, professional preparation as a nursing home administrator offers simultaneous preparation for becoming the administrator of a continuing-care retirement community (CCRC).

The original CCRCs (often called life care communities) were usually set up and managed by religious communities. In return for all their worldly possessions, participants were promised care for the rest of their life. Today the typical resident pays a one-time entrance fee plus monthly fees.

The CCRC that offers life care is, in essence, an insurance pooling. The entry fees and monthly fees are set based on actuarial calculations to cover the expected lifetime costs of each resident. In exchange for the entry and monthly fees, residents are guaranteed care no matter how long they live, even if their personal funds run out. Not every resident will need expensive nursing facility care, but the fees paid by all residents pay for those who do. As with an insurance annuity, those who live longer receive more benefits than those who die earlier.

Normally, the new resident initially occupies either a detached (garden) apartment or moves into an apartment building. As the need arises for more protected or more assisted living, residents may move progressively from a detached unit to an attached apartment to "sheltered" care (assisted living) and, as needed, into full-time nursing care.

In 1990, CCRCs served some 230,000 residents whose average age was 82, 79% of whom were women. The average age at entering was 77 (a second retirement for most). The average age in CCRC nursing centers was 86. Currently, the number of CCRCs is estimated between 1,200 and 1,800.

The CCRC is predominantly a middle-class housing phenomenon—the wealthy get assistance in their homes. Entry fees usually are set to collect 25% of projected lifetime costs, with monthly service fees accounting for the remaining 75%. Few if any facilities place a cap on monthly service fees: These must fluctuate to account for inflation and other costs. CCRC administrations prefer to admit only persons capable of independent living. The relationship between the resident and the administration is lengthy—24 hours a day for 12 to 14 years. The administrators guarantee a service package with no time constraints and no limit on cost in the full-featured CCRC.

Array of Facilities

A broad array of financial arrangements has emerged. Three types of CCRCs are identified in the literature.

Type A or *all-inclusive* CCRCs (about 33% of facilities) guarantee fully paid nursing care for as long as needed at no extra cost beyond the resident's monthly fee. Many services are bundled or included in the monthly fee (e.g., two or more meals each day, cleaning, laundry, linen, utilities, and recreation facilities). Fees vary by geographical area and size of living unit, averaging $70,000 to well over $200,000 for entry fees and $900 to well over $2,000 for monthly fees.

Type B or *modified* CCRCs (about 26% of facilities) usually offer nursing care at no substantial increase in monthly fees, but include fewer services. Fees, for example, may be charged for cleaning or laundry and only one or two meals may be included. Residents in this type community assume some of the financial risk of extended nursing-care costs. Entry and monthly fees are commensurably reduced.

Type C or *fee-for-service* CCRCs (about 38% of facilities) usually offer no meals or personal care service in the monthly fee. Access to nursing care, on-site (usually) or off-site, is normally guaranteed, but the resident using the service bears the full costs.

Originally entry fees were usually nonrefundable. Competition for residents has spawned an array of approaches varying from no refund to

100% refund upon resale of one's unit.

Eighty to 90% of all CCRCs are not-for-profit, most of them also having a church affiliation. However, for-profit corporations have been eager to enter the field.

Regulation

Resident contracts vary. By 1990, 31 states had some type of regulation in effect, but little uniformity existed among them. Some states regulate through the insurance department, others through the health department, offices on aging, or even departments that supervise securities and corporations.

Successfully building and operating a CCRC is a complex business venture. The most common reason for failure is low occupancy rate— major costs are fixed (see part 3 for a discussion of fixed and variable costs).

Hospitals

Hospitals and home health care agencies are vying for many of the same residents sought by the free-standing nursing facility. Hospitals are adding competing, hospital-based nursing facilities at an alarming rate. By 1991, 767 hospitals had 56,292 beds and were serving 51,897 patients.

Hospitals are building nursing facilities for several reasons. They want to ensure an immediately available nursing facility bed to place their patients. With this maneuver their DRG costs can be capped for each admission by means of an early discharge. Simultaneously, a new income stream from Medicare can begin by placing a new patient in a skilled-nursing bed. This trend is likely to intensify as long as hospitals are forced to seek new revenue streams to supplement the losses incurred on daily charges. A study by Lagoe (1984) showed a 53% decrease in hospital nonacute census when nursing home beds were made readily available, sensitizing hospitals to possible income losses. Hospitals themselves are moving toward increased specialization under pressures from the DRGs. Duke University Health System has begun referring to itself as a hospital offering "quarternary" care, one specialization level beyond the previous tertiary care level of sophistication (Duke Health, 1995).

There are only about 5,300 community hospitals in the United States, compared to more than 15,000 nursing facilities. Hospitals are seeking alternative sources of income because their occupancy rates and average length of stay continue on a downward trend. Between 1989 and 1993, median occupancy rates decreased from 49% to 47%, and average length of stay decreased from 4.34 days to 3.83 days (Lutz, 1994).

ROLE OF THE NURSING FACILITY IN THE LONG-TERM-CARE CONTINUUM

Institutional nursing care is prescribed by physicians for persons in a stable or unstable condition who require continuing medical supervision and the services of licensed nursing personnel around the clock.

OUTSIDE RESOURCES OF THE NURSING FACILITY

The nursing facility staff alone is physically and emotionally incapable of meeting the complete psychosocial and medical needs of its residents. Churches, schools, and other community groups, along with individual volunteers, are necessarily a part of caregiving in a nursing facility.

Outliving one's peers is one of the more difficult adjustments in advanced age. For persons living to the age of 80 and beyond, the deaths of most of one's friends and peer family members is a sad reality. In every facility a portion of the resident/patient population is left with no one who is interested in their welfare.

There is simply not enough money in the average nursing home budget to staff at a level sufficient to provide all the human contact and caring that is needed by the residents/patients. Even in those few instances where there are funds, there remains a qualitative difference between care offered by a paid staff member and what a volunteer from the community brings to the situation. If the nursing home experience is to be fully humanized, it will occur only when there is sufficient contact between the residents/patients and the community.

MAJOR ORGANIZATIONS IN THE LONG-TERM-CARE FIELD

The following are some of the outside groups and organizations that will directly or indirectly impact the lives of nursing home administrators.

American Association of Homes and Services for the Aging (AAHSA)—The national not-for-profit industry group. Represents approximately 5,000 nursing homes, life-care communities, assisted living and senior housing, and community services organizations. *www.aahsa.org*

American Association of Retired Persons (AARP)—over 33 million Americans aged 50 and over. Represents aging Americans' interests on a number of issues. *www.aarpwebplace.org*

American College of Health Care Administrators—the professional organization for nursing home administrators. About 6,000 members (of about 40,000 administrators). *www.achca.org*

American College of Healthcare Executives—28,000 members, mainly hospital executives. *www.ache.com*

American Federation for Aging Research—national voluntary organization focusing on biomedical research in aging. *www.afar.org*

American Geriatrics Society—major society for aging interests. About 6,000 members *www.americangeriatrics.org*

American Health Care Association—the for-profit national nursing home association. Has 50 state affiliates, 12,000 members, mostly representing the for-profit nursing home interests. *www.ahca.org*

American Society on Aging—broadly representative of professionals interested in the field of aging. *www.asaging.org*

Assisted Living Federation of America—over 6,500 members and growing rapidly as the major national professional association of assisted living facilities. *www.alfa.org*

Gerontological Society of America—broad array of 6,500 persons interested in aging *www.geron.org*

Gray Panthers—8,000 active, 40,000 membership organization to further the interests of older women. Chapters in 35 states (Maddox et al., 2001). *www.graypanthers.org*

U.S. Administration on Aging—a major resource on legislation, policy, and funding. *www.aoa.gov*

National Institute on Aging maintains an informational Web site at *www.nih.gov/nia*

National Association of Boards of Examiners for Long-term care Administrators—the required national nursing home administrator exam is offered by NAB, as well as a new assisted living national exam. *www.nabweb.org*

National Citizens' Coalition for Nursing Home Reform—the major national coalition for new legislation in the long-term care field. *www.nccnhr.org*

National Council of Senior Citizens—4.5 million members in 4,500 local clubs. *www.ncsinc.org*

National Council on Aging—nonprofit group helping community service organizations to enhance lives of older adults. *www.ncoa.org*

4.2 The Social Security Act: Medicare and Medicaid

4.2.1 THE SOCIAL SECURITY ACT: MEDICARE

The nursing home industry is molded by the Social Security Act and owes the larger part of its economic existence (passing the $100 billion per year mark in 2000) to the original legislation and its later amendments. This one act is mainly responsible for generating the financial support for older persons that has enabled the nursing home industry to become the second largest segment of the health care industry, after hospitals.

ORIGINS OF THE SOCIAL SECURITY ACT

When the Social Security Act came into existence in 1935, it was a response to a fundamental societal change in American life: our evolution from an agrarian to a highly industrialized form of society. Growing old suddenly became visible nationally during the shift from an agricultural society, in which the aged were normally cared for by the family in the home, to a society where the workplace was a factory. Workers in an industrialized society are controlled by economic conditions beyond their influence. Urbanization and industrialization brought increased problems to the aged, such as unemployment and economic survivorship of the dependents when the wage earner died.

The event that brought these problems to the attention of America in dramatic terms was the Great Depression of the 1930s. By 1935, 50% of older Americans were indigent. Within 5 years, the proportion had grown to 66% (Clement, 1985).

IMPACT OF THE SOCIAL SECURITY ACT

Although additional factors are involved, a comparison of the number of aged persons receiving Social Security checks and the percentage of them living at the poverty level reveals a clear association. By 1959, the proportion of older Americans who were indigent had fallen to 35%. Although this reflected some improvement, it still constituted a major social problem. As Social Security benefits during the 1950s and 1960s continued to expand, the percentage of aged persons living in poverty declined to 14% by 1978 (Kaplan, 1985). According to the United States Census Bureau, during the inflation and recession period from 1979 to 1982, older persons receiving Social Security checks based on cost of living adjustments (COLAs), which began in 1975, were the only group studied whose poverty rate did not increase.

In 1985, the President's Council of Economic Advisors declared that older Americans were no longer disproportionately poor and that the percentage of the general population in poverty (15.2%) was slightly higher than that of the same segment of the older population (Kaplan, 1985). Today nearly all Americans are covered by Social Security, although on occasion a person will apply for admission to a nursing home who has no Medicare eligibility. In 1950, only 1 of 4 persons received Social Security checks, but by 1977 9 out of 10 did.

Many factors, such as the political activism of aged persons, general improvements in the economy, the Older Americans Act of 1965, and related actions have led to general improvement in their economic condition. Even so, while direct measurement is not feasible, it appears that a significant number of older Americans have little more than their Social Security check for income—a poverty-level income.

ASPECTS AFFECTING THE NURSING HOME INDUSTRY

The nursing home industry owes its size to Social Security checks and reimbursement of Medicare and Medicaid bill for residents/patients.

The Original Social Security Act and its Amendments

The original Social Security Act, as passed in 1935, consisted of 11 titles enacting the program, authorizing the necessary taxes, and establishing the administrative mechanisms of the act. Numerous amendments have been added to the Social Security Act over the years. Only those more directly affecting the nursing home industry are mentioned here

In 1950, persons who were permanently and totally disabled who might at some time need nursing home care were added as beneficiaries. In that same year, federal matching funds were made available to states to pay for medical care for persons on public assistance—a precursor of Medicaid, which was to come in 1965. States were required to establish licensing programs for nursing homes. Some already had done so.

By 1956, the Social Security program was known as OASDI: old age, survivors, and disabled insurance. It was not until 1960 that an *H* (for health) was added, and it became OASDHI. The next step toward the Medicaid program, so critical to the nursing home industry, came in 1960 with the Kerr-Mills Act, which amended the Social Security Act to provide Medical Assistance to the Aged (MAA). This amendment offered 50% to 84% in matching funds to states, depending on the per capital income of each state. However, during the following 5 years, only 25 states implemented this program.

The major amendments affecting the nursing home industry were added in 1965, with the passage of Title 18, known as Medicare, and one year later, Title 19, known as Medicaid.

Amendments in 1967 called for the licensure of nursing home administrators and recognized the category "intermediate care facility." The 1972 amendments established the definition of the skilled nursing facility (SNF) and dropped the term "extended care facility" (ECF), which had been causing some confusion. In 1990, the federal designation "intermediate care nursing facility" (ICF) and "skilled nursing facility" (SNF) were replaced by the single term "nursing facility."

Title 20 was added in 1974, supporting, among other things, in-home services to older persons. In 1977 antifraud amendments were passed to minimize abuse of the program. Numerous additional amendments were passed during the 1980s. The primary focus has been containment of costs, rather than expansion of services since the mid-1970s.

In general, it appears that from 1935 to about 1975 the federal government sought to expand benefits under the Social Security Act, whereas since 1975 the thrust has been to reduce the rate of cost increases and the units of service for which payment is made.

CONDITIONS OF PARTICIPATION

After an extended implementation period and several additional amendments (described further on), the Social Security Administration prepared an extensive set of rules, or minimum conditions, which it required any nursing facility receiving federal funds to meet (Freymann, 1980; Miller, 1982, Rosenfeld, Gaylord & Allen, 1983; Smith, 1981).

Proposed rules were published in the *Federal Register* on July 12, 1973. So many comments were received that the usual 30-day period for public comment was extended to 60 days, ending September 13, 1973. Officials made several changes in response to public comments and on January 17, 1974, published the final rules.

Importance to the Nursing Home Industry

Federal rules are of overriding importance to the nursing home industry because, directly or indirectly, most nursing homes must comply with them, especially if they expect to be reimbursed for services to Medicare or Medicaid patients (Boling, Vroom, & Sommers, 1983; Freymann, 1980; Miller & Barry, 1979).

Nursing homes are licensed by the states (Wilson, 19??). However, most states relied very heavily on these earlier federal conditions of participation in drawing up their own standards for licensing nursing homes (Smith, 1981). The net effect is that nearly every nursing home, directly or indirectly, is obligated to comply with the federal standards (Miller & Barry, 1979).

These new rules did bring some clarity to the industry. Nomenclature (what to call something) for the various levels of nursing care facilities had been a source of confusion at the federal level (and still is at the state level). States use different designations for nursing home levels of care. To further complicate matters, the development of continuing care retirements communities and the concept of assisted living, which is used in a number of states, suggests that we may be moving into a period of multiple designations for nursing home and nursing home–like services.

Using federal money in part, states conduct on-site inspections of nursing home facilities to determine whether it meets state, and usually, federal requirements.

Not many months after the 1974 conditions were published, the Department of Health, Education, and Welfare (now the Department of Health and Human Services) commissioned "Operation Common Sense," which involved a group of federal regulation writers who committed themselves "to revise and recodify [these] regulations to produce clear, readable and helpful documents" (Center for Medicare and Medicaid Services [CMS], 1974, p. 7042). In the process of making the regulations more easily understandabl3, these federal employees attempted to introduce "needed" policy changes at the same time.

By 1976, a drive called the "Long-Term Care Facility Improvement Campaign," was on within the Department of Health Education and

Welfare. It began by issuing a monograph supporting the idea of a comprehensive patient-assessment mechanism.

Out of this grew a 3-year project called the Patient Care Evaluation Project (PACE). PACE staff-tested two versions (PACE I and PACE II). Criticisms were that the instrument brought "burdensome paperwork," that it put "too much emphasis on the medical model" (for the nursing home), and that "evidence was lacking that PACE produced either cost effectiveness or benefit." However, the federal government was preparing to move.

In response to grumblings from its regional offices, state agencies, and the general public, the Centers for Medicare and Medicaid Services (the federal agency that administers Medicare and Medicaid) published a general notice in the June 8, 1978, *Federal Register* that it planned to revise these federal regulations. It invited public comment.

The response by 1,200 organizations, individuals, and providers was impressive. Hearing were held in California, Georgia, the District of Columbia, Maryland, and Illinois. In addition, 620 written comments were received. "Most commentators," CMS reports, "urged us to find ways to ease the burdens of regulation." In the summer of 1980, CMS published what it assumed to be the new requirements destined to replace the long-criticized 1974 amendments.

CMS officials ran into heavy seas. President Jimmy Carter, during whose administration all these changes had been proposed, lost the election to Ronald Reagan, who rejected the proposed revisions, using the Tax Equity and Fiscal Responsibility Act of 1981 as his vehicle.

Several years of unrest followed. To deflect Congressional criticism, the executive branch suggested that the Institute of Medicine appoint a 20-person panel to study nursing home care. This panel issued a 400-page report in the summer of 1986. They found the quality of care and quality of life in nursing homes to be "unsatisfactory" and called for a new federal government regulation effort (Committee On Nursing Home Reform, 1986). The panel members sought a strengthening of the federal requirements, with a new emphasis on inspections based more on the quality of patient care actually delivered, that is focus on outcomes of care mentioned in part 1. Patients' rights, they argued, should be given more attention.

A coalition of more than 40 concerned long-term-care organizations successfully lobbied for new legislation that embodied much of the 200-page Institute of Medicine report. Medicare and Medicaid long-term-care amendments were passed in the 1987 Omnibus Budget Reconciliation Act (OBRA). This legislation, and new federal requirements proposed by the federal Centers for Medicare and Medicaid Services in the February 2, 1989, *Federal Register,* were implemented during 1989 and 1990. This ended a 15-year period during which the federal regulations

(Conditions of Participation) remained static despite constant attempts at reform.

We turn now to an examination of the basic components of the Medicare and Medicaid legislation after which we will examine several other pieces of legislation that affect and constitute what may be called the long-term-care continuum.

MEDICARE

As of this printing, these were the basic Medicare and Medicaid coverages and we use the past tense although they may still be current. See also the current edition of *Federal Requirements and Guidelines to Surveyors* from Springer Publishing Company for any changes. Attempts have been made to modify them during each session of Congress and these attempts continue.

Part A

Everyone receiving Social Security was automatically covered under Part A.

Hospital Costs. Covered hospital-related costs were paid on the following basis: During the first 60 days of hospitalization for each period of illness (defined below), the patient pays the equivalent of the 1st day, and Medicare pays for the other 59. Since 1965, the years of Medicare coverage, the cost of 1st-day coverage rose from nearly $100 to almost $1,000.

During days 61 to 90 of hospitalization, the patient paid for about 25% of the daily rate and Medicare picked up the remaining costs. Inpatient days were covered only during the first 90 days of any spell of illness. Each Medicare recipient had a lifetime reserve of 60 days, which could be used after the 90th day of hospitalization. During days 91 to 150, the patient paid for about 50% of the daily rate. In addition, each Medicare recipient was eligible for up to 190 days of inpatient psychiatric care during his or her lifetime.

Prospective Payment: The Era of DRGs. Beginning with federal fiscal year 1984, the federal government began to pay hospitals for Medicare patient costs on the basis of 467 diagnostic/reimbursement categories (Prospective payment, 1983). Each year Medicare officials decided prospectively (ahead of time) on the amount of reimbursement for each Medicare hospital admission based on the principal diagnosis, that is, the condition established after study to be chiefly responsible for admission of the patient.

DRG stands for diagnostically related group (of diseases). There are 9,000 disease codes listed in a book called *International Classification of Diseases*. Using the ninth edition's clinical modifications (called ICDM-9CM), the federal government identified 467 diseases for reimbursement to hospitals for care of Medicare patients based on their principal diagnosis and the severity of the disease for which the Medicare patient was admitted.

The theory was that some patients' length of stay was shorter than average and some were longer. Medicare reimbursed on the average length of stay for each disease, based on the level of severity experienced by the patient. At the end of each year, Medicare made adjustments, using up to approximately 6% of its total funds to reimburse hospitals for especially expensive cases (called outliers).

Payments varied for each of the nine United States geographical regions established by Medicare and by whether the hospital was rural or urban. For example, a hospital in New York City would be reimbursed at a higher rate than a hospital in rural Georgia for treating a patient with the same principal diagnosis. The amount of each hospital's reimbursement rate was based 25% on whether it was rural or urban and 75% on the cost experience of that hospital during the first year it was in the program, called the base year. New base years were designated as time passed.

One impact for the long-term-care industry was that because payment was by disease (no matter how extended the length of stay of each patient) hospitals sought to place Medicare patients in a nursing home, home health care agency, or "nursing home bed equivalent" for what is currently called "subacute" care. This is the phenomenon of hospitals' discharging Medicare patients "quicker and sicker." As has already been seen, hospitals often opened their own "nursing home equivalent" (i.e., Medicare-certified beds) in the hospital itself, in order to start up a new stream of cash income for themselves for that same patient.

Nursing Facility Costs. For each spell of illness, Medicare paid 100% of "reasonable costs" during the first 20 days. During days 21 to 100 the patient co-paid a required amount, usually set at well over half the daily cost. Medicare paid nothing beyond 100 days of nursing facility care during any one spell of illness.

Home Health Care Costs. Medicare paid 100% of all home health care costs associated with any one spell of illness (care provided for a diagnosed illness for which 3 or more days of hospital care was given).

It is important to realize that Medicare was intended to cover brief periods of illness; it provided short-term acute care and was not intended to cover long-term-care patients. (Medicaid is the vehicle for covering long periods of illness, but only after the individual has spent all but about $2,000 of his or her total resources; this is discussed in more detail later).

Eligibility for Nursing Facility Care. To be eligible for inpatient nursing facility care, at least four conditions had to be met. The Medicare patient had to (a) have spent 3 consecutive days in a hospital (not including the day of discharge); (b) be transferred to a nursing facility because treatment for the original cause of hospitalization is required; (c) be admitted within 14 days of hospital discharge (leeway is generally allowed up to 30 days); and (d) be certified by a physician to be in need of and receiving nursing care or rehabilitation services on a *daily* basis.

Part B

Part B Was Voluntary. The Medicare recipient had to pay a small monthly premium, determined every 2 years and based on the benefits paid and administration costs of Part B. General funds from the United States Treasury paid one half of the costs of Part B and the participants paid the other half.

Three major expenses were covered under Part B:

1. Medical expenses (including physician services, inpatient and out-patient medical services and supplies, physical and speech therapy, ambulance, diagnostic X-ray, laboratory and other tests, dressings, splints, medical equipment)
2. Outpatient hospital treatment
3. Home health care

Payments under Part B. After the recipient paid an annual deductible amount, Medicare Part B paid 80% of Medicare-determined reasonable charges for medical expenses, outpatient hospital treatment, and home health care. If home health care qualified under Part A posthospital care, 100% of home health care costs were paid under Part A.

Excluded from coverage. Many health care costs associated with older persons were excluded from payment by Medicare Parts A and B. Neither plan would pay for

- routine physical and related tests
- eyeglasses or eye examinations
- hearing examinations or hearing aids
- immunizations (except for pneumococcal shots)

- routine foot care
- orthopedic shoes or other supportive devices for the feet
- custodial care
- preventive care, filling, removal or replacement of teeth

DEFINITIONS

Approved Charges. Under Part B, approved charges were those determined as follows: The carrier in each geographic area annually reviewed the charges made by physicians and suppliers during the previous year. Suppliers were persons or organizations other than physicians who furnished equipment or services, such as ambulance transportation laboratory tests, and medical equipment such as wheelchairs.

To calculate an approved charge, the carrier determined the customary charge, that is the one most frequently made by each physician and supplier during the previous year. The carrier then found the prevailing charge for each service and material supplied during that year. The prevailing charge was an amount sufficient to pay for the customary charges in three out of every four bills that were submitted in the previous year for each service and supply (limited by an economic index ceiling). When a claim was received from a physician or supplier, the carrier compared the actual charge with the customary and prevailing charges for that service or supply and paid 80% of the lowest of the three. The Medicare recipient paid the remaining 20%, either out of pocket or through a small insurance policy (called Medigap insurance), which was designed to pay the remaining 20%.

Assignment. When a physician or supplier accepted an assignment of the medical insurance payment under Part B, he or she agreed that the total charge to the patient would be the one approved by the carrier. In this case, Medicare paid the physician or supplier directly, after subtracting any part of the annual deductible that was not met.

Assignment was voluntary and had to be agreed to by both the provider and the patient. It guaranteed that the physician or supplier would not charge the patient more than the 20% of approved charges not paid by the carrier.

Intermediaries and carriers. Medicare payments were actually made by private insurance organizations that had contracted with the federal government to do so. Organizations handling claims from nursing facilities, hospitals, and home health care agencies were called intermediaries. Organizations dealing with claims from doctors and other medical suppliers covered under the medical insurance (Part B) were called carriers.

4.2.2 TITLE 19: MEDICAID

Medicaid and Medicare were both passed as amendments to the Social Security Act. Medicare has been essentially an insurance program for recipients of Social Security benefits. Medicaid, as designed, literally has been medical aid for persons receiving welfare and for comparable groups of persons who were defined as medically indigent.

Whereas Medicare was a federally run program, Medicaid was a program of federal grants to the states to enable them to provide medical assistance to persons in the following five categories:

- families with dependent children (AFDC)
- the aged—persons receiving Old Age Assistance (OAA)
- persons who are blind—Aid to the Blind (AB)
- persons with permanent and total disabilities (that is, persons receiving federally aided public assistance)
- comparable groups of medically indigent persons not currently on welfare but who fall into the preceding categories. Such persons are considered medically needy when medical expenses reduce their income below the Medicaid eligibility level.

"Spend Down"

Using a community simulation model research by Sloan and Shayne (1985) suggests that the majority of nursing home residents/patients were at entry either already financially qualified for Medicaid or would have been so immediately had they been institutionalized. After undertaking similar research Adams, Meiners and Burwell (1993) concluded that (a) one in four persons admitted as private paying stayed long enough to become Medicaid recipients, (b) approximately one in three persons eventually covered by Medicaid were not eligible when admitted, and (c) about 30% to 40% of Medicaid expenditures on nursing home care is attributable to individuals who spent down. Different studies come up with different conclusions, depending on the original assumptions and geographical locations of research. Estimates from a National Nursing Home Survey were that 14% of nursing home residents were admitted as already receiving Medicaid (Short, Kemper, Llewellyn, & and Walden, 1992).

The federal share ranged between 50% to 83% of costs, depending on the state's per capita income. Each state determined its coverage above a basic minimum of at least some of each of the following services: inpatient hospital, outpatient hospital, other laboratory and X-ray, nursing, and medical.

In addition to these basic services, a state could include any medical care recognized under state law if it chose. No residency requirements could be established for eligibility for services. Medicaid recipients have not been subject to deductible payments, as in the case of Medicare, but states have been allowed to require some co-payments for recipients for care. Some states, for example, charged co-payments for prescriptions (usually 50 cents per prescription), dental visits, eye visits, and similar services, charging a $1 to $2 co-payment per visit (Muse & Sawyer, 1982).

Changing Congressional Goals

Originally the federal government set July 1, 1975, as the date by which all participating states were to be offering comprehensive services to all eligible persons. As cost soared under the program, Congress scaled down this goal and in the 1980s and following years moved toward containing Medicaid costs rather than expanding its services. Congress has been concerned because Medicaid has no ceiling on annual expenditures. The federal government was committed to pay its share of services that the states provided Medicaid recipients.

Buy-in Agreements

To maximize the contribution of federal dollars to state programs, participating states have signed buy-in agreements under which the state pays for Part B costs for Medicaid recipients. The buy-in obligated the federal government to pay entirely for medical costs that might have been shared by the states' Medicaid programs, thus reducing the total dollar costs to the states (Muse & Sawyer, 1982). So intense has been the states' effort to shift costs from state budgets to the federal budget that several states placed a special tax on nursing homes, then used the taxes collected to help pay for Medicaid-assisted health care for older persons, thereby shifting an even larger dollar burden to the federal government.

To further contain costs, some states have obliged county governments to use their own funds to pay for a portion (usually about 3% to 5%) of Medicaid costs. Medicaid dollars, initially committed by county social workers, thus became more carefully supervised by the county governments.

Eligibility for Medicaid has been generally determined at the county level by a social worker, and the program was usually administered by the local department of social services, which assigned recipients as part of the case load of its social worker.

As mentioned elsewhere, older persons have traditionally benefited to a great extent under the Medicaid program; they represent approximately 15% of all recipients, but received slightly more than one third of the benefits paid out (Muse & Sawyer). Spending in 1997 was over $160 billion with 30% of that going to care for older persons (Maddox et al., 2001).

Unmarried persons appeared to be five times more likely than married persons and Medicaid enrollees ten times more likely than those without Medicaid to use nursing homes (see Feinleib, Cunningham, & Short, 1994).

Both the federal and state governments have been seeking ways to reduce expenditures under Medicare and Medicaid. Consequently, details of the payment plans change constantly. The reader should obtain current information and check with the local Medicare and Medicaid offices for the latest coverages and payment mechanisms.

In 1997, the Program of All-Inclusive Care for the Elderly (PACE) was formalized as an integrated Medicare-Medicaid for managed care for older persons (Maddox et al., 2001).

FACILITY BEDS BY CERTIFICATION CATEGORY

Licensed nursing facilities may apply to be certified for participation in the Medicare and/or Medicaid program on a voluntary basis. Facilities may participate in the Medicaid only (Title 19) program, the Medicare only (Title 18) program, or the Medicare-Medicaid dually certified (Title 18 and 19) program. Since 1991, the Medicare program classified facilities as skilled nursing facilities (SNFs) while the Medicaid-certified facilities are designated as "nursing facilities" (NFs). Federal Medicare certification allows for all or part of a facility to be certified.

Over the years 1993 to 1999, about 3% of facilities were certified Medicare only and 50% certified Medicaid only with an increasing trend toward dual certification, which increased from 34% in 1993 to 43% in 1999 due to a relaxing of Medicare reimbursement rules that reduced payment for unfilled Medicare beds.

RESIDENTS BY PAYER SOURCE

The typical nursing facility profile is about 68% Medicaid, 24% Medicare, and 8% private paying residents. The profile varies among the multifacility chains and stand-alone facilities. Many facilities have Veterans Administration beds, some contract with local hospitals to reserve beds, some have managed care, some workers' compensation, and the like. On the whole, facilities resemble this profile with some variations one way or the other. It is a complex picture inasmuch as any single patient may be consecutively on Medicare, then private paying while in Medicaid spend-down, then become a Medicaid resident.

Currently the federal government is attempting to control Medicare and Medicaid costs by supply restrictions, reimbursement limitations, and tightened eligibility requirements. The Balanced Budget Act of 1997 mandated the use of a prospective payment system for both skilled nursing facilities and home health care and by permitting states to allow mandated enrollment in a managed care organization as a condition of receiving Medicaid assistance (Giacalone, 2001). This led to the Balanced Budget Refinement Act of 1999 in which some of the draconian Medicare and Medicaid cuts mandated by the Balanced Budget Act of 1997 were mitigated. This process will continue over the next decades as the need for nursing home care rises and funds for care are curtailed by the federal government and state legislatures.

4.3 Older Americans Act, 1965

The Older Americans Act (OAA) can be characterized as Congress's response to noninstitutional, primarily nonhealth-care needs of older persons. Medicare and Medicaid provide primarily for their institutionalized health care needs (home health care, for example, being the exception). Title 20 of the Social Security Act is also a response to the primarily noninstitutional needs of older persons.

The Older Americans Act authorizes payment for almost any activity that may lead to an improved quality of life for persons 60 years and over (with some programs, for instance, "reemployment" programs for persons 55 and over). The funds and agencies authorized and generated by the Older Americans Act play major roles in shaping the long-term-care industry in the United States. For this reason some of its more important features are explored in the text that follows.

PRECURSORS OF THE OLDER AMERICANS ACT

Events that laid the foundation for the passage of the Older Americans Act in 1965 began about 1945, when Connecticut set up a commission concerned with the needs of older individuals. By 1961, all states had established similar commissions or aging units. That same year a White House Conference on Aging was held, at which heavy pressure for a federal role in addressing the needs of older individuals was brought to bear by lobbyists. Two years later President John F. Kennedy sent a message to Congress entitled "Elderly Citizens of Our Nation." He recommended federal help for older individuals who did not need institutional care but who were encountering increased difficulty in successfully performing the activities of daily living. Continued lobbying for federal aid for the functional older person led to passage of the Older Americans Act in 1965.

GRAND OBJECTIVES: TITLE 1

Title 1 states the goals of the Older Americans Act: equal opportunity of every older individual to the full and free enjoyment of

- adequate income
- the best possible physical and mental health that science can offer, without regard to economic status
- affordable, suitable housing
- full restorative services for those needing institutional care
- employment
- retirement with health and dignity
- pursuit of the widest civic, cultural, educational, and recreational opportunities
- efficient community services: low-cost transportation, choices in living arrangements, coordinated social service assistance
- immediate benefit of technologic developments
- freedom, independence, and the free exercise of individual initiative in planning and managing one's own life

Other portions of the Older Americans Act authorize the Commissioner on Aging, who is the administrator of the Older Americans Act, to pay for virtually any service or activity that will foster these broadly stated goals. The goals and authorizations are sweeping; however, the economic realities of the level of funding have prevented implementing large-scale programs to achieve these goals.

OTHER TITLES

Title 2 established the Administration on Aging (AOA) within the Office of Human Development Services (OHDS), which is in the federal Department of Health and Human Services (DHHS). The Commissioner on Aging, appointed by the President and confirmed by the Senate, is empowered to administer the Older Americans Act and reports directly to the Secretary of Health and Human Services.

Title 3 authorized grants to the states to create planning and service areas within which the local Area Agencies on Aging (AAAs) function. Title 3b is concerned with social services, Title 3c1 with congregate nutritional services for those 60 or over as well as their spouses, and Title 3c2 with home-delivered meals. Title 4 deals with research and training. Title 5 creates the Senior Community Services Employment Program (SCSEP) for those 55 or older with limited incomes (usually 125% of poverty). Title 6 addressed grants to American Indian tribes. Title 7, passed in 1984, authorized a health education and training program for older individuals.

AMENDMENTS

The Older Americans Act was substantially amended in 1967 and 1969, annually from 1972 to 1975, and again in 1977, 1978, 1981, 1984, and 1992. Most of the significant amendments focused on expanding and repositioning the various programs, especially those under Title 3. The amendments of 1978 are of special interest to the nursing home industry. They require state plans to include a long-term-care ombudsman program that will

- investigate and resolve complaints by or on behalf of long-term-care patients
- monitor, develop, and ensure implementation of federal, state, and local laws that govern long-term-care facilities
- give public agencies information about the problems of older individuals residing in long-term-care facilities
- train volunteers and enlist and develop community citizen organizations

To accomplish these goals the states had to initiate procedures allowing ombudspersons to have access to any long-term-care facility records and patient records without disclosing the plaintiff's identity, without his or her written consent, or a court order. Further, each state has had to set up a statewide complaint-recording system to spot problems over time and report them to the state agency that licenses and certifies the long-term-care facilities, and to report to the federal Commissioner on Aging.

Finally, under the 1978 amendments, the state has to ensure that the ombudspersons' files are secure, meaning accessible only to the ombudspersons themselves, unless the inquiring person, such as a concerned nursing home administrator, has written permission from the person who lodged the complaint or has a court order. In short, the state agency is to serve as a watchdog over the nursing facilities, and although it cannot take legal action against a facility, it is expected to go to the state licensing and certification agency, which is empowered to do so. Amendments in 1992 again addressed and expanded provisions for ombudspersons (Cherry, 1993; Sharma & Fallavolleta, 1992).

Beyond the ombudsperson program itself, the state agency and the local Area Agencies on Aging have been authorized to serve as advocates in their areas. This is interpreted to mean that they ensure that the nursing facilities observe the laws and give good quality resident/patient care.

COMPREHENSIVE SERVICES SYSTEM

Another major assignment to the states and their local Area Agencies on Aging is to foster the development of comprehensive and coordinated service systems for all older individuals. This is to be accomplished primarily through establishing numerous supportive services, nutrition programs, and multipurpose senior centers.

Definition of Supportive Services

The local Area Agency on Aging has legislative approval to engage in all the following wide-range activities:

- health services, including education, training, welfare, information, recreation, homemaker, counseling, and referral to specialists
- transportation to and from supportive services
- services to encourage older persons to use supportive services
- help for older persons to obtain housing, repair and renovate to minimum housing standards, adapt homes to individual's disabilities and introduce modifications to prevent unlawful entry
- services to avoid institutionalization, including preinstitutional evaluation and screening, and legal services, including tax and financial counseling
- physical exercise services
- health screening
- career counseling
- ombudsperson services for long-term-care complaints
- unique disabilities services
- job counseling
- other services necessary for the welfare of older individuals

In sum, the local Area Agency on Aging is empowered to engage in a wide variety of activities on behalf of older persons in the community. Generally, however, funding has been at a modest level.

EFFECTIVENESS OF THE ACT

The extent to which the Older Americans Act has achieved its goals is debatable. Clearly, the local Area Agencies on Aging have been given a mandate that could cost billons of dollars if implemented and has been awarded a shoestring budget to accomplish the task. Whether the services under the Older Americans Act would be available without a means test of every older person is also in question.

One of the greatest burdens of growing old is the loneliness resulting from loss of friends and family members of the same generation (Maddox et al., 2001). For many individuals, regardless of their income level, participating in the congregate meal is a primary source of social contact with other people.

Have the Area Agencies on Aging been successful in establishing a coordinated service system for long-term care in their communities? Generally, no. They have had neither the funds nor the organizational authority to bring together and organize the long-term-care providers in the communities. Despite the meager funding levels and lack of authority, however, there is a network of services in place for all older Americans who need assistance to remain outside an institution. This is a major improvement over the decades before the 1960s, when such services did not exist at all. This network and the nutritional assistance to all older Americans have become integral to the long-term-care system in which nursing facilities are active participants.

Still, much need remains unmet. In a 1994 *Wall Street Journal* article, Michael McCarthy, a staff reporter, reviewed some unsettling data. In 1993, as many as 827,000 Americans had received Meals on Wheels and 2.5 million had received subsidized meals at community centers. Even so, the Urban Institute (a private nonprofit research group in Washington, D.C.) estimated that in 1994, 4.9 million older persons were either malnourished or hungry—about 16% of the population over 60. The Urban Institute found that two thirds of needy older persons are not being reached by food assistance projects. In New York State, 2,500 older persons are on waiting lists for home-delivered meals. About 62,000 of its older residents are in the program, but officials estimate about 10,000 more are starving to death in urban high-rise buildings. The funding levels for the Older Americans Act have fallen behind with each succeeding year as inflation and a dramatically increasing older population outstrip funding. This is not surprising since the government funds available amounted to about 53 cents per person according to a 1992 Government Accounting Office study.

4.4 Labor and Management

What rights do nursing home administrators have when employees in the facility are seeking to form a union? What rights do the employees have? What are the basic laws and regulations governing the managers' dealings with employees?

This section provides a framework to enable the reader to begin to answer these questions.

4.4.1 Early Management–Labor Relations in the U.S.

During most of the earlier years of its history, the United States government strongly supported management in its dealings with employees. It was not until 1935 that American workers won government sanction of the right to form trade unions.

The passage of the National Labor Relations Act (also known as the Wagner Act) in 1935 was the first nationwide American labor legislation to favor the growth of trade unions. It was the culmination of a long slow process.

MANAGEMENT PREFERENCES

Most managers would prefer not to have to deal with organized labor. Unionization is perceived as intensifying the difficulty of the administrator's responsibilities. There is a natural tendency for what organizational theorists call the "we–they" phenomenon to occur in the relationship between labor and management. Workers often perceive their interests as different from those of managers, whose task is to operate cost effectively, that is, to produce the best results for the least cost.

The administrator would be happy to pay nurses and nurses' aides the premium wages that will attract the most competent workers available, but pressures to keep costs down do not often permit this. As discussed in part 2, the result is that most nursing home workers, especially the nurses' aides and the kitchen and housekeeping staffs, are paid at prevailing rates in the particular geographical area, which are usually close to the required minimum wage levels. Understandably, these workers, many of whom hold a second full-time job to make ends meet, seek to increase their personal incomes from the nursing facility and obtain the best working conditions on their jobs. Tensions between managers and workers are inevitably built into the situation. How do they deal with them? What are the manager's rights? What rights do the employees have?

THE COLONIAL PERIOD

So powerful were the managers in the Colonial period that workers contented themselves with forming "fraternal unions" to help one another cope with personal economic adversity, but certainly not to act collectively for improved working conditions and more pay (U.S. Department of Labor, 1976). Employers were able to prevent effective unionization. Employers could, at their own discretion, fire any worker seeking to organize a union, refuse to negotiate with any union representative, and require each new employee to sign a "yellow-dog" contract, by which the worker agreed not to join a union (Chruden & Sherman, 1980).

During the nineteenth century, the United States courts consistently sided with management. In 1806, a federal court ruled that workers who sought to unite to exert pressure on managers were participating in a "conspiracy in restraint of trade," which in effect meant that such activity was to be treated as criminal activity (Ivancevich & Glueck, 1983). The first hint of rights for workers did not appear until 1842, when the Massachusetts Supreme Court ruled that unions that did not resort to illegal tactics were not guilty of criminal conspiracy (Chruden & Sherman, 1980). Still, managers could fire any worker at will for union activity, impose yellow-dog contracts, and when all else failed obtain a court injunction against threatened strikes. The managers still retained nearly all of the power (Ivancevich & Glueck, 1983). Despite this, the union movement grew. By 1886, skilled workers such as machinists, bricklayers, and carpenters formed the American Federation of Labor (AFL).

It was not until 1935 that another major labor force, the Congress of Industrial Organizations (CIO), emerged (Raskin, 1981) and in 1955 merged with the American Federation of Labor. The growth of unionization was a slow process because the government did not substantially back labor until the Wagner Act was passed in 1935.

The federal government had actually given American workers some negotiating rights earlier in the century in order to deep the nation's railroads running. The Railway Labor Act of 1926 was the first federal legislation that sanctioned union organization and the right to bargain collectively with management (Chruden & Sherman, 1980).

The first national effort to define workers' and managers' respective rights came just 6 years later. In 1932, the Norris-LaGuardia Act, also called the Anti-Injunction Act, limited the powers of federal courts to side with management through the issuing of injunctions, that is, court decrees that stopped or limited union efforts to picket, boycott, or strike. Yellow-dog contracts were prohibited (Ivancevich & Glueck, 1983).

4.4.2 Major Legislation Affecting Employer-Employee Relationships

THE WAGNER ACT, 1935

The Wagner Act of 1935 is the landmark law that for the first time in federal legislation defined the rights of workers (Boling et al., 1983). The Wagner Act limited the freedom of employers to state their views on proposed unionization. The Wagner Act also guaranteed employee bargaining rights: "Employees shall have the right to self-organization, to form, join, or assist labor organizations, to bargain collectively through representatives of their own choosing, and to engage in concerted activities, for the purpose of collective bargaining or other mutual aid or protection" (Chruden & Sherman, 1980).

Proportion of Workers in Unions

In 1933 there were 3 million unionized workers in this country. By 1947 they numbered 15 million, representing about 31% of the work force.

Union membership increased until about 1956, representing about 35% of employees (Noe et al., 2000), then declined until 1963, when it resumed a slow growth. In 1980, about 20 million workers were in unions, approximately 20% of the total work force and 29% of nonagricultural workers (Ivancevich & Glueck, 1983). Today unions represent about 10% of private sector employees and some analysts foresee membership continuing to trend down to 5% (Noe et al., 2000). One estimate is that the percentage of nursing home employees in unions declined steadily from 17% in 1983 to 11% in 1998 (Giacalone, 2001).

The period from 1935 to 1947 was one of dramatic growth in union membership. The power given to unions through the Wagner Act resulted in what Congress in 1947 viewed as abuses. This led to the Taft–Hartley Act, which placed limitations on unions, just as the Wagner Act had placed limitations on managers 12 years earlier.

THE TAFT–HARTLEY ACT, 1947

In the provisions of the Taft–Hartley Act, unions were prohibited from the following actions (Chruden & Sherman, 1980; Ivancevich & Glueck, 1983)

Prohibitions Against Unions:

1. Restraining or coercing employees in the exercise of their right to join a union or not (unless an agreement existed with management that every worker must be a union member). Union members could not physically prevent other workers from entering a facility, nor act violently toward nonunion employees, nor threaten employees for not supporting union activities.

2. Causing an employer to discriminate against an employee for antiunion activity, nor could unions force employers to hire only workers acceptable to the union.

3. Bargaining with an employer in bad faith. They could not insist on negotiating "illegal" provisions, such as the administration's prerogative to appoint supervisors.

4. Participating in secondary boycotts or jurisdictional disputes. Unions may not picket a nursing home in an attempt to force it to apply pressure on a subcontractor (e.g., a food service contractor) to recognize a union, nor can a union force an employer to do business only with others, such as suppliers, who are unionized; nor can one union picket for recognition when another union is already certified for a nursing home.

5. Charging excessive or discriminatory membership fees. They may not charge a higher initiation fee to employees who did not join the

union until after a union contract was negotiated.

6. Coercing or restraining employees in the selection of the parties to bargain on management's behalf. The manager is free to hire the best labor lawyer available to represent the facility.

7. Forcing managers to hire employees when they are not needed (called featherbedding).

However, when the Wagner Act was amended by the pro-management Taft–Hartley Act, certain employee's rights were retained (Ivancevich & Glueck, 1983).

Prohibitions Against Management

1. Management may not interfere with, restrain, or coerce employees in the exercise of their rights. Managers may not, for example, give wage increases that are timed to discourage employees from joining a union or threaten with loss of their jobs employees who vote for a union.

2. It cannot interfere with or attempt to dominate any labor organization, or contribute financial or other support to a labor organization. For example, managers cannot take an active part in union affairs, or permit a nursing home supervisor to participate actively in a union, or show favoritism toward one union over another.

3. It cannot discriminate in hiring or giving tenure to employees or set any terms for employment so as to encourage or discourage union membership. For example, they cannot fire an employee who urges others to join a union or demote an employee for union activity.

4. Management may not fire or discriminate against any employee who files charges or gives testimony under the Wagner Act.

5. It cannot refuse to bargain collectively with the duly chosen representatives of its employees. For example, the nursing home administrator must provide financial data to a union if the facility claims to be experiencing financial losses, must bargain on mandatory subjects such as hours and wages, and must meet with union representatives duly appointed by a certified bargaining unit.

An important consideration for nursing home administrators is the denial of legal protection to supervisors seeking to form their own unions, thus keeping the management roles of these persons (usually department heads in nursing homes) clearly managerial in function and identification.

Probably the single most important provision of the Taft–Hartley Act for nursing home administrators is the restoration of the right of managers to express their views regarding unions and unionizing efforts. This means that administrators are free to express their opinions about their employees' voting for a union in the workplace and judgements about unions in general. Administrators are still prohibited from threatening, coercing, or bribing employees concerning their union membership or their decision to join or not to join a union.

THE NATIONAL LABOR RELATIONS BOARD

A major aspect of the Taft–Hartley Act was its creation of the National Labor Relations Board (NLRB), which plays a dominant role in United States labor-management relations. It has the following responsibilities (Chruden & Sherman, 1980):

• to determine what the bargaining unit or units within an organization shall be. (A unit contains those employees who are to be represented by a particular union and are covered by the agreement with it.)
• to conduct representation elections by secret ballot for the purpose of determining which, if any, union shall represent the employees within a unit
• to investigate unfair labor practice charges filed by unions or employees and to prosecute any violations revealed by such investigations

The board is empowered to initiate action against illegal strikes or unfair labor practices by unions. In a typical month, as many as 4,000 new cases are filed with the NLRB.

One of the more controversial features of the Taft–Hartley Act is a provision allowing the president of the United States, through the office of the attorney general, to seek an injunction for a period of 80 days against strikes or walkouts affecting the nation's welfare or health. Some labor leaders have called this "slave labor" (Chruden & Sherman, 1980).

THE LANDRUM–GRIFFIN ACT, 1959

Officially designated the Labor-Management Reporting and Disclosure Act of 1959, the Landrum-Griffin Act seeks to protect the interests of the individual union member against possible union abuses. Specifically the act confers several rights to each union member (Ivancevich & Glueck, 1983).

Each union member has a right to

• nominate candidates for union office
• vote in union elections
• attend union meetings

• examine required annual financial reports by the union to the secretary of labor.

In addition, employers are required to report any payments or loans made to unions—its officers or any members—to eliminate what were called "sweetheart contracts," under which union officials and the managers benefited but the rank and file of union members did not.

SETTLING DISPUTES IN THE HEALTH CARE INDUSTRY

The NLRB had jurisdiction over health care institutions. However, until 1974 the board was expressly forbidden by the original Taft–Hartley law to hear cases in the nonprofit sector. Because the vast majority of nursing homes and hospitals operating in the 1950s and 1960s were nonprofit, this meant that most of the health care industry was not subject to these labor laws.

In 1973 Congress began talking of having the law apply to not-for-profit nursing homes and hospitals. Nursing homes and hospitals pressed for the following benefits (American Hospital Association, 1976; Rosmann, 1975):

• special protection against strikes
• priority for rapid NLRB action on disputes
• mandatory mediation requirements (Johns & Saks, 2001)
• limit on the number of bargaining units to one each for professional, technical, clinical, and maintenance and service workers

The nursing homes and hospitals were successful on the whole.

In 1974 Congress amended the Taft–Hartley Act to bring nursing homes and hospitals under its regulations (Non-Profit Hospital Amendments, 1974) (Wilson & Neuhauser, 1982). However, special provisions were made (Pointer & Metzger, 1975):

• A nursing home, hospital or union must give to the other party 90 days' notice of a desire to change an existing contract (this is 30 days more notice than required of others).
• The Federal Mediation and Conciliation Service (FMCS) must be given 30 days' notice if an impasse occurs in bargaining for an initial contract after the union is first recognized.
• A nursing home or hospital union may not picket or strike without 10 days' prior notice, in order to allow the facility to make provisions for continuity of care (no prior notice is required of other unions).

• The FMCS may appoint a board of inquiry to mediate the dispute if it decides a strike would imperil the welfare or health of the community. Neither the nursing home nor the union is obliged to accept the board's recommendations, but they must provide any witnesses or information sought by the board.

For-profit nursing homes benefited from the 1974 amendment to the Taft–Hartley Act because of these special labor relations rules (Miller, 1982).

THE BARGAINING UNIT

Labor unions must seek recognition as representing the majority of persons in a specific bargaining unit of a nursing home. As indicated earlier, nursing homes and hospitals sought to limit the number of bargaining units in negotiations to one each for professional, technical, clinical, and maintenance and service workers.

During most of the decade after the 1974 amendments to the Taft–Hartley Act, the NLRB ruled that in nursing homes and hospitals, service and maintenance workers, clerical staff, licensed practical nurses, registered nurses, and security guard units constitute appropriate bargaining units (Miller, 1982).

In 1984, the NLRB issued a new ruling. In *St. Francis Hospital v. International Brotherhood of Electrical Workers Local 474,* the NLRB ruled that a group of 39 maintenance workers did not constitute an appropriate bargaining unit. Health care workers thereafter had to represent either "all professionals" or "all nonprofessionals" rather than the particular interest groups allowed during the previous decade.

The effect of this NLRB ruling is to make union organization of nursing facility employees much more difficult. A far more diverse group of workers must be approached than before for purposes of union representation in elections. At that time, the Service Employees International Union argued that this made it extremely difficult for health care workers to unionize (Washington Report on Medicine and Health, 1984).

Decisions favoring either labor or management reflect the political administration in power. Nursing homes and hospitals had originally wanted to keep the number of bargaining units to no more than four. According to Miller, the NLRB, under more liberal (i.e., pro-labor) auspices in Washington, had permitted five. Under more management-oriented administrations, the number of allowable bargaining units was cut back to two, which could ease matters considerably for nursing home administrators.

The unionization of nursing facilities is a complicated affair. Vigorous attempts to unionize nursing homes have been undertaken by several unions in recent years. A study by the AFL-CIO and data from 1983 to 1986 showed that 15.9% of nursing home facilities were unionized. By the beginning of the 1990s, about 20% of United States nursing facilities were believed to have unions (Long-Term Care News, 1990).

All regions of the country have unionized nursing facilities. From "most unionized" to "least unionized" are the mid-Atlantic region, followed by the West Coast, New England, the Midwest, Southeast, and South Central states. The Service Employees International Union (SEIU), for example, had organized 225 of the 1,832 nursing homes in California by 1990.

Since 1990 the SEIU has been the most active union seeking to organize nursing home workers. Beginning in the mid-1990s it waged a campaign against a number of the major nursing chains including numerous attacks on the quality of care provided by nursing facilities and arguing that nurses in particular are overworked, stressed-out and sick ("Caring Till it Hurts," 1995; "Falling Short," 1995; *National Nurse Survey,* 1995). In some cases SEIU claimed harassment (Scott, 1994), in others it attempted to prevent mergers of nursing home chains (Shriver, 1995). Strikes have been called to draw attention to "patient care and demands for a new contract" (Moore, 1995).

The largest proportion of nursing homes with unions are in the Service Employees International Union, which is an AFL-CIO member with a membership of over 600,000 (Health Care Labor Manual, 1983). The membership in SEIU increased from 762,000 members in 1989 to more than 1 million in 1997 (Noe et al., 2000). In the mid-1990s, the SEIU represented 60,000 RNs, 30,000 LPNs, and 400,000 health care workers overall. In 1989, the National Union of Hospital and Health Care Employees, which had about 74,000 members, merged with two other unions. About two thirds of their members joined the SEIU, and the remaining one third joined the American Federation of State County and Municipal Employees. However, to complicate the picture, nursing homes have been organized by numerous other unions such as the United Food and Commercial Workers, the Teamsters, and the Federation of Nurses and Health Professionals, which is an offshoot of the American Federation of Teachers.

Normally, employees in nursing, dietary, housekeeping, and laundry are the most likely to be unionized. A growing number of employers, particularly the larger chains, attempted to prevent unionization of nurses by arguing that all nurses (RNs and LPNs) are statutory supervisors and are thereby excluded from labor law protection to join a union. The employers insisted that all nurses supervise nurses' aides, hence all nurses are supervisory personnel and therefore not covered by labor laws. In a setback for unionization of nursing home workers, the United States Supreme Court, by a 5-4 decision, agreed and ruled in 1994 that nurses who supervise lesser-skilled employees are not protected by the National Labor Relations Act (Burda, 1993; *NLRB v. Health Care and Retirement Corporation of America*).

On May 29, 2001, the U.S. Supreme Court in *NLRB v. Kentucky River Community Care, Inc.* again confirmed that professional employees such as nurses who direct other employees are supervisors and thus ineligible for union membership.

Conventional wisdom in the nursing home industry is that facilities are subject to being unionized when employee management–employee communication is low and focuses more on dissatisfaction with working conditions than on pay levels.

NONUNION WORKERS

At least 75% of the total labor workforce in this country is not unionized. What of their rights?

Over the years the federal government has enacted legislation establishing and protecting the rights of all workers in general. Three of these laws are the Civil Rights Act of 1964, the Equal Employment Opportunities Act of 1972, and the Americans With Disabilities Act of 1992.

EQUAL PAY ACT, 1963

This act requires that men and women performing equal jobs receive equal pay, covers all facilities, in effect, and is enforced by the Equal Employment Opportunities Commission (EEOC) (Noe et al., 2000).

CIVIL RIGHTS ACT, 1964

Title VII of the Civil Rights Act of 1964 prohibited employers and others from discriminating against employees on the basis of race, color, religion, sex, or national origin. Title VII also prohibits discrimination with regard to any employment condition including hiring, firing, promotion, transfer, and admission to training programs.

CONSUMER CREDIT PROTECTION ACT, 1968

Title III of this act limits the amount of an employee's earnings that may be garnisheed and protects employees from being discharged for any one debt. In general, the amount of an employee's earnings that may be garnisheed is the lesser of 25% of disposable earnings or the amount by which disposable earnings are greater than 30 times the federal minimum wage. Other conditions apply. The Department of Labor's Wage Hour Division administers and enforces Title III. Violations can require back pay, reinstatement, and fines up to $1,000 or imprisonment for not more than 1 year, or both.

EQUAL EMPLOYMENT OPPORTUNITIES ACT, 1972

The Equal Employment Opportunities Act (EEOA) amended Title VII of the Civil Rights Act. EEOA strengthened enforcement of the original act and expanded its coverage to additional groups, such as state and local government workers and private employers of more than 15 persons.

What Is Discrimination?

Congress did not define discrimination in its legislation. Over the years the courts have established three definitions (Noe et al., 2000):

• During World War II, discrimination was defined as harmful actions motivated by personal animosity toward the group of which the target person was a member.
• Later this was redefined as unequal treatment. Accordingly, a practice is illegal if it applies different standards or different treatment to different groups of employees or applicants. For example, minorities may not be kept in less desirable departments (different treatment); rejecting women with preschool-age children is not permissible (different standards). Point: The administrator may impose any standards so long as they are applied equally to all groups or individuals and do not result in any intended or unintended adverse treatment of any group.
• In *Greggs v. Duke Power Co.* (1971), the United States Supreme Court defined employment discrimination as unequal impact. In this case Duke Power was using employment tests and educational requirements that screened out a grater proportion of Blacks than whites (Ivancevich & Glueck, 1983). This is also called *adverse impact.*

For the purposes of Title VII cases adverse impact is often measured when the selection rate for a protected minority group is less than 80% of the selection rate for a majority group, as mentioned in part 2.

Although the practice in the Duke Power case was not motivated by prejudice against Blacks and the tests were all applied equally, they had the result of adverse impact, that is, unequal impact on Blacks. The job involved was that of shoveling coal into a furnace. Duke failed to prove that passing employment tests and requiring a level of education were related to success on the job. The burden of proof is on the employer to show that a hiring standard is job-related.

Minority groups that are specifically protected under the Civil Rights Act are Blacks, Hispanics, American Indians, Alaskan natives and Asian Pacific Islanders.

Discrimination Based on Gender. Few situations exist that justify discrimination based on gender. In the current cultural setting, perhaps it is justifiable to employ women as a wet nurse or to model women's clothes or as an attendant in a women's locker room. In the final analysis, the only legitimate basis for discrimination based on sex may be that the employee must use body organs specific to his or her gender to accomplish the job requirements, e.g., wet nursing or providing semen for a sperm bank.

Sexual Harassment. Sexual harassment has been defined in the EEOC guidelines as follows:

> Unwelcome sexual advances, request for sexual favors, and other verbal or physical conduct of a sexual nature, constitutes sexual harassment when (1) submission to such conduct is either explicitly or implicitly a term or condition of an individual's employment, (2) submission or a rejection of such conduct by an individual is used as a basis for employment decisions affecting such individual, or (3) such conduct has a purpose or effect of reasonably interfering with an individual's work performance, or creating an intimidating, hostile, or offensive working environment.

In recent years, two general categories of cases have emerged: quid pro quo and hostile work environment. In quid pro quo, the harassment is not only a demand for sexual favors, but also the adverse employment decision that results from the rejection of those demands. A hostile-work-environment case requires evidence of pervasive offensive conduct of a sexual nature, such as, proof that obscenities and sexual gestures, remarks, or touching were commonplace. Some cases have involved the presence of nude or partially nude women as part of the proof of discrimination (*Robinson v. Jacksonville Shipyards*, 1991).

The facility can be held strictly liable for the acts of department managers who are found to be sexually harassing employees. A written policy against sexual harassment containing procedures available to employees is an advisable step for facility management to take. It has been pointed out that sexual harassment laws apply equally to women and men of every sexual orientation (Argenti, 1994). Sexual harassment laws generally are aimed at superior-subordinate relationships, but apply to peer relationships and those between residents/patients and employees. The number of sexual harassment charges rose from 7,000 in 1991 to nearly 16,000 in 1997 (Noe et al., 2000).

PREGNANCY DISCRIMINATION ACT, 1978

The 1964 Civil Rights Act was amended in 1978 to end discrimination against pregnant women. The act makes it illegal to discriminate on the basis of pregnancy, childbirth, or related medical conditions in hiring, promoting, suspending, or discharging women who are pregnant. In addition, the employer is required to pay medical and hospital costs for childbirth to the same extent it pays for other conditions.

EQUAL EMPLOYMENT OPPORTUNITY COMMISSION: ENFORCING THE EEOC LAWS

The Equal Employment Opportunity Commission (EEOC) was established by the 1964 Civil Rights Act. The commission was empowered to interpret the act and resolve charges brought under it. The 1972 amendments gave the commission additional authority to bring lawsuits against employers in the federal courts. Since 1979 the EEOC has enforced the Age Discrimination in Employment Act (ADEA) of 1967, the Equal Pay Act (EDA) of 1963, Section 501 of the Rehabilitation Act of 1973, and the Americans With Disabilities Act of 1990. On average, about 17,000 age-discrimination complaints were filed each year during the 1990s (Noe et al., 2000, p80). Employers have been generally successful in finding creative ways to successfully shed older workers without being prosecuted.

Even so, the commission still cannot directly issue enforceable orders as do other agencies such as the Environmental Protection Agency. Hence, the EEOC cannot order an employer to discontinue discriminatory practices, nor can it order back pay to victims of discrimination. It must seek action through the courts.

The average backlog of cases for the EEOC runs upwards of approximately 20,000. It is not possible to handle all of them, of course. Only a small percentage of charges are eventually resolved by the EEOC or by the courts (Ivancevich & Glueck, 1983). Nevertheless, legal history is being made by the EEOC, and its presence is felt in employment practices. (Noe et al., 2000).

EEOC Procedures

Step 1. The EEOC has the power to require employers to report employment statistics on federal forms.

Step 2. If the EEOC feels charges are justified, it authorizes its preinvestigation division to review the complaints.

Step 3. The investigation division then interviews all parties concerned.

Step 4. If there is substance to the case, the EEOC seeks an out-of-court settlement.

Step 5. If the parties cannot be reconciled, the EEOC can sue the employer.

In cases settled by court decisions, the courts have required such actions as back pay, reinstatement of employees, immediate promotion of employees, hiring quotas, abolition of testing programs, and creation of special training programs. Some settlements have cost in the millions of dollars.

Specifically, the EEOC may seek any or all of the following relief under the acts noted:

- back pay (all acts)
- hiring, promotion, reinstatement, benefit restoration, front pay, and other affirmative relief (Title VII, ADA, ADEA)
- actual pecuniary loss other than backpay (Title VII, ADA)
- liquidated damages (ADEA, EPA)
- compensatory damages for future monetary losses and mental anguish (Title VII, ADA
- punitive damages when employer acts with malice or reckless disregard for federally protected rights (Title VII, ADA)
- posting of a notice to all employees advising them of their rights under the laws EEOC enforces and their right to be free from retaliation (all acts)
- corrective or preventive actions taken to cure the source of the identified discrimination and minimize the chance of its recurrence (all acts)
- reasonable accommodation (ADA)
- stopping the specific discriminatory practices involved in the case (all acts).

LAWS AFFECTING FEDERAL CONTRACTORS AND SUBCONTRACTORS

Several laws and executive orders (orders issued by the president of the United States) govern hiring and job practices of firms that hold federal contracts of more than $50,000. While it is unlikely that any nursing facility would be directly affected by these regulations, many contractors doing construction work for them are subject to these regulations (Noe et al., 2000).

EXECUTIVE ORDER 11246

This order by President requires written affirmative action programs of all contractors with 50 or more employees and $50,000 or more in federal contracts. To enforce this order, the Office of Federal Contract Compliance Programs (OFCCP) was established and was later given responsibility for administering laws protecting veterans. (Noe et al., 2000).

THE VOCATIONAL REHABILITATION ACT, 1973

This act requires federal government contractors to mount affirmative action programs for those with disabilities. It is enforced by the OFCCP. The act also provides a measure of federal support for programs to assist in training those with disabilities. By 1980, approximately half of the 15 million Americans with disabilities who were of working age had been able to find employment (Ivancevich & Glueck, 1983).

VIETNAM ERA VETERANS READJUSTMENT ACT, 1974

This act requires firms with more than $10,000 in federal contracts to have affirmative action programs for employment and advancement of Vietnam veterans.

THE AMERICAN WITH DISABILITIES ACT, 1990

Title I of the Americans With Disabilities Act of 1990 (ADA) prohibits facilities from discriminating against qualified individuals with disabilities in job application procedures, hiring, firing, advancement, compensation, job training, and other terms, conditions, and privileges of employment.

A individual with a disability is a person who

- has a physical or mental impairment that substantially limits one or more of the major life activities (e.g., walking, lifting, seeing, learning, doing manual tasks)

- has a record of such an impairment (e.g., has been treated for a mental illness); or
- is regarded as having such an impairment (e.g., a person who has extensive scars from burns).

The act applies to any qualified individual with a disability who can perform the essential functions of the position with or without reasonable accommodation. Individuals who are HIV positive or have AIDS are considered to have disabilities within the meaning of the ADA. (Current users of illegal drugs are not similarly protected.) In 1999, about 1.4% of AIDS cases occurred among persons 65 and older, with the ratio of men to women of 7:1 (Maddox et al., 2001). Residents with AIDS are now common occurrences in U.S. nursing facilities. The facility may not limit, segregate, or classify job applicant or employee with disabilities in any way that adversely affects his or her opportunities. Facilities may not fire or refuse to hire such persons for any cause that could be eliminated by reasonable accommodation.

Reasonable Accommodation

This may include making existing facilities freely accessible to persons with disabilities, supplying readers or interpreters, modifying policies, examinations or training manuals, restructuring jobs or changing work schedules, reassigning the individual to a vacant position, or acquiring or modifying equipment for their use.

Undue Hardship.

The facility is required to make an accommodation to the known disability of a qualified applicant or employee if it would not impose an undue hardship on the facility. *Undue hardship* is defined as an action that requires significant difficulty or expense when considered in light of factors such as a company's size, financial resources, and the nature and cost of the proposed accommodation.

Standards

The facility is not required to lower quality or production standards to make an accommodation nor to provide personal use items such as glasses or hearing aids.

Medical Examinations

The facility may not ask job applicants about the existence, nature, or severity of a disability. Applicants may be asked about their ability to perform specific job functions. A job offer may be conditioned on the results of a medical examination if the examination is required for all entering employees in similar jobs. Medical examinations of employees must be job related and consistent with the employer's business needs. (EEOC, 1994). Medical tests must contain only "normal" medical test aspects given to all preemployment applicants and contain no features that could be construed to be testing for or testing a disability. The EEOC notice describes a number of scenarios and illustrations concerning preemployment medical examinations around which the facility should build its medical examination policies.

If an applicant is not hired because of post-offer medical exam results, the reason must be given and a statement made that no reasonable accommodation was available that would have enabled the applicant to perform the essential job functions or that accommodation would impose an undue hardship.

Employee/Applicant Rights

Employees and applicants are entitled to apply to the Equal Employment Opportunity Commission. If the applicant is successful the EEOC may require that the person be placed in a position as if the discrimination had never occurred. This might entitle the applicant to hiring, promotion, reinstatement, back pay or other remuneration, or reasonable accommodation including reassignment. The successful complainant may also be entitled to damages for future money losses, mental anguish, and inconvenience. Punitive damages may also be imposed on the facility if the EEOC feels it acted with malice or reckless indifference. The complainant may also be entitled to recover attorney's fees. Charges can be filed at any field office of the EEOC, which are located in 50 cities.

Unanticipated Results

Through the 1990s, approximately 90,000 complaints were filed, with about 50% found to have merit (Noe et al., 2000). Surprisingly few (10%) concerned failure to hire. Half of these complaints dealt with firings, about one third with failure to make reasonable accommodation. According to the National Organization on Disability, a private citizens group, fewer persons with disabilities (31%) were employed in 1993 than in 1986 before the act (33%) (Noe et al., 2000). Of significance to nursing homes is that the largest identifiable category of complaints allege back problems (Noe et al., 2000). Lower back disability accounts for about 25% of all lost workdays and is estimated to cost nearly $30 billion each year (Noe et al., 2000).

PATIENT SELF-DETERMINATION ACT, 1990

The Patient Self-Determination Act (PSDA) of 1990 was technically an amendment to the federal Medicare and Medicaid law passed as part of the 1990 Omnibus Budget Reconciliation Act. It is usually referred to, however as the Patient Self-Determination Act.

Requirements

The act requires that all health care facilities accepting Medicare or Medicaid money do the following things:

• Provide written information to residents/patients at the time of admission concerning an individual's right under State law (whether statutory or as recognized by the courts of the State) to make decisions concerning . . . medical care, including the right to accept or refuse medical or surgical treatment and the right to formulate advance directives.
• Maintain written policies and procedures with respect to advance directives (e.g., living wills and health care power of attorney) and to inform residents/patients of the policies (Maddox et al., 2001).
• Document in the individual's medical record whether or not the individual has executed an advance directive.
• Ensure compliance with the requirements of state law (whether statutory or as recognized by the courts of the state) respecting advance directives at facilities of the provider.
• Provide (individually or with others) for education for staff and the community on issues concerning advance directives.

The facility may not "condition the provision of care or otherwise discriminate against an individual based on whether or not the individual has executed an advance directive."

A signed copy of each resident/patient's acknowledgment of receipt of information and the opportunity to act under the provisions of the PSDA should be in the resident/patient's file. Relevant advance directives should be prominently located in the resident/patient's medical record.

SAFE MEDICAL DEVICES ACT, 1990

Under the Safe Medical Devices Act of 1990 nursing homes must report to the Food and Drug Administration and/or the manufacturer all incidents in which a medical device caused or contributed to a resident's death, serious injury, or illness.

A medical device is any instrument, implement, machine, implant, or related article intended for use in diagnosing, treating, or preventing disease. Drugs are not medical devices. Nursing home examples are items such as blood glucose devices, blood pressure devices, catheters, hearing aids, infusion pumps, pacemakers, restraints, scales, thermometers, and wheelchairs (Carley, 1991).

All incidents that suggest a reasonable probability that a medical device has caused or contributed to a resident or patient's death, serious illness, or injury must be reported. Reports are to be made as soon as possible, but no later than 10 days after incident.

CLINICAL LABORATORY IMPROVEMENT ACT

The Clinical Laboratory Improvement Act (CLIA) requires that any medical facility that conducts named tests meet stringent CLIA requirements. Most nursing facilities do not conduct laboratory tests that do not come under the waived test list; for example, the use of glucometers is waived. Changes to the list of waived tests have occurred periodically, see for example, in the May 15, 1995, *Federal Register.* However, all nursing facilities must obtain a certificate of waiver from the Food and Drug Administration.

CIVIL RIGHTS ACT, 1991

This act expanded the 1964 Civil Rights Act. The 1964 Civil Rights Act only permitted back pay and perhaps attorney's fees. The 1991 act permitted compensatory damage such as money lost, emotional pain and suffering, and loss of enjoyment of life. Punitive damages which are meant to discourage other employers from similar practices, were also allowed by providing payments to the plaintiff beyond actual damages suffered. This applied to the Civil Rights Act of 1964, the Americans With Disabilities Act, and the Age Discrimination in Employment Act of 1967. Maximum punitive damages per incident were set at between $50,000 for smaller employers to $300,000 for employers with more than 500 employees (Noe et al., 2000).

FAMILY AND MEDICAL LEAVE ACT, 1993

Under the Family and Medical Leave Act (FMLA), a covered employer (one with 50 or more employees) must allow up to 12 weeks per year of unpaid leave connected with pregnancy, childbirth, and recovery, or a serious health condition affecting an employee or his family member (Maddox et al., 2001). To be eligible, the employee must have worked for at least 12 months (a minimum 1,250 hours) prior to the leave. The 12 months need not be consecutive.

Benefits

A person is entitled to benefits in connection for (a) the birth of a son or daughter, (b) adoption or foster care, (c) caring for a spouse, son, daughter, or parent with a serious health condition, or (d) a serious health condition that prevents the employee from performing his or her job functions. A serious health condition does not normally include any short-term condition that could be covered under regular sick-leave policies. Absence for substance abuse without a treatment program is not within the definition of a serious health condition for the purposes of this act.

Options

The employee may request the leave in reduced work hours or any combination of modified work schedule to accommodate covered reasons for unpaid leave under the act.

Return

Generally, the employee is entitled to return to his or her former job or its equivalent at the same pay, benefits, and other equal working conditions.

In practice, only 3.7% of workers have taken advantage of this act according to one study (Maddox et al., 2001). The rate may be higher in nursing facilities, but the workers who most need the act's benefits (the nurses' aides) can least afford to take leave without pay.

HEALTH INSURANCE PORTABILITY AND ACCOUNTABILITY ACT EFFECTIVE 2001

Effective April, 2001, the Department of Health and Human Services issued privacy standards facilities must ensure for their residents in order to continue to be eligible for Medicare funds. Included are such requirements as

- a policy against e-mailing patient records
- a written information security plan

- assurance that third-party vendors and contractors are compliant with HIPAA
- a written record that all patients in the facility are informed about all the ways their records are being used
- a written record that all patients have been given the opportunity to refuse to allow the facility to share their medical information

4.4.3 Regulation of Compensation

Most states and the federal government have passed laws that regulate compensation for work performed. Federal jurisdiction covers only those workers engaged in producing goods for interstate and foreign commerce. Technically, the federal government does not have authority to regulate worker compensation within states.

More than 40 states have their own wage and hour laws and also regulate other conditions of employment, such as hours allowed per week before overtime must be paid.

The practical effect of having both federal and state regulations governing compensation is that both prevail. In reality, the federal laws are applied to most workers regardless of whether they are producing goods for interstate or foreign commerce. This breadth of application of the federal wage laws is achieved by including persons whose work (loosely defined) is closely related to any production for interstate or foreign commerce.

On a day-to-day basis, this means that nursing home employee compensation and other work conditions must meet both federal and state regulations.

The original goals of federal wage and hour regulations were to encourage spreading work among as many wage earners as feasible and to establish a floor for wages for any worker regardless of the job. Requiring a rate of 1½ times the regular pay rate for all overtime has helped to accomplish spreading the work. Requiring a minimum wage for all persons has accomplished the second goal.

FAIR LABOR STANDARDS ACT

The Fair Labor Standards Act (known as the Wage and Hour Act) was originally passed in 1938, but like the Social Security Act of 1935, it has been amended many times. The four primary foci of the act are minimum wage rates, overtime, child labor, and equal rights (Noe et al., 2000).

Minimum Wage Rates

When first instituted, the minimum wage was 25 cents per hour. Over the decades it has risen nearly 15-fold as the value of the dollar has declined.

The new minimum wage must be calculated on the actual earning wage before any additional payments are added. For example, if the employee works a 46-hour week, he or she received the minimum wage for the first 40 hours and is paid at 1½ times that rate for the additional 6 hours. Generally, the employee must be paid in cash or in a "negotiable instrument payable at par" (a check) except that board, lodging, and other facilities regularly furnished to employees may be provided in lieu of cash wages or the cost deducted from cash wages (Noe et al., 2000).

What is work? Preparatory activities integral to the employee's job may be considered work time. If an employee performs work that is prohibited with the knowledge and or acquiescence of management, the employee must be paid, even if the work is away from the facility as long as the employer has reason to believe the work is being performed. On-call or waiting time may be considered work if the employee is engaged by the employer to wait for the work. Travel associated with or required by the job is compensable. Bona fide meal periods are not compensable, must be 30 minutes in duration and totally free the employee from performing any work. If meal periods are frequently interrupted, as happens often in a nursing facility setting, the whole meal period may be considered compensable work time. Rest periods and coffee breaks are compensable.

The minimum wage rates are especially important to nursing homes because many of them pay nurses' aides and housekeeping and maintenance employees at or just above the minimum wage.

Overtime

The Fair Labor Standards Act requires overtime for all hours over 40 hours per week, to be paid at 1½ the regular rate of pay. Hospital and nursing home employees are entitled to an exception in that overtime may be calculated on the basis of a 14-day period if overtime is paid for hours worked in excess of 8 daily and in excess of 80 during the 14 day period. There must be an agreement to this arrangement between employee and employer. Overtime must be calculated on the basis of a single work week and not be averaged over 2 or more weeks. A fluctuating work week is permitted under certain circumstances.

Whenever compensatory time is given for overtime hours worked, the employee must be given 1½ hour off for every hour of overtime worked. Employees may not accumulate more than 240 hours, however.

If bonuses are paid for some other period—a month or a quarter, for example—the base for overtime wage must be recalculated to add any additional remuneration to the base rate for that period in calculating the time-and-a-half rate for all hours worked over 80 hours in each 2-week period.

Because of their exemption from coverage by the Fair Labor Standards Act, management personnel are referred to as exempt employees. Nonmanagement employees are considered nonexempt. A number of complicated definitions apply to this area.

Congress amends this act frequently, so it is important to check with the Department of Labor to keep abreast of current and upcoming regulations and changes.

Exempt/Nonexempt

Executive, professional, administrative, and outside sales occupations are exempt from FSLA coverage. Nonexempt occupations are covered and include most hourly employees such as the nurses and nurses' aides. It is estimated that about 20% of employees are in the exempt category (Noe et al., 2000).

Enforcement of FSLA

Records may be subpoenaed without a warrant at off-site locations. Normally a warrant is required for on-site inspections. Violations are subject to a penalty of up to $1,000 per violation. Injunctions may be issued regarding minimum wage, overtime, child labor, and record-keeping violations. Criminal proceedings may be brought by the Department of Justice. First offenders may be fined not to exceed $10,000. Second offenders may be so fined and a maximum prison sentence of 6 months imposed. Wage and hour inspectors are liable to show up unannounced. In general, the word of the employee is taken most seriously by these inspectors. If an employee said she worked 2 hours per week "off the clock" for the previous year, the facility may be required to pay that employee for 2 hours of overtime per week for that past year.

Child Labor

Minors under 16 may not be employed except under a temporary permit issued by the Department of Labor. Many states have regulations concerning the employment of persons between ages 16 and 18 in certain industries, such as nursing homes, where the worker can be exposed to disease or other hazardous conditions. Generally, special temporary work permits must be obtained.

EQUAL PAY ACT

In 1963, the Fair labor Standards Act was amended by the Equal Pay Act. Under that amendment

> No employer shall discriminate between employees on the basis of sex by paying wages to employees less than the rate at which he (*sic*) pays wages to employees of the opposite sex for equal work on jobs which require equal skill, effort and responsibility, and similar working conditions. (Quoted by Chruden & Sherman, 1980)

Progress has been slow in this area. Department of Labor, Bureau of Labor Statistics studies have shown that women earn slightly over 60 cents for every dollar men earn in comparable positions.

The equal-pay provision of the Fair Labor Standards Act is of special concern to nursing home operators, who may employ male and female nurses, male and female aides, and male and female maintenance and laundry persons.

4.4.4 Workers' Compensation

Workers' compensation laws are based on the principle that employees themselves should not have to pay costs associated with injuries that occur at work. On-the-job injuries, the lawmakers have reasoned, are a cost of doing business and should be passed on to the consumer.

In New Jersey, Texas, and South Carolina, workers' compensation insurance is voluntary. In all other states it is compulsory for employers to participate in a state-sponsored or state-approved program.

Under most state laws, workers are paid a percentage of their regular wages while recovering from an injury on the job. States normally set limits to benefits and specify how long they must be paid.

Hospitalization and other medical costs are also normally covered by workers' compensation insurance funds, and there are usually death benefits for the worker's family. States establish commissions that handle any claims that are in dispute. Generally, the result is little cost to the injured worker and reasonably rapid assistance.

States usually take one of two basic approaches to funding workers' compensation insurance. Sometimes the state operates its own insurance system in which employers are usually obliged to participate. In other states, employers are allowed either to self-insure or to join a private insurance company program.

One characteristic of most workers' compensation plans is that the amount the employer must pay per month is experience-based. Under this system, employers with good safety records pay less than those with large numbers of claims. In some states, benefits to the injured worker are reduced if the worker is willfully negligent in following safety procedures.

4.4.5 Unemployment Compensation

In 1993 alone, 216,400 employees in nursing and personal-care facilities suffered work-related illnesses and injuries, an incident rate of 16.9 nonfatal injuries and illnesses per 100 full-time employees (Burda, 1995). This was 50% higher than the hospitals' 10.9 rate. The nursing and personal-care homes injury rate in 1993 was the second highest among all industries with 100,000 or more total injuries and illnesses. Only the rate for motor vehicle and equipment-makers was higher (17.7).

Employees who participate in the Social Security Act program are eligible for unemployment compensation when they are laid off by their employer. Nearly all nursing home employees are covered by the Social Security Act.

Unemployment compensation is available for up to 26 weeks through the state employment agency if the worker registers and is willing to accept any suitable comparable work offered through the agency.

Unemployment compensation is funded by a federal payroll tax based on the wages of each employee up to a certain maximum. The federal government turns these monies over to the states for disbursement.

A separate record is kept for each employer. Once a company has paid an account equivalent to the required reserve, its rate of taxation is reduced. In actual practice, this means that nursing facilities with few unemployment compensation claims against them pay at a lower tax rate than those with a large number of such claims.

Experience has shown that although an employee may be discharged or let go for valid reasons (unrelated to lack of work), unless the facility has extremely good documentation on the circumstances of the dismissal the employee may be successful in claiming unemployment compensation. When this happens the costs of the unemployment compensation paid by the state is allocated to the individual nursing facility's account.

4.4.6 Retirement

AGE DISCRIMINATION EMPLOYMENT ACT, 1967

This act, which was amended in 1978, protects employees from being discriminated against on the basis of age. It is intended to prevent companies from replacing older employees with younger ones, whether to achieve a younger average among the working force or to avoid paying pension benefits. There are some exceptions, such as certain occupational groups and employers with fewer than 20 employees, but the practical effect is that no employees in the typical nursing facility can be forced to retire against their wishes solely on the basis of their age.

THE EMPLOYEE RETIREMENT INCOME SECURITY ACT, 1975

During the 1960s, Congress investigated pensions for American workers and discovered that for a variety of reasons, up to one half of American workers covered by pension plans would never receive any benefits. The largest problem was a failure of businesses to fund their pension plans adequately. The basic problem for the worker was loss of any pension benefits when leaving the company for almost any reason before retirement.

In response to this problem, Congress passed the Employee Retirement Income Security Act (ERISA) of 1975. The EEOC is the primary agency responsible for enforcing this act, which act sets minimum funding levels for pension funds, requires certification every 3 years of the actuarial soundness of the plan, and requires vesting of the employee's equity in the pension fund. Employers are *not* required under ERISA or any other law to provide a private pension fund for their employees (Noe et al., 2000).

Among its regulation, ERISA set up the Pension Benefit Guaranty Corporation in 1974, which is supported by premiums from employers to ensure that employees will eventually receive retirement funds. Companies that decide to withdraw from the plan must make substantial payments into the corporation before being permitted to do so. This and other elements of the act create hardships for employers who otherwise are committed to providing pension benefits for employees.

One major drawback to the ERISA legislation is that its rules are so demanding that many employers choose not to offer pension plans at all. Also, upon implementation of the act, many employers chose to withdraw their plans rather than try to comply with the law when it went into effect. Another unfortunate result is that many employers are electing to receive their accumulated retirement benefits when they leave the organization. Studies have documented that all to often these pension benefits never find their way into 401k or similar retirement mechanisms (Noe et al., 2000).

In place of regular company-created and company-maintained pension plans, a number of employers have opted to offer employees participation in what are known as 401k and similar plans under which employees contribute money on a tax-deferred basis for retirement purposes. The major drawback for the employee is that upon leaving the company she often receives her 401k contributions in a lump sum. Employees can roll these 401k funds over to similar tax-deferred investments within a specified number of days and retain them for eventual retirement purpose; but as with regular lump-sum pension proceeds given to an employee at termination, the temptation to use the funds for current expenses is often too great (Maddox et al., 2001)

4.5 Workplace Safety: Occupational Safety and Health Act

ORIGIN AND PASSAGE

For the first seven decades of the twentieth century state governments were responsible for safety in the workplace. During that period, organized labor became less and less satisfied with enforcement of state laws, variation in laws among the states, and often the absence of any safety laws. In the 5 years before the passage of federal legislation, job-related accidents were causing up to 2.5 million disabilities and 14,000 deaths annually (U.S. Department of Labor, 1976).

After 3 years of intense lobbying by employees and the unions, Congress passed the Occupational Safety and Health Act (OSHA) in 1970. OSHA applies to nearly all employees and includes all of those working in nursing homes.

FEDERAL IMPLEMENTATION

Two federal agencies have been set up to implement OSHA. The act is administered by the Occupational Safety and Health Administration in the Department of Labor, and the National Institute of Occupational Safety and Health (NIOSH) was established to conduct research and develop standards.

A major goal of the act has been to turn workplace safety enforcement back to the states with a strengthened work-safety law. States have been encouraged to establish their own inspection programs and industrial safety laboratories.

In addition to requiring that all standards are met, OSHA imposes on employers a general duty to provide each employee a safe workplace, free from recognized hazards that cause or are likely to cause death or serious physical harm. For example, pending the publication of final regulations regarding the control of infections (such as AIDS), OSHA invoked the "general duty" obligation when inspecting nursing facilities.

THREE OSHA IMPACT AREAS

OSHA directly affects the operations of nursing care facilities in at least three main areas:

1. meeting the standards set by OSHA
2. cooperating in OSHA inspections of the facility
3. keeping the necessary records on job-related accidents and illnesses

SOURCES OF STANDARDS

OSHA standards may originate from a variety of sources. The secretary of labor may issue and revise standards at will. This may be done on the secretary's own initiative, on recommendation of the National Institute of Occupational Safety and Health, or at the urging of interested parties such as labor unions or groups of affected employees.

Adopting Standards of Other Organizations

OSHA has adopted several national consensus standards that were developed by other groups, including the National Fire Protection Association's *Life Safety Code* (1985) and the *Standards for the Physically Handicapped* of the American National Standards Institute (1980).

DEFINITION OF *STANDARD*

OSHA safety standards are "practices, means, operations or processes, reasonably necessary to provide safe . . . employment" (Ivancevich & Glueck, 1983; Noe et al., 2000). Each employer is responsible for knowing OSHA standards (either federal or federal and state) for his or her facility.

The original standards ran to 350 pages of small print in the *Federal Register*. Subsequently, supplementary volumes of standards have been published. Some annual volumes have been over 700 pages in length. Even so, each manager is responsible for knowing applicable standards and is subject to both fines and imprisonment if found to be in violation of them.

OSHA REQUIREMENTS

OSHA bulletins have listed the following as just some of its requirements.

Employers

Every employer must furnish a workplace free from recognized hazards that are causing or are likely to cause death or serious harm to employees and shall comply with OSHA standards, displaying the OSHA poster that informs employees of their rights and responsibilities, and compiling annual figures on work-related illnesses and accidents

Employees

Each employee shall obey all OSHA requirements. However, the facility is held responsible for worker violation of OSHA standards. The employer has the choice of dismissing such a worker, but there are no punishments for the worker who willfully ignores OSHA requirements. Willful disregard of OSHA rules is, however, grounds for termination under federal law.

Any employee may lodge a complaint with OSHA. The complaint must be in writing and signed with a description of the hazardous condition. The signed complaint is submitted to the OSHA regional director and to the employer, unsigned if the employee wishes to remain anonymous.

Inspections

OSHA inspectors will visit at times of their own choosing or at the invitation of any employer, union, or employee. Employees requesting an inspection need not be identified.

The employer and the employees must each designate a representative to accompany the OSHA inspector(s). If the employees do not do so, the

OSHA compliance officer must consult several employees during the visit. This officer must hold an opening conference to discuss the scope and reason for the inspection and a concluding conference in which findings are presented to the employer.

Employers must not discriminate against any employee(s) who asks for an OSHA safety or health inspection. Any employee may file a complaint with the nearest OSHA office within 30 days for any such alleged discrimination.

OSHA inspectors examine *the premises* for compliance with regulations and *the records* of illnesses and injuries to employees.

Citations

Citations may be issued at the end of the inspection itself or later by mail. Any citation issued must be posted at or near the site of violation for 3 days or for the duration of the violation, whichever is longer. One citation must be issued for each serious and nonserious violation found and a time limit specified for its correction.

OSHA compliance officers may categorize employer violations as

1. *imminent danger*—can close operations down
2. *serious*—calls for a major fine
3. *nonserious*—a violation in which a direct and immediate relationship exists between the condition and occupational health, but not such as to cause death or serious physical harm
4. *de minimus*—small violation—notification is given, but no fine imposed; a violation of a standard that is not directly or immediately related to occupational safety or health.

In every case, a time period is specified within which the violation must be corrected. A fine of $7,000 per day per violation may be imposed after the time limit set for abatement (correction) of the violation.

Fines

Fines, some mandatory under OBRA 1990, are to be imposed for the following:

1. *willful or repeated violations*: up to $70,000 per violation (mandatory); may double after first conviction
2. *serious violation*: mandatory penalty up to $7,000 for each violation
3. *nonserious violation:* optional penalties up to $7,000 each
4. *failure to correct* within proposed time period: up to $7,000 per day
5. *willful violation*: minimum fine $5,000

Employers have the right to appeal fines or citations within the OSHA structure or in the courts. Notice of contest must be filed within 15 days.

Record Keeping

The area that most directly affects nursing home administrators on a daily basis is keeping standardized records of illnesses and injuries from which ratios must be calculated. This record is an OSHA form called "Log and Summary of Occupational Injuries and Illnesses," which must be kept by each facility.

Accidents and illnesses that do not have to be reported are those that require only first aid and do not result in any work time lost. Accidents and illnesses that do have to be reported are those that result in death(s), disabilities that cause the employee to miss work, and injuries that require treatment by a physician. Reporting requirements were tightened on May 2,1994. Fatal or serious multiple cases (three or more hospitalized) must be reported to the OSHA regional director orally, by telephone, within 8 hours, which begins as soon as any facility representatives become aware of the situation. Also, such incidents must be reported if death or hospitalization occur within 30 days of the incident. Other cases must be recorded within 6 days and reported on routine forms as requested by OSHA.

Occupational illness is a definition of special relevance to the nursing home setting. An occupational illness is any abnormal condition or disorder, other than one resulting from an occupational injury, caused by exposure to environmental factors associated with employment. It includes acute and chronic illnesses or diseases that may be caused by inhalation, absorption, ingestion, or direct contact (Chruden & Sherman).

OSHA defines an occupational injury as any injury, such as a cut, fracture, sprain amputation, that results from a work accident or from an exposure involving a single accident in the work environment (Chruden & Sherman).

Each time a recordable case is entered in the log mentioned above, a "Supplementary Record of Occupational Injuries and Illnesses" must be completed, giving information on what the employee was doing, which part of the body was affected, and the identity of the employee.

OSHA Form 102, "Summary of Occupational Injuries and Illnesses," must be submitted annually and posted where employees can easily see it, e.g., above the time clock, at least during January and February of every year.

The Current and Emerging Situation

Completing, submitting, and posting accident and illness forms as required will remain a continuing requirement for nursing home administrators, but the inspection issue is another matter. After years during which few, if any, nursing facilities were being inspected in the various states, OSHA inspectors have begun showing up to perform routine inspection of nursing facilities. In many locales OSHA inspectors will, at the invitation of the facility, perform dry-run inspections for an employer, advising on any "violations" and providing an opportunity for correction before any official inspection.

Since OSHA was enacted, fatalities in the work force are estimated to have decreased by 10% and total injuries to have decreased by 15% (Ivancevich & Glueck, 1983; Noe et al., 2000).

4.6 Fire Safety: The *Life Safety Code*®

The National Fire Protection Association is a private, nonprofit organization with headquarters in Quincy, Massachusetts. It is not a government agency, nor does it write federal regulations. However, because the regulations for licensing nursing homes include adherence to the *Life Safety Code*® these fire safety standards have, in effect, the force of law for nursing homes.

The National Fire Protection Association has more than 150 committees, one of which, the Committee on Safety to Life, establishes and revises these standards. The committee has met since 1913 and currently has several standing subcommittees.

The code has evolved over the years, benefiting from the hindsight gained from the experience of many tragic fires. This code represents the collected wisdom on fire prevention and fire containment.

The regulations passed in the *Federal Register* in 1974 required nursing facilities to "meet such provisions of the *Life Safety Code*® of the National Fire Protection Association as are applicable to nursing homes" (405.1134A). These regulations have been revised regularly with new editions approximately every 3 years. The ones described in the following sections are from the 1994 edition of *Life Safety Code*®.

Note: The materials on the Life Safety Code® in this section are reprinted with permission from NFPA 101-1994, *Life Safety Code*®, sixth edition, © 1994, National Fire Protection Association, Quincy, MA 02269. This reprinted material is neither the actual wording nor the complete and official position of the National Fire Protection Association on the referenced subject, which is represented only by the standard in its entirety. This material is intended to apprise persons in the nursing home field of the general nature and functions within the facility of *The Life Safety Code*®.

The actual wording of the *Life Safety Code®* is not used in the following pages. The major concepts and a number of the essential features of the code presented below are summaries of the code presented for study purposes. The code itself is not directly quoted, only paraphrased. Under no circumstances, then, should the reader treat this material as a substitute for obtaining the actual *Life Safety Code®*.

The sixth edition, edited by Ron Cote, (1994) offers highly useful interpretations of the *Life Safety Code®*. The National Fire Protection Association's *Health Care Facilities Handbook®*, edited by (1993) Burton R. Klein, P.E., (4th ed., 1993) and copies of the code itself may be ordered from National Fire Protection, Inc., Batterymarch Park, Quincy, MA 02269, telephone 1-800-344-3555.

HEALTH CARE OCCUPANCIES (SECTION 31-4 OF THE FIRE SAFETY CODE)*

A-31-4 Compromised Health

Due to the compromised health and mobility of residents a primary emphasis is placed on superior construction, quick discovery of fire, quick notification of the fire department, and early extinguishment.

31-4.1 Emphasis. Emphasis must be placed on removing patients from the room of fire origin and anyone directly exposed to the fire. The current emphasis is on moving occupants themselves rather than on having movable beds (an earlier now deleted requirement).

31-4.1.1 Fire Plan. Every administration must have written copies of a fire plan available to all supervisory personnel and an evacuation plan to areas of refuge. All employees must receive periodic in-service training and drill practice for their specific individualized duty assignments. A copy of the plan must be at the security center or telephone operator location.

31.4.1.2 Fire drills with actual transmission of a fire alarm signal and a simulated emergency condition (e.g., placement of an object in a room or area designated as the fire origin, which must be quickly located and transmitted by staff). All personnel in the facility, including administrators, maintenance, etc. must be trained. Quarterly drills for each shift must be conducted (9:00 p.m. to 6:00 a.m. drills may use a coded

---

*Life Safety Code® and 101® are registered trademarks of the National Fire Protection Association, Inc., Quincy, MA 02269.

announcement rather than an audible alarm). Infirm and/or bedridden patients do not have to be physically moved to safe areas or the exterior.

To reduce patient anxiety, doors to patient rooms in the area of planned fire origin may be closed. Drills must be on a random basis, at least once every 3 months for every employee. Empty wheelchairs may be used to simulate relocation of residents to adjacent safe smoke compartments.

31-4.1.3 Training. All employees must be trained in life safety procedures and devices.

31-4.2 Procedures in Case of Fire

31-4.2.1 Minimum response must include all personnel, removing all patients directly involved in the fire area, quick transmission of an alarm signal, confinement of the fire by closing doors to isolate the fire, and all duties assigned in the fire safety plan.

Upon discovering a fire, the discoverer must come to the aid of any person involved while calling aloud an agreed-upon code phrase; any individual within hearing must activate an alarm at the nearest manual fire station (if no person is endangered, the discoverer must activate the nearest manual alarm). All personnel must immediately undertake their assigned duties. The telephone operator, who must be immediately notified of the fire location, must notify the fire department and alert all building occupants.

31-4.2.2 The written fire safety plan must include: using alarm devices, transmitting alarms to the fire department, how to respond to alarms, how to isolate the fire, how to evacuate the fire area, preparation for building evacuation and extinguishing the fire.

31-4.2.3 The goal is to close as many doors as possible to prevent smoke from spreading and, to the extent feasible, to confine the fire to the room of origin. No or low loss of life occurs when staff close the doors, according to studies conducted. Closing the doors has the most significant effect on limiting the spread of fire and smoke and limiting or eliminating any loss of life.

31-4.3 Maintenance of Exits

All exits must be maintained. If locks exist on any exits, sufficient staff must be available 24 hours a day to ensure prompt release of any locks in fire or any emergency situation.

31-4.4 Smoking

Many, if not most, nursing facilities are adopting a no-smoking policy. For those that do not universally prohibit smoking in the building, the following requirements must be met. Smoking is not permitted in any location with flammable liquids, combustible gases, or where oxygen is being used or any other location designated as hazardous. Such areas must post No Smoking signs. Any smoking by nonresponsible patients must be prohibited except under strict supervision. Ashtrays must be safely designed and of noncombustible material, and metal closable containers must be available.

A-31-4.4 In cases where a ban on all smoking is not possible or not enforced, it is important to train staff and to exercise full control over all smoking. Smoking in bed and placing smoking materials in improper waste containers lead the causes of fire in nursing homes.

31-4.5 Furnishings, Bedding, and Decorations

31-4.5.1 Draperies and any similar hanging material including bed cubicle curtains must not interfere with the operations of smoke detectors and sprinklers. One option (12-3.5.3) is to hang curtains 18" below the sprinkler or detector or use a thin mesh that will not inhibit their functioning. Or (13-3.5.6) have a minimum vertical distance meeting NFPA 13 Standard for the Installation of Sprinkler Systems, which assumes occupants are basically nonambulatory, with sufficient staff 24 hours each day. Draperies, furniture with upholstery, and mattresses must be tested to meet heat release standards.

31-4.5.4 Combustible decorations are prohibited. Photographs and paintings in limited quantities are permitted.

31-4.5.5 Soiled linen and trash collection containers must be limited to a capacity of 32 gallons within any 64-square-foot area. Mobile soiled linen and trash collection receptacles of 33 gallons and more must be mobile and in an area or room protected as a hazard area when unattended. Housekeeping staff, for example, who must leave an area for whatever reason must store mobile containers in such a hazard-protected area.

31-4.6 New engineered smoke control systems must meet standards of NFPA 92A, *Recommended Practice for Smoke-Control Systems* and NFPA 92B, *Guide for Smoke Management Systems in Malls, Atria, and Large Areas.*

31-4.7 portable space-heating devices are prohibited except for use in nonsleeping staff and employee areas where the heating elements do not exceed 212° F.

SECTION 12-1 NEW HEALTH CARE OCCUPANCIES

(Only certain sections applying directly to nursing facilities are mentioned here. Numerous exceptions are cited in the full document to which the reader should refer when planning any new building.)

General Requirements (Section 12-1)

New nursing facilities must either meet the standards stipulated here or demonstrate equivalent safety. Alternative designs are allowed as long as they provide equivalent safety as based on chapter 3 of NFPA 101M, *Manual on Alternative Approaches to Life Safety.*

These requirements apply to new buildings or sections used as health care occupancies.

12-1.1.2 Objective. To limit the development and spreading of a fire to the room of fire origin and reduce the need for evacuation, except from the room of fire origin. These are achieved partially through requirements aimed at prevention of ignition, fire detection, controlling fire development, confinement of the fire effect, the fire's extinguishment, provision of evacuation facilities, and staff action.

12-1.1.3 Total concept. It is believed that evacuation between floors in a facility is too time-consuming (up to 30 minutes being required), hence the basic approach is to defend in place.

12-1.1.4.1 Additions. Additions not meeting these standards must be separated by a fire barrier having at least a 2-hour fire-resistance rating and of required construction materials.

12-1.1.4.2 Communicating openings. Shall be limited to corridors protected by approved self-closing fire doors. These doors, when necessary, may be held open by automatic release devices. These doors are normally kept closed.

A-12-1.1.4.5 Automatic sprinkler protection. Required of all new health care occupancies.

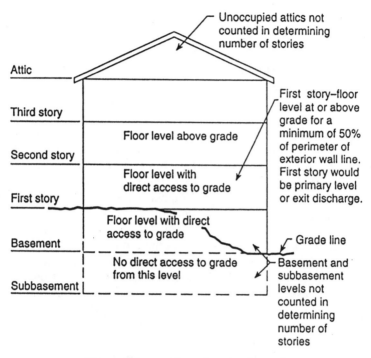

Determining number of stories for application of minimum construction requirements. Because of sloping grade, the primary level of exit discharge is not obvious. The fifty percent perimeter guideline of 12-1.6.1 clarifies that for the arrangement illustrated, the first story is the primary level of exit discharge. Number of stories includes primary level of exit discharge and all occupiable floors located above. This is an example of a three-story building.

FIGURE 4-7. Building section view illustrating grade line and story designation.

Reprinted with permission from *NFPA Life Safety Code® Handbook,* 6th Ed., Ron Cote, P.E., Edidtor, 1994, p. 374.

12-1.6.1 Construction requirements. The primary level of exit discharge of a building is the lowest story with a floor level at or above finished grade on the exterior wall with 50% or more of its perimeter. Figure 4-7 is a figure of a three-story building

12-1.6.2 Construction and multistory buildings. Constructions types are specified for a variety of buildings. All multistory health care facilities must be constructed of noncombustible materials. In three-story or more-buildings the major construction elements must be protected by a 2-hour fire resistance rating.

12-1.6.4 Openings for pipes, etc. All penetrations of walls must be protected with such means as metal plates, masonry fill, or similar approved product to prevent the spread of fire and smoke.

12-1.7 Occupant load. Means of egress must be provided for one person for each 120 sq. ft. of gross floor area in health care sleeping areas and for one person each 240 sq. ft. of gross floor area in inpatient treatment areas, such as physical therapy. If the actual count of persons exceeds these numbers, the actual number of persons becomes the minimum occupant load for determining required egress.

12-2.2.2-7 Doors. Locks are not permitted on patient sleeping room doors. An exception is permitted for using a device that locks a door so that staff can unlock it from the corridor and the patient can exit the room without use of any key. Such an approach would prevent patients from accidentally wandering into an isolation room, but the patient in the isolation room would be able to exit the room without use of a key or tool. Also, for patients who might endanger themselves, for example, Alzheimer patients, a lock may be installed, provided staff carry keys at all times or other provision for remotely unlocking all such doors. Doors in a required means of egress may not be equipped with a latch or lock that requires the use of a tool or key from the egress side. At maximum, only one delayed egress device may be used along the length of any egress.

5-2 Means of Egress

Interior stairs, in general, must have a minimum clear width of 44" except for handrails not exceeding 3½" at or below handrail height on each side. Riser maximum height is 7", minimum height of risers is 4". Minimum tread depth is 11", minimum headroom is 6' 8". Maximum height between landings is 12'.

Handrails are required on both sides and must be not less than 34" nor more than 38" above the surface of the tread measured vertically to the top of the rail from the leading edge of the tread. Handrail clearance must be at least 1½" when smooth surfaces are used, more if rough surfaces. Handrails must be graspable firmly with a comfortable grip so the hand can slide along the rail without encountering any obstructions.

5.2.3 Smokeproof enclosures. >A smokeproof enclosure is a set(s) of enclosed stairs designed to limit the infiltration of heat, smoke, and fire gases from a fire in any part of a building that limits entry of the products of combustion into the stairway. Such stairwells must have a 2-hour fire-resistance and a door with a 1 1.2 hour fire protection rating.

5-2.4 Horizontal exits. A horizontal exit is a passage from one area of a building to another, separated by a fire barrier, space, or other protection enabling each area to be a fire compartment independent of the one in which a fire exists. It can be a bridge to another building. No stairs or ramps are normally involved. At least 30 sq. ft. per patient must be provided within the aggregated area of corridors, patient rooms, treatment rooms, lounge dining area and other low hazard areas on each side. A single door may be permitted, provided the exit serves one direction only and is at least 41.5" wide. If separating two fire areas, two doors swinging opposite directions, each at least 41.5" is required.

5.2.5 Ramps. The usual definition is

- 20° to 50° = a stairway
- 7°–20° = a stairway and landings
- under 7° = a ramp

Nearly horizontal landings are required at both ends of ramps. Ramps are to be slip resistant and have a clear width of at least 44". The maximum rise for a single ramp run is 30".

12-2.3.3 Aisles, corridors, and ramps used for exit must be at least 8' in width clear and unobstructed.

12-2.4 Number of exits. At least two exits located remotely from each other must be provided for each floor and fire section of a building. At least one exit from each floor or fire section must lead directly outside, to a stair, a smokeproof enclosure, a ramp, or an exit passageway. At no time can an exit passageway require return through the compartment of origin.

12-2.5 Arrangement of means of egress. Every patient room must have an exit access door leading directly to an exit access corridor (some exceptions exist, e.g., a door opening directly to the outside).

12-2.6.2 Travel distance to exits. Travel distance between the door in any room and an exit access and an exit must not exceed 150' and travel from within any patient room to same must not exceed 200'. Travel distance within a room to an exit must not exceed 50'.

12-2.7 Discharge from exits. Each required exit ramp or stair must lead directly outside at grade or be an enclosed passage meeting all fire-resistance regulations at grade.

12-2.8 Illumination of means of egress. Must be continuous with all exit floor surfaces illuminated at the level of 1 foot-candle, measured at the floor of the exit access, the exit, and the exit discharge. Failure of any single light source (electric bulb) must not leave any area in darkness, hence the need for overlapping light sources, separately wired.

5-9 Emergency lighting must have automatic transfer between normal poser and an emergency source. Storage batteries are acceptable if they meet the candlelight requirements for a period of 1½ hours. Automotive type batteries are not acceptable. An on-site generator normally is required as the second source of emergency lighting.

5-10 Exit marking. Exit signs must be readily visible from any direction of exit access. Tactile signage is required at each door into an exit stair enclosure. No point in the exit access route may be more than 100'. Exit signs must have letters at least 6" high and not less than 3/4" wide and be of contrasting color.

Emergency power. Most facilities have an emergency electrical generator. This generator must go on within 10 seconds of a power failure. Such a generator is not required, however, in a freestanding building in which the management precludes the provision of care for any patient who may need to be sustained by electrical life-support equipment such as a respirator or suction apparatus, and in which battery-operated systems or equipment are provided to maintain power to exit lights and means of egress, stairways, medicinal preparation areas, and the like for a minimum of 1½ hours. Battery power is also required to operate all alarm systems. Separate power supplies controlled by separate switches that are protected from fire threat are required.

12-3 Protection

12-3.1 Vertical openings. Any stairway, ramp, elevator, hoist or chute (e.g., for laundry) between stories must be enclosed with protective construction, for example, fire resistance of 1 hour in buildings required to have 1-hour protection, one hour fire resistance for buildings of not more than three stories, and of 2 hours for enclosures in buildings of over three stories.

12-3.2 Protection from hazards. Hazardous areas are spaces with contents that are flammable or combustible and represent a higher than normal hazard. Hazardous areas must be protected by fire barriers with a fire-resistance rating of 1 hour or a completely automatic extinguishing system. Hazardous areas include

- mechanical equipment rooms
- laundry
- kitchens, repair shops
- handicraft shops
- employee locker areas
- gift shop

The following must have both 1 hour fire resistance and a compete extinguishment system: soiled linen rooms, paint ships, trash collection rooms, and rooms or spaces, including repair shops, used for the storage of combustible supplies and equipment in quantities deemed hazardous by the authority having jurisdiction.

Cooking facilities. Numerous regulations govern cooking facilities. A major focus is the requirement for a regularly serviced, fixed, automatic fire-extinguishing system for cook stoves. Small appliances such as equipment for food warming or limited cooking (such as a small microwave) are exempted from cooking regulations for commercial cooking equipment.

12-3.3 Interior finish. A number of requirements specify the type of wall materials usable and the degree of flame spread, smoke development, and similar characteristics so as to ensure that walls do not contribute to the spread of fire. No specific requirements pertain to floor finishes.

12-3.4 Detection, alarm, and communications systems. This is an extensive section with numerous provisions and exceptions. The following are some of the more salient requirements. A manually operated fire alarm system, electrically monitored, is required. This means that when any component part of the fire alarm system malfunctions, a continuous trouble alert indication is sent electronically to a continuously attended location.

The fire alarm system must be designed to notify all building occupants when any alarm station is activated. The local fire department (or its equivalent) must be automatically notified whenever any fire alarm station is activated. Codes for identifying fire zones are permitted.

Emergency control. Activating any fire alarm station must automatically activate all appropriate devices (e.g., the sprinkler system, alarms, door releases).

New nursing homes must have an automatically operated smoke detection system. Smoke detectors must be located no farther apart than 30' and not more than 15' from any wall.

The automatic smoke detection and fire detection systems must both be connected electrically. Manual pull stations should be located so no employee has to leave the fire area to activate the alarm. A distinct supervisory signal must be provided to a constantly attended location in the event of any malfunction or action that would reduce sprinkler system performance. The main nursing station is often chosen for such a location.

12-3.5 Extinguishment requirements. *A supervised automatic sprinkler system must be installed.* Quick response sprinklers must be used in the smoke compartment. Some exceptions may be made regarding sprinkler type.

Portable fire extinguishers meeting NFPA and local codes must be installed. Hand fire extinguishers are required on every floor and in every hazardous area. The travel distance to any extinguisher may be no more than 75' to a Class A extinguisher, 50' to a Class B or C extinguisher. Short persons must be able to reach the extinguisher. Every extinguisher must be in operating condition at all items Fire extinguishers must be checked quarterly by a qualified person and be serviced annually by a qualified examiner who must show the date that the inspection and servicing was accomplished on an attached tag.

12-3.6 Corridor doors. Doors protecting openings in corridor partitions must be able to resist the passage of smoke but need not have a fire-protection rating. Doors must have a positive latch that cannot be held in the retracted position. Roller latches are not permitted. The latch must be able to hold the door in a closed position.

12-3.7 Subdivision of building spaces. Smoke barriers are required to meet the following specifications:

1. divide every story used by patients for sleeping or treatments into at least two smoke compartments
2. divide every story having an occupant load of 50 or more persons, regardless of use, into at least two smoke compartments
3. limit the size of each smoke compartment required above to no more than 22,500 sq. ft.
4. limit the travel distance in the required smoke barrier to 200'.

Doors shall be 1¾" thick, solid bodied wood core or of construction of 20-minute resistance-fire rating. Vision panels must be provided in swinging doors.

12-3.8 Outside window or door. Each patient sleeping room shall have an outside window or outside door. The maximum allowable sill height is 36" above the floor. The window does not have to be operable.

CONCLUDING OBSERVATIONS

The administrator who is planning new construction must meet all state and local codes as well. Many areas of the Life Safety Code® have been left uncovered. There are, for example, additional sections on utilities, heating, ventilation, air conditioning, elevators, rubbish chutes, incinerators, laundry chutes, and so on, that have not been discussed.

The reader realizes, of course, that this is an introduction to only a few of the more salient aspects of the Life Safety Code®. The reader is strongly urged to purchase the *Life Safety Code® Handbook* for the year containing the requirements that he or she must meet.

The *Life Safety Code® Handbook* is an essential tool for administrators. It is the administrator's job to understand the code and its basic requirements in order to ensure that the facility is in basic conformity with regulations and to work intelligently with engineers, architects, and state building code officials in planning and pursuing any nursing facility construction project.

4.7 Americans with Disabilities Act: Accessibility Guidelines for Facilities

On Friday, July 26, 1991 the U.S. Department of Justice, Office of the Attorney General issued the following final rule (Part III 28 CFR Part 36) for the purpose of achieving nondiscrimination on the basis of disability. These requirements apply to nursing facilities that are newly built or renovated and are available from the Americans With Disabilities Act's Architectural and Transportation Barriers Compliance Board, U.S. Department of Justice, Civil Rights Division (Washington, D.C.). They can also be found in the *Federal Register,* Vol. 56, No. 144 (Friday, July 26, 1991, pages 35544—35691).

The following pages provide an overview of these requirements, most of which are based on the standards developed and approved by the Council of American Building Officials/American National Standards Institute, Inc., entitled *American National Standard Accessible and Usable Buildings and Facilities.*

Any administrator who is planning, building, or renovating a nursing facility should obtain and use both of the following documents:

• *American National Standard Accessible and Usable Buildings and Facilities* (CAB0/ANSI A117.1-1992) which is available from Buildings Officials and Code Administrators International, 4051 West Flossmoor Road, Country Club Hill, IL, 60477

Note: The following information, figures, and tables are reproduced here with the permission of the Council of American Building Officials, Executive Offices, 5203 Leesburg Pike, #708, Falls Church, VA 22041. As indicated in each figure and table, however, ordering address for copies of American National Standard Accessible and Usable Buildings and Facilities is located in Country Club Hill, IL, as noted in text. The information provided in this textbook is designed provide only an introduction to the reader of the nature and importance of the directions of these requirements. Under no circumstances may the following pages be utilized in actual planning, construction or renovating of a nursing facility.

• Americans With Disabilities Act of 1990, Accessibility Guidelines for Facilities, *Federal Register,* Vol. 56, No. 144 (Friday, July 26, 1991), Final Rule Part III CFR 28, Part 36, which is available from the Americans With Disabilities Act's Architectural and Transportation Barriers Compliance Board, 1331 F Street, N.W., Suite 1000, Washington, DC 20004.

STANDARDS FOR ACCESSIBLE DESIGN (APPENDIX A TO PART 36)

The following is an overview of the following standards.

1. PURPOSE

To set guidelines for accessibility for individuals with disabilities. Are to be applied during the design, construction and alteration of facilities.

2. GENERAL

Departures from these guidelines are permitted where equivalent access is provided.

3. MISCELLANEOUS INSTRUCTIONS AND DEFINITIONS

Graphic conventions. These are illustrated in Table 4-8.

Selected Definitions

Access aisle. An accessible pedestrian space between elements, such as parking spaces, seating, and desks, that provides clearances appropriate for use of the elements.

Accessible. Describes a site, building, facility, or portion thereof that complies with these requirements.

Accessible element. An element specified by these requirements (e.g., telephone, controls, and the like)

Accessible route. A continuous unobstructed path connecting all accessible elements and spaces of a facility. Interior accessible routes may include corridors, floors, ramps, elevators, lists and clear floor space at fixtures. Exterior accessible route may include parking access aisles, curb ramps, crosswalks at vehicular ways, walks, ramps and lifts.

Accessible space. A space that complies with these requirements.

Addition. An expansion, extension, or increase in the gross floor area of a facility.

Area of rescue assistance. An area, which has direct access to an exit, where people who are unable to use stairs may remain temporarily in safety to await further instructions or assistance during emergency evacuation.

Assembly area. A room or space accommodating a group of individuals for recreational, educational, or amusement purposes or for consumption of food and drink.

Table 4-8. Americans With Disabilities Act Graphic Conventions

Convention	Description
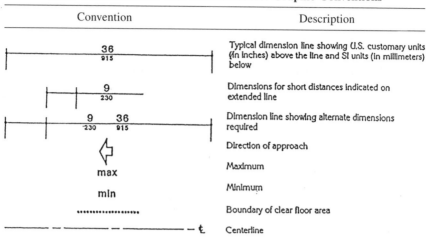	Typical dimension line showing U.S. customary units (in inches) above the line and SI units (in millimeters) below
	Dimensions for short distances indicated on extended line
	Dimension line showing alternate dimensions required
	Direction of approach
	Maximum
	Minimum
	Boundary of clear floor area
	Centerline

Americans with Disabilities Act of 1990, Accessibility Guidelines for Facilities. FederaL ,~zster Vol. 56, No. 144 / Friday, July 26, 1991 / Rules and Regulations, p. 35622. Final Rule Part III CFR 2&Part 36. A copy of the final federal rule should be obtained from American with Disabilities Act's Architectural and Transportation Barriers Compli.ance Board, U.S. Department of Justice, Civil Rights Division (Washington, DC). A copy of American National Standard Accessible and Usable Bu4#~ CABO/ ANSI A117.1-1992 should be obtained from American National Standards Institute, 11 West 42nd St., New York, NY, 10036.

Clear. Unobstructed.

Clear floor space. The minimum unobstructed floor or ground space required to accommodate a single, stationary wheelchair and occupant.

Egress, means of. A continuous and unobstructed way of exit travel from any point in a facility to a public way.

Element. An architectural or mechanical component of a facility, space or site (e.g., telephone, curb ramp, door, drinking fountain, seating, or toilet).

Signage. Displayed verbal, symbolic, tactile and pictorial information.

Space. A definable area (e.g., room, toilet room, hall, assembly area, entrance, storage room, alcove, courtyard, or lobby).

Tactile. Describes an object that can be perceived using the sense of touch.

Walk. An exterior pathway with a prepared surface intended for pedestrian use.

4. ACCESSIBLE ELEMENTS AND SPECIFICATIONS OF SECTION 6 MEDICAL FACILITIES

(6)(3) Long-term-care facilities, nursing homes—at least 50% of patient bedrooms and toilets and all public use and common use areas are required to be designed and constructed to be accessible. (Author's note: Given the nature of the patient mix in the typical nursing facility, it seems illogical to build any resident/patient rooms and toilets that are not accessible to persons with disabilities.)

4.1 Minimum requirements

Accessible sites must provide at least one accessible route that complies with 4.3 within the boundary of the site from public transportation stops, accessible parking spaces, passenger loading zones, if furnished, and public streets or sidewalks to an accessible building entrance.

Accessible routes must have at least one complying with 4.3 connecting accessible buildings, accessible facilities, accessible elements, and accessible spaces that are on the same site.

Several other minimum requirements are stated, most of which are outlined below.

4.2 Space Allowance and Reach Ranges

Wheelchair passage width. 36" continuously, 32" at any one point (see Figure 4-8).
Width of wheelchair passing. 60" (see Figure 4-9).
Wheelchair turning space (to make 180° turn). Clear space of 60" or T-shaped space (see Figure 4-10).
Relationship of maneuvering clearances to wheelchair spaces. One unobstructed side adjoining an accessible route (see Figure 4-11).
High forward reach. Generally 48" (demonstrated in Figure 4-12).
Side reach. Between 9" and 54" off the floor (see Figure 4-13).

4.3 Accessible Route

Must meet definition above, be at least 36" wide (32" at doors), allow for turns around objects (see Figure 4-14), have passing spaces 60" wide at least every 200', 80 inch turn room, stable, firm and slip-resistant surface texture, and meet change of level requirements.

4.4 Protruding Objects

Objects located between 27" and 80" above the floor must protrude no more than 4" into any hall or passageway or walk. Objects with their leading edge 27" high or less may protrude any amount from the wall. Freestanding objects mounted on posts or pylons may overhang 12" when mounted between 27" and 80" above the floor (e.g., a telephone booth). In no case may protruding objects reduce the clear width of an accessible route or maneuvering space (see Figure 4-15).

4.5 Ground and Floor Surfaces

In general the ground must be stable and firm, the floor slip-resistant. Changes in level.

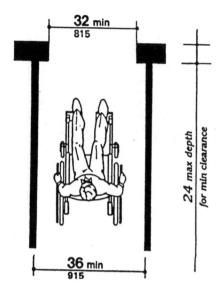

FIGURE 4-8. Minimum clear width for single wheelchair.
Americans with Disabilities Act of 1990, Accessibility Guidelines for Facilities. *Federal Register* / Vol. 56, No. 144 / Friday, July 26, 1991 / Rules and Regulations, p. 35622. Final Rule Part III CFR 28 Part 36. A copy of the final federal rule should be obtained from American with Disabilities Act's Architectural and Transportation Barriers Compliance Board, U.S. Department of Justice, Civil Rights Division (Washington, DC). A copy of *American National Standard Accessible and Usable Buildings and Facilities,* CABO/ANSI A117.1–1992 should be obtained from American National Standards Institute, 11 West 42nd St., New York, NY, 10036.

- Up to ¼" may be vertical and without edge
- Between ¼" and ½" beveled edge required
- Over ½": ramp treatment required.

Carpet. Must be securely attached, firm or no pad, with maximum pile height of ½", level cut, and trimmed along exposed edge that conforms to changes in level in paragraph above (see Figure 4-16a).

Gratings. Maximum width of openings: ½". If in walkways, the ½" openings must be perpendicular to dominant direction of travel (see Figure 4-16b and c).

4.6 Parking and Passenger Loading Zones

Number of Parking Spaces	Minimum Accessible Spaces
1–25	1
26–50	2
51–75	3
76–100	4
101–150	5

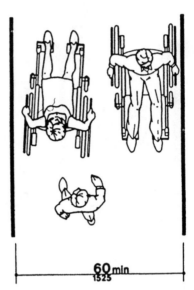

FIGURE 4-9. Minimum clear width for two wheelchairs.
Americans with Disabilities Act of 1990, Accessibility Guidelines for Facilities. *Federal Register* / Vol. 56, No. 144 / Friday, July 26, 1991 / Rules and Regulations, p. 35622. Final Rule Part III CFR 28 Part 36. A copy of the final federal rule should be obtained from American with Disabilities Act's Architectural and Transportation Barriers Compliance Board, U.S. Department of Justice, Civil Rights Division (Washington, DC). A copy of *American National Standard Accessible and Usable Buildings and Facilities,* CABO/ANSI A117.1–1992 should be obtained from American National Standards Institute, 11 West 42nd St., New York, NY, 10036.

Number of Parking Spaces	Minimum Accessible Spaces
151–200	6
201–300	7
301–400	8

Spaces shall be at least 96" wide with an accessible aisle at least 60" wide (two spaces may share one aisle). A van space must be provided and designated by signage (see Figure 4-17, 4-18).

The standard handicapped symbol must be places so that it is not obscured by a parked vehicle. A passenger loading zone at least 60" wide and 20' long adjacent and parallel to the vehicle pull-up space must be provided.

4.7 Curb Ramps

Location. Wherever an accessible route crosses a curb (see Figure 4-19 and 4-20).

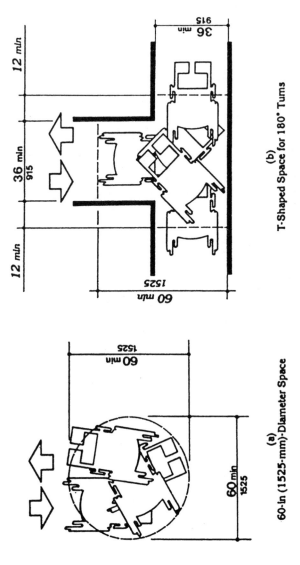

(a)
60-In (1525-mm)-Diameter Space

(b)
T-Shaped Space for 180° Turns

FIGURE 4-10. Wheelchair turning space.

Americans with Disabilities Act of 1990, Accessibility Guidelines for Facilities. *Federal Register* / Vol. 56, No. 144 / Friday, July 26, 1991 / Rules and Regulations, p. 35622. Final Rule Part III CFR 28 Part 36. A copy of the final federal rule should be obtained from American with Disabilities Act's Architectural and Transportation Barriers Compliance Board, U.S. Department of Justice, Civil Rights Division (Washington, DC). A copy of *American National Standard Accessible and Usable Buildings and Facilities*, CABO/ANSI A117.1–1992 should be obtained from American National Standards Institute, 11 West 42nd St., New York, NY, 10036.

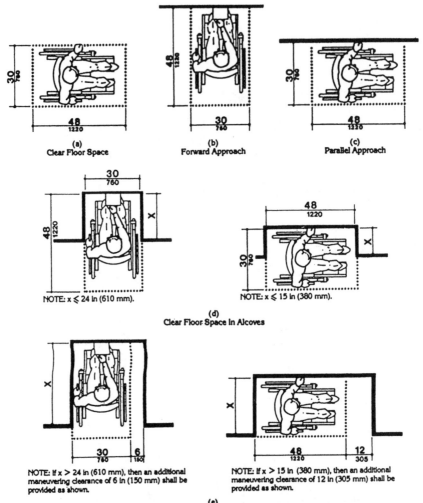

FIGURE 4-11. Minimum clear floor space for wheelchairs.
Americans with Disabilities Act of 1990, Accessibility Guidelines for Facilities. *Federal Register* / Vol. 56, No. 144 / Friday, July 26, 1991 / Rules and Regulations, p. 35622. Final Rule Part III CFR 28 Part 36. A copy of the final federal rule should be obtained from American with Disabilities Act's Architectural and Transportation Barriers Compliance Board, U.S. Department of Justice, Civil Rights Division (Washington, DC). A copy of *American National Standard Accessible and Usable Buildings and Facilities,* CABO/ANSI A117.1–1992 should be obtained from American National Standards Institute, 11 West 42nd St., New York, NY, 10036.

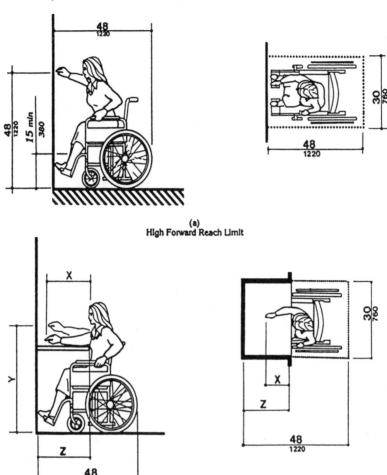

(a)
High Forward Reach Limit

NOTE: x shall be ≤ 25 in (635 mm); z shall be ⩾ x. When x < 20 in (510 mm), then y shall be 48 in (1220 mm) maximum. When x is 20 to 25 in (510 to 635 mm), then y shall be 44 in (1120 mm) maximum.

FIGURE 4-12. Forward reach.

Americans with Disabilities Act of 1990, Accessibility Guidelines for Facilities. *Federal Register* / Vol. 56, No. 144 / Friday, July 26, 1991 / Rules and Regulations, p. 35622. Final Rule Part III CFR 28 Part 36. A copy of the final federal rule should be obtained from American with Disabilities Act's Architectural and Transportation Barriers Compliance Board, U.S. Department of Justice, Civil Rights Division (Washington, DC). A copy of *American National Standard Accessible and Usable Buildings and Facilities,* CABO/ANSI A117.1–1992 should be obtained from American National Standards Institute, 11 West 42nd St., New York, NY, 10036.

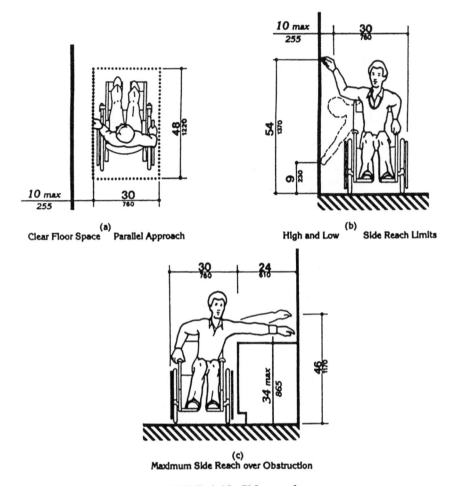

(a)
Clear Floor Space   Parallel Approach

(b)
High and Low   Side Reach Limits

(c)
Maximum Side Reach over Obstruction

FIGURE 4-13. Side reach.
Americans with Disabilities Act of 1990, Accessibility Guidelines for Facilities. *Federal Register* / Vol. 56, No. 144 / Friday, July 26, 1991 / Rules and Regulations, p. 35622. Final Rule Part III CFR 28 Part 36. A copy of the final federal rule should be obtained from American with Disabilities Act's Architectural and Transportation Barriers Compliance Board, U.S. Department of Justice, Civil Rights Division (Washington, DC). A copy of *American National Standard Accessible and Usable Buildings and Facilities,* CABO/ANSI A117.1–1992 should be obtained from American National Standards Institute, 11 West 42nd St., New York, NY, 10036.

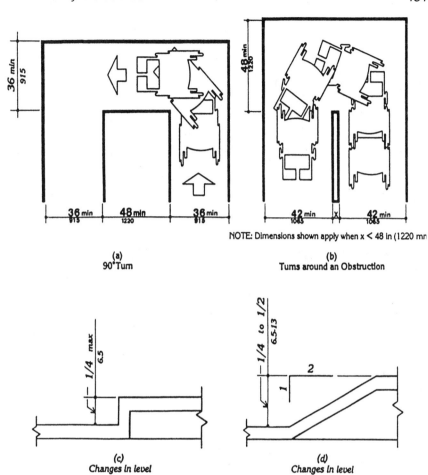

FIGURE 4-14. Accessible route.
Americans with Disabilities Act of 1990, Accessibility Guidelines for Facilities. *Federal Register* / Vol. 56, No. 144 / Friday, July 26, 1991 / Rules and Regulations, p. 35622. Final Rule Part III CFR 28 Part 36. A copy of the final federal rule should be obtained from American with Disabilities Act's Architectural and Transportation Barriers Compliance Board, U.S. Department of Justice, Civil Rights Division (Washington, DC). A copy of *American National Standard Accessible and Usable Buildings and Facilities,* CABO/ANSI A117.1–1992 should be obtained from American National Standards Institute, 11 West 42nd St., New York, NY, 10036.

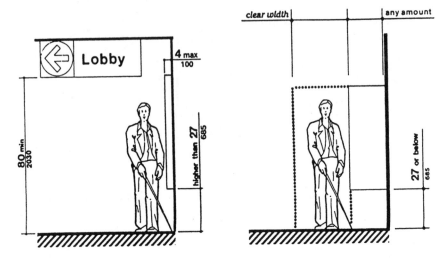

FIGURE 4-15. Protruding objects. (a) Walking parallel to a wall.
Americans with Disabilities Act of 1990, Accessibility Guidelines for Facilities. *Federal Register* / Vol.
56, No. 144 / Friday, July 26, 1991 / Rules and Regulations, p. 35622. Final Rule Part III CFR 28
Part 36. A copy of the final federal rule should be obtained from American with Disabilities Act's
Architectural and Transportation Barriers Compliance Board, U.S. Department of Justice, Civil
Rights Division (Washington, DC). A copy of *American National Standard Accessible and Usable
Buildings and Facilities,* CABO/ANSI A117.1–1992 should be obtained from American National
Standards Institute, 11 West 42nd St., New York, NY, 10036.

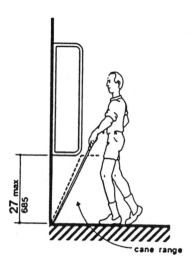

FIGURE 4-15(b). Walking perpendicular to a wall.

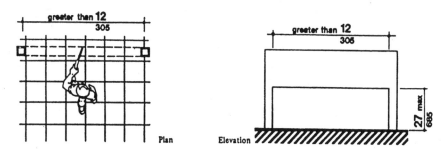

FIGURE 4-15(c). Free-standing overhanging objects.

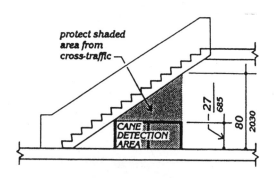

FIGURE 4-15(c-1). Overhead hazards.

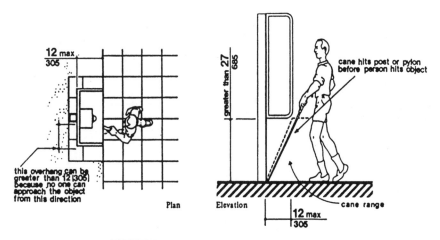

FIGURE 4-15(d). Overhanging objects.

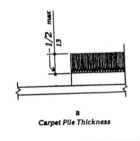

a
Carpet Pile Thickness

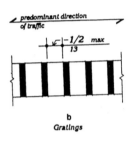

b
Gratings

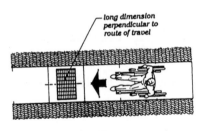

c
Grating Orientation

FIGURE 4-16. Protruding objects. (a) Carpet pile thickness, (b) gratings, and (c) grating orientation.

Americans with Disabilities Act of 1990, Accessibility Guidelines for Facilities. *Federal Register* / Vol. 56, No. 144 / Friday, July 26, 1991 / Rules and Regulations, p. 35622. Final Rule Part III CFR 28 Part 36. A copy of the final federal rule should be obtained from American with Disabilities Act's Architectural and Transportation Barriers Compliance Board, U.S. Department of Justice, Civil Rights Division (Washington, DC). A copy of *American National Standard Accessible and Usable Buildings and Facilities,* CABO/ANSI A117.1–1992 should be obtained from American National Standards Institute, 11 West 42nd St., New York, NY, 10036.

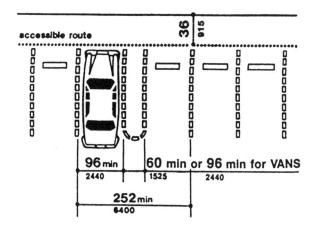

FIGURE 4-17. Dimensions of parking spaces.
Americans with Disabilities Act of 1990, Accessibility Guidelines for Facilities. *Federal Register* / Vol. 56, No. 144 / Friday, July 26, 1991 / Rules and Regulations, p. 35622. Final Rule Part III CFR 28 Part 36. A copy of the final federal rule should be obtained from American with Disabilities Act's Architectural and Transportation Barriers Compliance Board, U.S. Department of Justice, Civil Rights Division (Washington, DC). A copy of *American National Standard Accessible and Usable Buildings and Facilities,* CABO/ANSI A117.1–1992 should be obtained from American National Standards Institute, 11 West 42nd St., New York, NY, 10036.

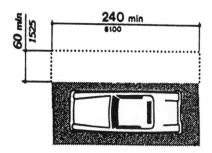

FIGURE 4-18. Access aisle at passenger loading zones.
Americans with Disabilities Act of 1990, Accessibility Guidelines for Facilities. *Federal Register* / Vol. 56, No. 144 / Friday, July 26, 1991 / Rules and Regulations, p. 35622. Final Rule Part III CFR 28 Part 36. A copy of the final federal rule should be obtained from American with Disabilities Act's Architectural and Transportation Barriers Compliance Board, U.S. Department of Justice, Civil Rights Division (Washington, DC). A copy of *American National Standard Accessible and Usable Buildings and Facilities,* CABO/ANSI A117.1–1992 should be obtained from American National Standards Institute, 11 West 42nd St., New York, NY, 10036.

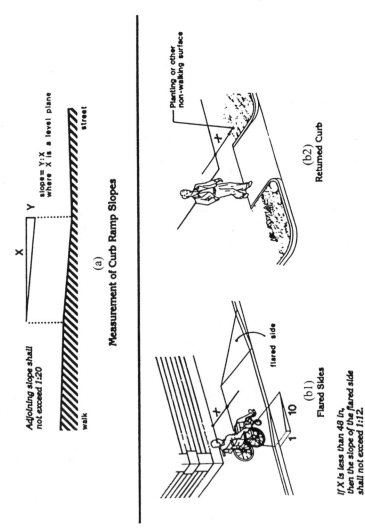

FIGURE 4-19. Measurement of curb ramp slopes (a), sides of curb ramps (b).
Americans with Disabilities Act of 1990, Accessibility Guidelines for Facilities. *Federal Register* / Vol. 56, No. 144 / Friday, July 26, 1991 / Rules and Regulations, p. 35622. Final Rule Part III CFR 28 Part 36. A copy of the final federal rule should be obtained from American with Disabilities Act's Architectural and Transportation Barriers Compliance Board, U.S. Department of Justice, Civil Rights Division (Washington, DC). A copy of *American National Standard Accessible and Usable Buildings and Facilities*, CABO/ANSI A117.1–1992 should be obtained from American National Standards Institute, 11 West 42nd St., New York, NY, 10036.

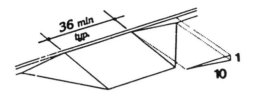

FIGURE 4-20. Built-up curb ramp.
Americans with Disabilities Act of 1990, Accessibility Guidelines for Facilities. *Federal Register* / Vol. 56, No. 144 / Friday, July 26, 1991 / Rules and Regulations, p. 35622. Final Rule Part III CFR 28 Part 36. A copy of the final federal rule should be obtained from American with Disabilities Act's Architectural and Transportation Barriers Compliance Board, U.S. Department of Justice, Civil Rights Division (Washington, DC). A copy of *American National Standard Accessible and Usable Buildings and Facilities*, CABO/ANSI A117.1–1992 should be obtained from American National Standards Institute, 11 West 42nd St., New York, NY, 10036.

4.8 Ramps

Ramp. Any part of an accessible route with a slope greater than 1:20.

Rise and slope. Least possible slope is to be used. Maximum slope is 1:12, maximum rise 30".

Landings. Required at bottom and top of each run, as wide as widest ramp run leading to it (minimum of 60"). Minimum 60" x 60" if ramp changes direction at a landing.

Handrails. If there is a rise of more than 6" or a horizontal projection of greater than 72" it must have handrails on both sides (see Figure 4-21).

Cross slopes. Maximum of 1:50.

4.9 Stairs

Treads and risers. On any given flight of stairs, riser heights and tread widths must be uniform. Treads must be no less than 11" apart, measured from one riser to another. Risers must be a maximum of 7" high. Open risers are never permitted on an accessible route. Nosing must project no more than 1½" (see Figure 4-22).

Handrails. See "ramps" above. Also, at the bottom, the handrail shall continue to slope for the distance of one tread past the bottom riser, then extend parallel to the floor or ground surface for 12". Gripping surfaces must be uninterrupted by newel posts, other construction elements, or obstructions. Top of handrail gripping surface shall be mounted between 34 and 38" above stair nosings. Ends of handrails shall be either rounded or returned smoothly to floor, wall or post. Handrails must not rotate within their fittings (see Figure 4-23).

4.10 Elevators

Numerous detailed requirements are set forth.

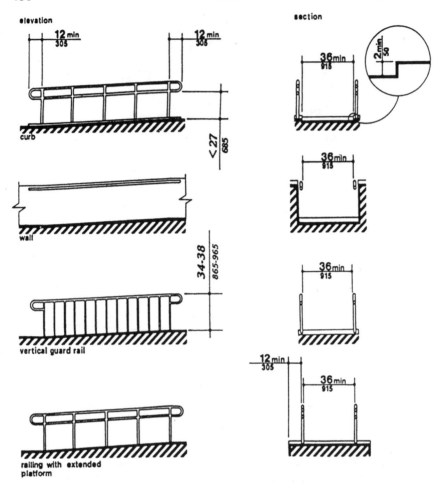

FIGURE 4-21. Examples of edge protection and handrail extensions.
Americans with Disabilities Act of 1990, Accessibility Guidelines for Facilities. *Federal Register* / Vol. 56, No. 144 / Friday, July 26, 1991 / Rules and Regulations, p. 35622. Final Rule Part III CFR 28 Part 36. A copy of the final federal rule should be obtained from American with Disabilities Act's Architectural and Transportation Barriers Compliance Board, U.S. Department of Justice, Civil Rights Division (Washington, DC). A copy of *American National Standard Accessible and Usable Buildings and Facilities,* CABO/ANSI A117.1–1992 should be obtained from American National Standards Institute, 11 West 42nd St., New York, NY, 10036.

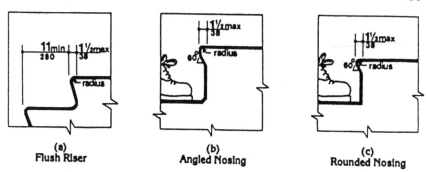

FIGURE 4-22. Usable tread width and examples of acceptable nosings.
Americans with Disabilities Act of 1990, Accessibility Guidelines for Facilities. *Federal Register* / Vol.
56, No. 144 / Friday, July 26, 1991 / Rules and Regulations, p. 35622. Final Rule Part III CFR 28
Part 36. A copy of the final federal rule should be obtained from American with Disabilities Act's
Architectural and Transportation Barriers Compliance Board, U.S. Department of Justice, Civil
Rights Division (Washington, DC). A copy of *American National Standard Accessible and Usable
Buildings and Facilities,* CABO/ANSI A117.1–1992 should be obtained from American National
Standards Institute, 11 West 42nd St., New York, NY, 10036.

4.11 Wheelchair Lifts

Lifts are permitted, must meet local requirements.

4.12 Windows

No requirements are set at this time.

4.13 Doors

Clear width. Must be 32" at openings which must be at an angle of 90°
to accessible route. Two doors in series must have at least 48" between them.

Thresholds at doorways. Shall not exceed ¾" in height for exterior
sliding doors or ½" for other types.

Hardware. Handles, pulls, latches, locks, and other operating devices on
accessible doors must have a shape that is easy to grasp with one
hand and does not require tight grasping, tight pinching, or twisting
of the wrist to operate. Lever operated mechanisms, push-type mechanisms, and shaped handles are acceptable designs, no more than
48" above the finished floor.

Door opening force. Five lbs. maximum for interior and sliding or folding doors.

Automatic doors and power-assisted doors. Should be slow-opening
and low-powered; not opening back to back faster than 3 seconds,
needing no more than 15 lbs. to stop movement.

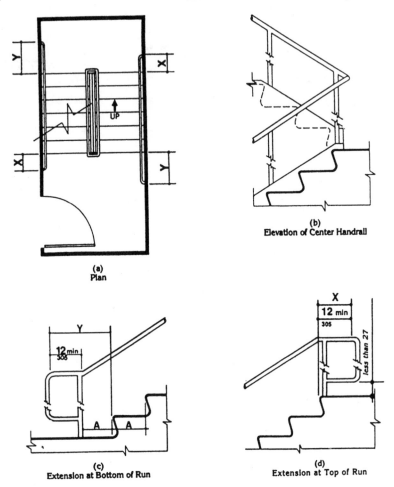

(a) Plan

(b) Elevation of Center Handrail

(c) Extension at Bottom of Run

(d) Extension at Top of Run

NOTE:
X is the 12 in minimum handrail extension required at each top riser.

Y is the minimum handrail extension of 12 in plus the width of one tread that is required at each bottom riser.

FIGURE 4-23. Stair handrails.
Americans with Disabilities Act of 1990, Accessibility Guidelines for Facilities. *Federal Register* / Vol. 56, No. 144 / Friday, July 26, 1991 / Rules and Regulations, p. 35622. Final Rule Part III CFR 28 Part 36. A copy of the final federal rule should be obtained from American with Disabilities Act's Architectural and Transportation Barriers Compliance Board, U.S. Department of Justice, Civil Rights Division (Washington, DC). A copy of *American National Standard Accessible and Usable Buildings and Facilities,* CABO/ANSI A117.1–1992 should be obtained from American National Standards Institute, 11 West 42nd St., New York, NY, 10036.

4.14 Entrances

Must be part of an accessible route and all accessible spaces and elements within a facility.

4.15 Drinking Fountains and Water Coolers

Spouts. Shall be no higher than 36", located at the front of the fountain, flowing parallel with the front of the unit and at least 4" high (to allow for a cup or glass to be inserted under the stream of water; (see Figure 4-24).

Controls. Shall be located at or near the front edge of the fountain, be operable with one hand, easily grasped, needing no more than 5 lbs. of pressure to operate.

4.16 Water Closets

Toilets not in stalls must meet clear floor space requirements and may have either right-handled or left-handled approach. Height of 17—19" to top of toilet seat, with grab bars on walls mounted 33–36" off floor on side and rear walls. Flush control to require no more than 5 lbs. of force to operate (see Figure 4-25).

4.17 Toilet Stalls

Toilet stalls must meet numerous dimension requirements (see Figure 4-26). They may be a specified standard or alternative size, must include grab bars, and if less than 60" in depth must provide 9" of toe clearance.

4.18 Urinals

Urinals may be wall-hung or stall type with elongated rim a maximum of 17" above the finished floor; clear floor space of 30" x 48" is required; hand operated flush lever (5 lbs. of force to operate at most) not more than 44" off floor.

4.19 Lavatories and Mirrors

Lavatories must be mounted with the rim or counter surface no higher than 24" above the finished floor, provide a clearance of at least 29" above the floor to the bottom or the apron (see Figure 4-27).

Hot water and drain pipes under lavatory. Shall be wrapped and any sharp or abrasive surfaces protected.

Faucets: Five lbs. of pressure maximum to operate.

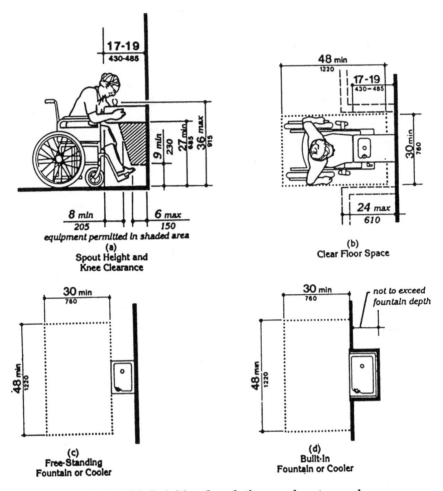

FIGURE 4-24. Drinking foundations and water coolers.
Americans with Disabilities Act of 1990, Accessibility Guidelines for Facilities. *Federal Register* / Vol. 56, No. 144 / Friday, July 26, 1991 / Rules and Regulations, p. 35622. Final Rule Part III CFR 28 Part 36. A copy of the final federal rule should be obtained from American with Disabilities Act's Architectural and Transportation Barriers Compliance Board, U.S. Department of Justice, Civil Rights Division (Washington, DC). A copy of *American National Standard Accessible and Usable Buildings and Facilities,* CABO/ANSI A117.1–1992 should be obtained from American National Standards Institute, 11 West 42nd St., New York, NY, 10036.

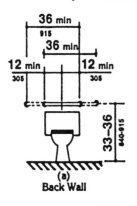

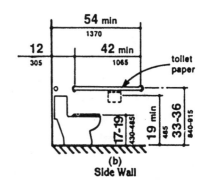

FIGURE 4-25. Grab bars at water closets.

Americans with Disabilities Act of 1990, Accessibility Guidelines for Facilities. *Federal Register* / Vol. 56, No. 144 / Friday, July 26, 1991 / Rules and Regulations, p. 35622. Final Rule Part III CFR 28 Part 36. A copy of the final federal rule should be obtained from American with Disabilities Act's Architectural and Transportation Barriers Compliance Board, U.S. Department of Justice, Civil Rights Division (Washington, DC). A copy of *American National Standard Accessible and Usable Buildings and Facilities,* CABO/ANSI A117.1–1992 should be obtained from American National Standards Institute, 11 West 42nd St., New York, NY, 10036.

Mirrors. Mounted with bottom edge of reflecting surface no higher than 40" above the finished floor. Must meet floor space requirements depending on arrangement of bathroom fixtures and have the following:

* an in-tub seat or a seat at the head of the tub
* grab bars and controls (5 lbs. of pressure maximum to operate) located on near side of tub enclosure
* a shower spray unit with hose at least 60" long that is usable as a hand-held shower or fixed shower spray

4.21 Shower Stalls

Must meet size requirements and have grab bars, controls, shower hand-held sprayer unit as required for tubs, and provide a seat.

4.22 Toilet Rooms

These must meet requirements as outlined above for doors, toilets, urinals, tubs, and so on. In addition, any medicine cabinet provided must be located so as to have a usable shelf no higher than 44" above the floor.

4.23 Bathrooms, Bathing Facilities, and Shower Rooms

Must meet all the above relevant requirements.

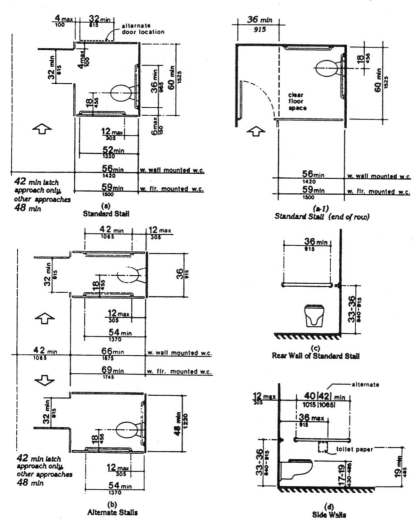

FIGURE 4-26. Toilet stalls.

Americans with Disabilities Act of 1990, Accessibility Guidelines for Facilities. *Federal Register* / Vol. 56, No. 144 / Friday, July 26, 1991 / Rules and Regulations, p. 35622. Final Rule Part III CFR 28 Part 36. A copy of the final federal rule should be obtained from American with Disabilities Act's Architectural and Transportation Barriers Compliance Board, U.S. Department of Justice, Civil Rights Division (Washington, DC). A copy of *American National Standard Accessible and Usable Buildings and Facilities,* CABO/ANSI A117.1–1992 should be obtained from American National Standards Institute, 11 West 42nd St., New York, NY, 10036.

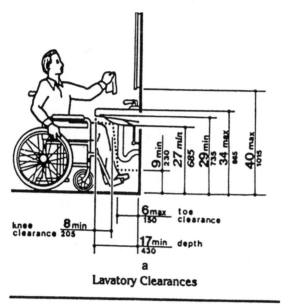

a
Lavatory Clearances

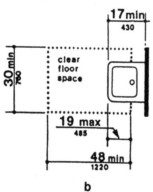

b

FIGURE 4-27. Lavatory clearances s(a): clear floor space at lavatories (b).
Americans with Disabilities Act of 1990, Accessibility Guidelines for Facilities. *Federal Register* / Vol. 56, No. 144 / Friday, July 26, 1991 / Rules and Regulations, p. 35622. Final Rule Part III CFR 28 Part 36. A copy of the final federal rule should be obtained from American with Disabilities Act's Architectural and Transportation Barriers Compliance Board, U.S. Department of Justice, Civil Rights Division (Washington, DC). A copy of *American National Standard Accessible and Usable Buildings and Facilities*, CABO/ANSI A117.1–1992 should be obtained from American National Standards Institute, 11 West 42nd St., New York, NY, 10036.

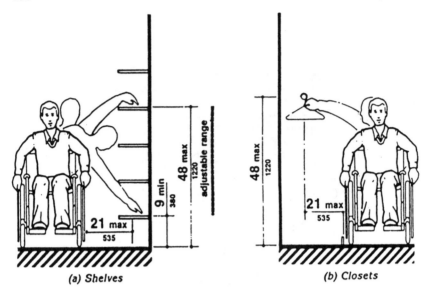

FIGURE 4-28. Storage shelves and closets.

Americans with Disabilities Act of 1990, Accessibility Guidelines for Facilities. *Federal Register* / Vol. 56, No. 144 / Friday, July 26, 1991 / Rules and Regulations, p. 35622. Final Rule Part III CFR 28 Part 36. A copy of the final federal rule should be obtained from American with Disabilities Act's Architectural and Transportation Barriers Compliance Board, U.S. Department of Justice, Civil Rights Division (Washington, DC). A copy of *American National Standard Accessible and Usable Buildings and Facilities,* CABO/ANSI A117.1–1992 should be obtained from American National Standards Institute, 11 West 42nd St., New York, NY, 10036.

4.24 Sinks

Must be accessible and mounted with counter or rim no higher than 34" above the finished floor. Knee clearance at least 27" high, 30" wide, and 19" deep under sink. Water depth maximum is 6½". Clear floor space of at least 30 x 48". All exposed pipes covered, faucets easily operated with maximum of 5 lbs. of pressure to operate.

4.25 Storage

A clear floor space of 30 x 48", within reach ranges of Figures 4-12 and 4-13, clothes rods a maximum of 54" above the finished floor (see Figure 4-28).

4.26 Handrails, Grab Bars, and Tub and Shower Seats

Handrails and grab bars must be 1¼ to 1½" or provide equivalent gripping surface. If wall-mounted, at least 1½" space between the grab bar and wall. The bending, sheer stress point must be 250 lbs. of pressure or greater. Fixtures must not rotate within fittings and have no sharp edges (minimum radius of edge = 1/8 inch, see ADA Figure 4-29).

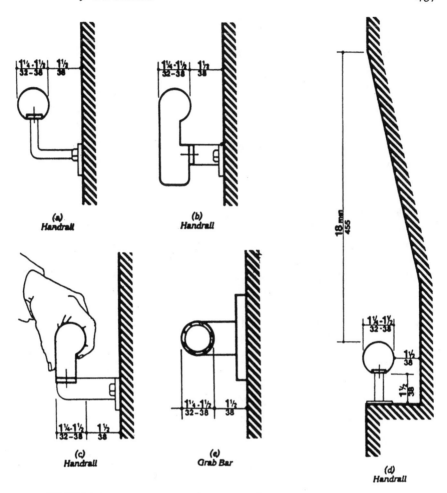

FIGURE 4-29. Sizes and spacing of handrails and grab bars.
Americans with Disabilities Act of 1990, Accessibility Guidelines for Facilities. *Federal Register* / Vol. 56, No. 144 / Friday, July 26, 1991 / Rules and Regulations, p. 35622. Final Rule Part III CFR 28 Part 36. A copy of the final federal rule should be obtained from American with Disabilities Act's Architectural and Transportation Barriers Compliance Board, U.S. Department of Justice, Civil Rights Division (Washington, DC). A copy of *American National Standard Accessible and Usable Buildings and Facilities,* CABO/ANSI A117.1–1992 should be obtained from American National Standards Institute, 11 West 42nd St., New York, NY, 10036.

4.27 Controls and Operating Mechanisms

Electrical switches must be located at least 15" above the floor. Clear floor space must allow a forward or parallel approach by a person in a wheelchair.

4.28 Alarms

At the least, **visual signal appliances** shall be provided in facilities in each of the following areas: restrooms and any other general usage areas (e.g., meeting rooms), hallways, lobbies, and any other area for common use.

Audible alarms. If provided, they shall produce a sound that exceeds the prevailing equivalent sound level in the room or space by at least 15 decibels or exceed any maximum sound level with a duration of 60 seconds by 5 decibels, whichever is louder. Maximum decibel level is 120.

Auxiliary alarms: Required in sleeping accommodations and connected to the building emergency alarm system and visible to all areas of the room.

Visual alarms. Must be provided and may be integrated into the facility alarm system. Must have following features:

- a xenon strobe-type lamp or equivalent
- color clear or nominal white
- .2 second maximum pulse duration
- minimum 75 candle intensity
- flash rate minimum of 1 Hz and maximum of 3 Hz
- 80" above highest floor level or 6" below ceiling, whichever is lower
- no more than 50' from all space in a room, 100' in large spaces such as auditoriums
- maximum 50' apart in hallways and common corridors

4.29 Detectable Warnings

On walking surfaces warnings shall be 0.9" in diameter and 0.2" in height with 2.35" spacing; they shall contrast visually and be of material similar to of that used on the surface. They shall be provided at hazardous vehicular areas that are without curbs and at edges of reflecting pools not having railings, walls, or curbs.

4.30 Signage

Letters must have a width-to-height ratio between 3:5 and 1:1 and a stroke-width-to-height ratio between 1:5 and 1:10.

Character height. Sized to viewing distance with a minimum of 3'.

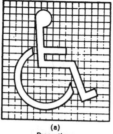

(a)
Proportions
International Symbol of Accessibility

(b)
Display Conditions
International Symbol of Accessibility

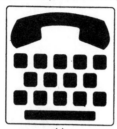

(c)
International TDD Symbol

(d)
International Symbol of Access for Hearing Loss

FIGURE 4-30. International symbols.

Americans with Disabilities Act of 1990, Accessibility Guidelines for Facilities. *Federal Register* / Vol. 56, No. 144 / Friday, July 26, 1991 / Rules and Regulations, p. 35622. Final Rule Part III CFR 28 Part 36. A copy of the final federal rule should be obtained from American with Disabilities Act's Architectural and Transportation Barriers Compliance Board, U.S. Department of Justice, Civil Rights Division (Washington, DC). A copy of *American National Standard Accessible and Usable Buildings and Facilities,* CABO/ANSI A117.1–1992 should be obtained from American National Standards Institute, 11 West 42nd St., New York, NY, 10036.

Raised and Braille characters and pictorial symbol signs must meet several size and type specifications.

Symbols of accessibility. International symbols shall be used and displayed for areas required to be identified as accessible (see Figure 4-30).

4.31 Telephones

Seating/location. At least 30" x 48" of clear floor space.

Mounting heights. Highest part shall be within ranges of 15 to 48" of forward reach and 54" to 9" above the floor for side reach.

Hearing-aid compatible and volume controllable. Both are required. Volume capable of a minimum of 12 decibels and a maximum of 18 decibels above normal; directories provided within reach and a 29 inch or longer cord. A text telephone may be required.

4.32 Fixed or Built-in Seating and Tables

Knee space of 27" high, 30" wide, and 19" deep must be provided.

Height. Tops of accessible tables and counters shall be from 28 to 34" above the floor or ground (see Figure 4-31).

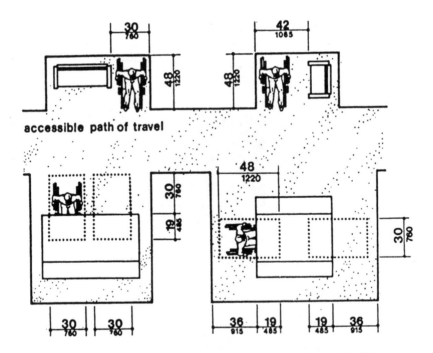

FIGURE 4-31. Minimum clearances for seating and tables.

Americans with Disabilities Act of 1990, Accessibility Guidelines for Facilities. *Federal Register* / Vol. 56, No. 144 / Friday, July 26, 1991 / Rules and Regulations, p. 35622. Final Rule Part III CFR 28 Part 36. A copy of the final federal rule should be obtained from American with Disabilities Act's Architectural and Transportation Barriers Compliance Board, U.S. Department of Justice, Civil Rights Division (Washington, DC). A copy of *American National Standard Accessible and Usable Buildings and Facilities,* CABO/ANSI A117.1–1992 should be obtained from American National Standards Institute, 11 West 42nd St., New York, NY, 10036.

4.33 Assembly Areas

Floor space requirements are provided in Figure 4-32. Wheelchair seating areas must allow a choice of admission prices and must lines of sight comparable to those for members of the general public, and adjoin an accessible route that serves as a means of egress in case of emergency. At least one companion fixed seat shall be next to each wheelchair space. Readily removable seats may be installed in wheelchair areas when not occupied. Floor surfaces of wheelchair areas must be level. Persons in wheelchairs must have full access to performing areas. Views of the stage must be complete. Assisted listening systems may be installed.

FACILITY COMPLIANCE WITH PHYSICAL ENVIRONMENT REQUIREMENTS

Table 3-12 demonstrates a compliance rate averaging over 95% and, in some cases 100%. Pest control and space and equipment were of concern to surveyors, though less so in 1999 than in 1993.

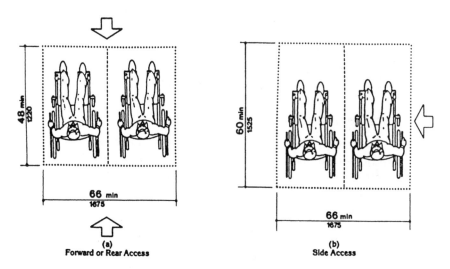

FIGURE 4-32. Space requirements for wheelchair seating spaces in series.
Americans with Disabilities Act of 1990, Accessibility Guidelines for Facilities. *Federal Register* / Vol. 56, No. 144 / Friday, July 26, 1991 / Rules and Regulations, p. 35622. Final Rule Part III CFR 28 Part 36. A copy of the final federal rule should be obtained from American with Disabilities Act's Architectural and Transportation Barriers Compliance Board, U.S. Department of Justice, Civil Rights Division (Washington, DC). A copy of *American National Standard Accessible and Usable Buildings and Facilities,* CABO/ANSI A117.1–1992 should be obtained from American National Standards Institute, 11 West 42nd St., New York, NY, 10036.

4.8 Expanding Facility Services: Health Planning

Health planning in America since the beginning of the twentieth century moved through three phases. During the first 50 years, it was mainly the concern of voluntary private groups. In the 1960s and 1970s, health planning leadership was assumed by the federal agencies. Since 1980, any formal health planning is carried out by each state.

PHASE 1: PRIVATE VOLUNTARY HEALTH PLANNING

The Local Health Council Movement

Consumers were the first to recognize a need to coordinate the planning of health organizations in the public and private sectors. Dissatisfaction about overlapping and duplication of services and lack of data collection efforts and a desire to lobby for health legislation proposals brought a number of private citizens together in the early 1920s in the local health council movement. By the 1950s, there were approximately 1,200 local health councils meeting in 32 of the 48 states.

Many professional health administrators equally deplored the lack of coordination and increasing costs in hospitals during those years and this gave rise to a number of hospital planning associations.

The Hill Burton Act

A new phase in health planning began shortly after the passage in 1946 of the Hill Burton Act, which over the next several decades was to fund the building of hundreds of hospitals, long-term-care facilities, and other related structures around the country.

Increasing Federal Involvement

During the 20 years following World War II, the federal government became actively involved for the first time in the financial support of almost every aspect of health care, from sponsoring research, building hospitals, and actually providing health care to the poor and older persons, to underwriting the education of nurses and physicians.

PHASE 2: FEDERALLY DOMINATED HEALTH PLANNING

Comprehensive Health Planning Act, 1966

In 1966, seeking to rationalize health planning and to give consumers a meaningful role in health care policy making, the federal government passed its first health planning law: the Comprehensive Health Planning Act.

This legislation mandated that all participating states set up state and local health planning entities called comprehensive health planning agencies (CHPs). The hospital planning associations often served as the nuclei for these agencies. Consumers were to constitute 51% of the boards and have an active voice in program planning.

Within 5 years it became evident that the Comprehensive Health Planning Agencies were all too often dominated by concerned health professionals. To counteract this trend, a new health planning law was passed in 1974, defining a "consumer" much more narrowly so as to ensure that professionals were not overrepresented on the local and state health planning agency boards.

The National Health Planning and Resources Development Act, 1974

The National Health Planning and Resources Development Act of 1974 was intended to rationalize health planning in the United States To accomplish this, 213 local health systems agencies were established. In many cases, the former comprehensive health planning agencies won the contracts to become the new health systems agencies (HSAs).

Each local health systems agency was made responsible for estimating the health needs in its geographical area for the prospective 5 years. This included the need, or lack of need, for nursing home beds. Based on this plan, the agency would attempt to determine whether the health care needs of its area were being met. It is this process that so directly affects nursing home operations in many states.

Certificate of Need

If the local health planning agency believed that there were insufficient nursing home beds in the area, it was willing to issue what is called a certificate of need (often referred to as a CON).

If the local health planning agency considered that there were enough or perhaps too many nursing home beds in the geographical area, it might refuse to issue a certificate of need. In effect, the agency could deny permission to build new long-term-care beds in that geographical region.

Capital Project Review

A second area in which local health systems agencies could affect nursing home administrators and owners was through review of capital projects. Each health systems agency was responsible for reviews of requests by nursing homes and other health providers to make capital expenditures for building new facilities or renovating existing structures.

PHASE 3: HEALTH PLANNING AS A STATE LEVEL ACTIVITY

Deemphasis of the Federal Role

Under President Ronald Reagan's leadership toward reducing federal government's role in health matters, Congress formally killed the National Health Planning and Resources Development Act in 1986. Health planning then became a state activity.

Increased Reliance on States

The certificate of need requirement is now addressed at the state level ("The State of Health Planning," 1984).

About half the states have dispensed with any certificate of need type of requirements, or are exempting all but the most expensive projects from requiring a certificate of need to build or renovate. In the several states that still retain some form of certificate of need, the rationale is that by controlling the number of new nursing home or hospital beds built or renovated, the state is able to exercise some control over health care costs.

4.9 Voluntary Operating Standards: Joint Commission on Accreditation of Healthcare Organizations

Long-term care facilities that meet certain requirements are eligible to apply for accreditation from the Joint Commission on Accreditation of Healthcare Organizations (JCAHO). Accreditation by JCAHO is voluntary, and currently less than 10% of long-term-care facilities have applied.

Some states are beginning to use JCAHO accreditation in lieu of state and/or federal inspections for meeting the federal and state requirements (Miller, 1982).

ORIGINS OF JCAHO

The JCAHO had its origins as a program for hospital evaluation established in 1918 by the American College of Surgeons (JCAHO). Its 22-member board consists of representatives from the American College of Physicians, the American College of Surgeons, the American Dental Association, the American Hospital Association, and the American Medical Association (JCAHO, 1982).

JCAHO MEMBERSHIP

Slightly more than 1,000 long-term-care facilities are members of JCA-HO. The Veterans Administration has traditionally required its long-term-care facilities to be JCAHO-accredited. As nursing home facilities seek to offer more medically complex care to the case managers of third-party payers, such as insurance companies and HMOs, these third-party payers frequently prefer that contracting nursing facilities have JCAHO accreditation because that is the accreditation process with which they are familiar.

Nearly all United States hospitals seek accreditation by JCAHO because the federal Medicare and Medicaid payers in effect "require" JCAHO accreditation to be eligible to receive Medicare and Medicaid payments. For nursing facilities to receive Medicare and Medicaid payments they must be certified by the federal Medicare and Medicaid officials and licensed by their individual state. Thus, JCAHO accreditation for hospitals has the same funding eligibility function as "certification" for nursing facilities. For nursing facilities, then, JCAHO accreditation is an extra, for hospitals it is a must until Congress permits others agencies besides JCAHO to accredit hospitals.

Trend Toward Seeking JCAHO Accreditation

A number of managed care organizations, more acquainted with the hospital accreditation process than with Medicare/Medicaid inspection in nursing facilities, are demanding that facilities seeking to offer subacute care or negotiating similar contracts with third-party private reimbursers acquire JCAHO accreditation as a quality control measure ("Quality Assurance," 1995).

ELIGIBILITY TO APPLY FOR JCAHO ACCREDITATION

An eligible long-term-care facility is one that is either hospital-based or freestanding and established "for inpatient care, that has an organized medical staff, or its equivalent, or a medical director, and that it provide continuous nursing service under professional nurse direction" (JCAHO, 1983b, p. 1).

The facility must also have been under the same ownership for at least 6 months, have a current unrestricted state license, and operate without restriction by reason of race, color, sex, or national origin. It must, in addition, submit a completed JCAHO application with all the information requested.

JCAHO ACCREDITATION PROCESS

The JCAHO offers a concise manual summarizing its accreditation requirements. After the application is accepted and processed, a survey team consisting of an administrator, a registered nurse, and a social worker visit the facility. The survey team report is evaluated by the JCAHO headquarters staff and a recommendation from the staff is forwarded to the Accreditation Committee of the JCAHO Board of Commissioners, who make the final decision. The entire process is normally completed in 100 days and costs between $6,000 and $11,000, depending on the number of team members and the number of days they are at the facility. A recent base fee was approximately $8,000 (Morrissey, 1995).

The JCAHO survey team examines the facility to discover if it is meeting the standards for the following (JCAHO, 1983b, p. v):

- building and grounds safety
- dental services
- dietetic services
- functional safety
- governing body and management
- infection/environment control
- laboratory, radiological, and other diagnostic services
- medical records, medical services, nursing services
- resident/patient activities, care management, rights and responsibilities
- pharmaceutical services
- quality assurance
- rehabilitation services
- social services
- spiritual services
- transfer agreements

In concert with the federal thrust on outcomes, the JCAHO accreditation process is increasingly focused on the quality of care actually being received by residents/patients. These JCAHO standards do not differ substantially from the federal requirements (see Allen, 1994, pp. 1–67).

The Quality of Life

In general, the JCAHO requires that each accredited organization have the equivalent of a continuous quality improvement program in place and functioning ("Quality Assurance," 1995, p. 11).

REFERENCES: PART FOUR

Abbott, A. (1991). Group long-term care. CNA group perspectives. *Continental Assurance Company, 12*(3), 3–4.

Adams, E. K., Meiners, M. R., & Burwell, B. O. (1993). Asset spend-down in nursing homes. *Medical Care, 31*(1), 1–23.

American Hospital Association. (1976). *Taft Hartley Amendments: Implications for the health care field. Report of a symposium.* Chicago: Author.

American Hospital Association. (1988). *Guide to the health care field.* Chicago: Author.

American Hospital Association. (1989). *Guide to the health care field.* Chicago: Author.

American National Standards Institute. (1980). *American National Standard specifications for making buildings and facilities accessible to and usable by physically handicapped people.* (ANSI A117.1–1980). New York: Author.

Argenti, P. A. (1994). *The portable MBA desk reference.* New York: Wiley.

Blake, J. B. (1959). *Public health in the town of Boston.* Cambridge, MA: Harvard University Press.

Boling, T. E., Vrooman, D. M., & Sommers, K. M. (1983). *Nursing home management.* Springfield, IL: Thomas.

Burda, D. (1995). Hospitals rank high as health hazard for employees. *Modern Healthcare, 25*(2), 24.

Burda, G. (1993). Long-term care facts must be addressed. *Modern Healthcare, 23*(44), 36.

Caring till it hurts: How nursing home work is becoming the most dangerous job in America. (1995). Washington, DC: Service Employees International Union-AFL-CIO.

Carley, M. M. (1991, December). New medical devices. Reporting requirements. *Contemporary Long-term care,* p. 66.

Cherry, R. L. (1993). Community presence and nursing home quality of care: The ombudsman as a complementary role. *Journal of Health and Social Behavior, 34,* 336–345.

Chruden, J. J., & Sherman, A. W., Jr. (1980). *Personnel management: The utilization of human resource* (6th ed.). Dallas, TX: South-Western.

Clement, P. F. (1985). History of U.S. aged poverty. *Perspectives on Aging, 9*(2), 4–7.

Committee on Nursing Home Regulation, Institute of Medicine. (1986). *Improving the quality of care in nursing homes.* Washington, DC: National Academy Press.

Council on Scientific Affairs. (1990). Home care in the 1990s. *Journal of the American Medical Association, 263,* 1241–1244.

Dainton, C. (1961). *The story of England's hospitals.* Springfield, IL: Thomas.

Duke health. (1995, Summer). Durham, NC: Duke University Medical Center Publication.

EEOC Notice 915.002. (1994, May 19). Enforcement guidance (rev. EEOC form 106 (6–91). Washington, DC: U.S. Government Printing Office.

Evans, J. G., Williams, T. F., Beattie, B. L., Michel, J-P., & Wilcock, G. K. (2000). *Oxford textbook of geriatric medicine* (2nd ed.). New York: Oxford University Press.

Expenditures and sources of payment for persons in nursing and personal care homes. (1994). (U.S. Department of Health and Human Services, Public Health Service, Agency for health Care Policy and Research Center for General Health Services Intramural Research, National Medical Expenditure Survey, Research Findings 19) (NTIS No. PB94–134764). Washington, DC: U.S. Department of health and Human Services.

Fair Labor Standards Act (1938). 29 U.S. Code §201, et seq.

Falling short. (1995, July). Austin, TX: SEIO.

Feinleib, S. E., Cunning, P. J., & Farley, P. F. (1994, August). *Use of nursing and personal care homes by the civilian population, 1987.* (AHCPR Pub. No. 94–0096). Rockville, MD: Public Health Service.

Freymann, J. G. (1980). *The American health care system: Its genesis and trajectory.* Huntington, NY: Krieger.

Giacalone, J.A. (2001). *The U.S. nursing home industry.* Armonk, NY: M.E. Sharpe.

Greene, V. L., Lively, M. E., & Ondrich, J. I. (1993). The cost-effectiveness of community services in a frail elderly population. *Gerontologist, 33*(2), 177–187.

Centers for Medicare and Medicaid Services (CMS). (1982). Conditions of participation for skilled nursing and intermediate care facilities (a proposed rule). In D. B. Miller (Ed.), *Long-term care administrators desk manual* (pp. 7042–7076). Greenvale, NY: Panel.

Harrington, C. H., Carrillo, M. S., Thollaug, S. C., Summers, P. R., & Wellin, V. (2000). *Nursing facilities, staffing, residents, and facility deficiencies, 1993 through 1999.* University of California at San Francisco: Department of Social and Behavioral Sciences

Health care labor manual: Vol. 1. (1983). Rockville, MD: Aspen.

care. Bowie, MD: Brady.

Hunter, R. J. (1955). *The origin of the Philadelphia General Hospital.* Philadelphia: Rittenhouse Press.

Ivancevich, J. M., & Glueck, W. F. (1983). *Foundations of personnel: Human resource management* (Rev. ed.). Plano, TX: Business Publications.

Joint Commission on Accreditation of Healthcare Organizations. (1989). *Quality assurance in long-term care.* Chicago: Author.

Joint Commission on Accreditation of Healthcare Organizations, Department of Publications. (1994). *Accreditation manual for long-term care, Vol. II: Scoring guidelines.* Oakbrook Terrace, IL: Author.

Joint Commission on Accreditation of Hospitals. (1979). *Accreditation manual for hospitals, 1980.* Chicago: Author.

Joint Commission on Accreditation of Hospitals. (1982). *Facts about JCAHO.* Chicago: Author.

Joint Commission on Accreditation of Hospitals. (1983a). *Accreditation manual for long-term care facilities-84.* Chicago: Author.

Joint Commission on Accreditation of Hospitals. (1983b). *JCAHO eligibility criteria.* Chicago: Author.

Kaplan, B. (1985). Social Security: 50 years later. *Perspectives on Aging, 9*(2), 4–7.

Lagore, R. J. (1994). Adding nursing facility beds: Impact on hospital nonacute care. *Hospital and Health Services Administration, 39,* 327–340.

Lathrop, J. K. (1985). *Life safety code handbook.* Quincy, MA: National Fire Protection Association.

Liu, F., Manton, K., & Allston, W. (1982). Demographic and epidemiological determinants of expenditures. In R. Vogel & H. Palmer (Eds.), *Long-term care* (pp. 81–132). Washington, DC: Health Care Financing Administration.

Long-Term Care News. (1990, January). p. 22.

Lutz, S. (1994). Hospitals' profit margins jump as costs are adjusted. *Modern Healthcare, 24*(43).

Maddox, G. L. (2001). *Encyclopedia of aging: Comprehensive resource in gerontology and geriatrics* (3rd ed.). New York: Springer.

Manton, K. G., Stallard, E., & Woodbury, M. A. (1994). Home health and skilled nursing facility use: 1982–90. *Health Care Financing Review, 16,* 155–183.

McCarthy, M. J. (1994, November 8). Frayed lifeless hunger among elderly surges: Meal programs just can't keep up. *Wall Street Journal,* p. 1811.

Miller, D. B. (Ed.). (1982). *Long-term care administrator's desk manual.* Greenvale, NY: Panel.

Miller, D. B., & Barry, J. T. (1979). *Nursing home organization and operation.* Boston: CBI.

Moore, J. D., Jr. (1995). Hillhaven nurses stage strike. *Modern Healthcare,* p. 12.

Morrissey, J. (1995). JCAHO decides against survey fee hike. *Modern Healthcare,* p. 21.

Muse, D. N., & Sawyer, D. (1982). *The Medicare and Medicaid handbook.* Washington, DC: Health Care Financing Administration.

National Fire Protection Association, Inc. (1985). *Life safety code 1985.* (NFPA 101 ANSI-NFPA 101). Quincy, MA: Author.

National Health Planning and Resources Development Act. (1974). Pub. L. 93–641.

National nurse survey. (1995). Washington, DC: Service Employees International Union.

Noe, R. A., Holelnbeck, J. R., Cerhart, B., & Wright, P. M. (2000). *Human resource management: Gaining a Competitive Advantage,* (3rd ed.). Boston: Irwin, McGraw-Hill.

Occupational Safety and Health Act (OSHA). (1970). Public Law 91–596.

Pegels, C. (1981). *Health care and the elderly* (p. 82). Rockville, MD: Aspen.

Pointer, D., & Metzger, N. (1975). *The National Labor Relations Act: A guidebook for health care facility administrators.* New York: Spectrum.

Prospective payment: DRG era dawns. (1983). *Medicine and Health,* p. 3.

Quality assurance in nursing facilities. (1995, May 16). *Nursing Home Law Letter.* Washington, DC: National Senior Citizens Law Center.

Raskin, A. H. (1981, December). From sitdowns to solidarity: Passage in the life of American labor. *Across the Board,* pp. 12–32.

Robinson v. Jacksonville Shipyards, 790 F. Supp. 1486 (M.D. Fla. 1991).

Rosenfeld, L. S., Gaylord, S. A., & Allen, J. E. (1983). *Introduction to long-term care for the aging.* Chapel Hill: The University of North Carolina Independent Study by Extension.

Rosmann, J. (1975). One year under Taft–Hartley. *Hospitals, 49*(24), 64–68.

Scott, L. (1994). NLRB order against Beverly voided. *Modern Healthcare, 24*(1).

Sharma, S. K., & Fallovolleta, B. S. (1992). *The Older American Act: Access to and utilization of the ombudsman program* (GAO-PEMD-92–21). Washington, DC: USGAO Program Evaluation and Methodology Division.

Short, P. F., Kemper, P., Llewellyn, J. C., & Walden, D. C. (1992). Public and private responsibility for financing nursing home care: The effect of Medicaid asset spend down. *Milbank Quarterly, 7,* 277–298.

Shriver, K. (1995, October 2). Union can't stop Vencor-Hillhaven deal. *Modern Healthcare,* p. 18.

Simon-Rusinowitz, L., & Hofland, B. F. (1993). Adopting a disability approach to home care services for older adults. *Gerontologist, 33,* 159–166.

Sloan, F. A., & Shayne, M. W. (1993). Long-term care, Medicaid, and impoverishment of the elderly. *Milbank Quarterly, 71,* 575–599.

Smith, D. B. (1981). *Long-term care in transition: The regulation of nursing homes.* Washington, DC: Association of University Programs of Health Administration.

Staff. (1984, October 1). Perspectives. *Washington Report on Medicine and Health,* pp. 1–4.

State of health planning. (1984, October 22). *Medicine and Health* (Insert).

Steinberg, R. M., & Carter, G. W. (1983). *Case management and the elderly.* Lexington, MA: Lexington Books.

Strahan, G. (1994). An overview of home health and hospice care patients. *Advance Data, 256,* Vital and Health Statistics, Centers for Disease Control, National Center for Health Statistics.

U.S. Department of Health, Education and Welfare. (1975). *Interpretive guidelines and survey procedures.* Washington, DC: American Health Care Association. (Originally published in the *Federal Register,* January 17, 1974.)

U.S. Department of Labor, Occupational Safety and Health Administration. (1976). *All about OSHA.* Washington, DC: U.S. Government Printing Office.

U.S. Department of Labor, Bureau of Labor Statistics. (1977). *U.S. Working women: A databook.* Washington, DC: U.S. Government Printing Office.

U.S. Department of Labor. (1976). *Brief history of the American labor movement.* (Bulletin 1000). Washington, DC: U.S. Government Printing Office.

Vladeck, B. C. (1980). *Unloving care: The nursing home tragedy.* New York: Basic Books.

Weissert, W. (1985, April). *Estimating the long term care population.* Report for the Office of the Assistant Secretary for Planning and Education, (p. 11). Washington, DC: U.S. Department of Health & Human Services.

Weissert, W. G. (1989). Models of adult day care. *Gerontologist, 29,* 648.

Wilson, F. A., & Neuhauser, D. (1982). *Health services in the United States* (2nd ed.). Cambridge, MA: Ballinger.

PART FIVE

Resident/Patient Care

5.1 The Aging Process

How many Americans die of old age each year? Depending on the definitions used, the answer could range from more than 1 million persons to zero. Our answer is, "zero." Old age is not a disease process.

It used to be customary to say that a person died of old age, but this is too imprecise an observation. It seems more functional to approach disease and disabilities and causes of death among older persons as one approaches these concerns in younger persons: to look for causes and seek either cure or relief.

Every older person, just as every younger one, dies of specific causes. Generally, one or more of the body systems (which are described later) become overwhelmed for some specific reason, such as a disease or an injury to the person, and death results (Kane, Ouslander, & Abrass, 1989). It is important, to understand that age changes are not in themselves diseases, but rather are natural losses of function (Hayflick, 1995).

RESEARCH ON AGING

The two groups who study aging individuals are identified by different names. Physicians who specialize in treating older individuals are called geriatricians. Professionals who study the problems of the aging population in society, and who usually are not physicians, are called gerontologists.

How much have the geriatricians and gerontologists learned about aging? With the development of clinical medicine over the past century, attention to the diseases of aging persons and the aging process itself have become increasingly active areas of scientific investigation. Much has been learned, and some of this knowledge will be discussed further along. However, a good deal of uncertainty remains. Much of the so-called knowledge about aging is still being tested and is not yet well established.

GENERAL OBSERVATIONS

One observation that seems safe to make is that aging is highly individualized. In the typical nursing home there are individuals whose chronological age is 90, yet their physiologic appearance and strong activity level are more characteristic of a 60-year-old person (Maddox, 2001). Similarly, there are those in their 60's and 70's in the same facility who appear to be more aged than the 90-year-old (Evans et al., 2000).

The extent to which this is due to genetic inheritance or is influenced by an individual's lifestyle and health behaviors remains a subject of lively debate.

A few additional general observations can be made about aging, none of them entirely safe, because for every such observation the reader may be able to produce valid exceptions.

Take, for example, the observations of Alexander Leaf (1973) who compared persons aged 75 with 30-year-olds and found that among those he studied, a person aged 75 has

92% of the former brain weight
84% of the former basal metabolism
70% of the former kidney filtration rate
43% of the former maximum breathing capacity

Those are impressive figures, but what do they mean? Does the progressive loss of cortical neurons (brain cells) mean that older persons are that much less smart? Apparently not. There is little substantial clinical evidence that reduction of mental competence accompanies reduction in brain weight.

If Leaf's data are correct—that, on average, when a person reaches 75 the brain weighs about 10% less, the body is burning calories at a reduced rate, the kidneys are filtering about three-fourths as fast, and the lungs process oxygen more slowly—what is the significance? Certainly this may be important for the physician and the pharmacist concerned about drug tolerance and dosages, but these data do not make the 75-year-old individual any more or less of a person than the 30-year-old (Evans, Williams, Beattie, Michel, & Wilcock, 2000).

The import of Leaf's data may be to confirm that, in general, aging is a continuous process that may begin at birth, that it is a gradual decline of at least some systems of the body that proceed at different rates in different individuals. Kane et al. (1989) suggest the 1% theory: that the majority of body organs lose function at the rate of 1% per year after age 30 (p. 5). They caution, however, that newer findings suggest that functional decreases observed in some groups of persons and not others may point to disease patterns among some groups rather than normal aging in the general population.

5.1.1 Overview of Appearance and Functional Changes Believed to Be Associated with Aging

The following observations are discussed at greater length under the headings of the 10 body systems described. By way of gaining an overall perspective, these are the phenomena that can be observed in aging individuals.

Change in collagen. Collagen is connective tissue that loses elasticity over time and appears to account for sagging of the skin often observed in the aging person. Sagging can occur around the eyes and jaws and can affect the general body tone of the muscles, especially in the arm.

Reduced reserve. Leaf's observation that the lungs' ability to process oxygen by age 75 is less than half their previous capacity tends to be true of several other body systems. One researcher believes that after age 20 the heart muscle, too, loses strength every year at the rate of 0.85% (Starr, 1964). Another concludes that at-rest heart output at age 75 is no more than 70% of at-rest heart output at age 30 (Leaf, 1973).

Gradual changes in the immune system. Usually, the body rejects foreign cells, but as the body ages, one theory holds that a progressive weakening of the immune response increases susceptibility to respiratory and other illnesses (Kane, et al., 1989; Maddox, 2001).

Temperature response changes. A reduction of capacity to maintain body temperature within a narrow range appears to lead to a diminished shivering and sweating response, allowing the body temperature of some older individuals to range dangerously. This can lead to their dying in heat waves and cold spells that do not so adversely affect younger people. Ten percent of those over 65, or 2.5 million Americans, are believed to be vulnerable to hypothermia (lowered body temperature) due to reduced heat production by the body (Reichel, 1983).

Postural imbalances. The balancing mechanisms appear to function less well, resulting in some persons aged 65 and over being progressively at risk of tripping (Redford, 1989).

Decalcification of the bones. Many older persons are at increased risk of bones breaking bones, especially if they fall (Glowacki, 1989).

Decreases in bowel function control. As the central nervous system tends to function less and less well in some older persons, the ability to control the bowels lessens.

Frequent anorexia. Anorexia (loss of appetite) among some older persons leads to their skipping meals and a reduced level of nutrition (Gibbons & Levy, 1989; Maddox, 2001).

Skin. With the loss of some subcutaneous fat, an older person may feel colder, and the skin may wrinkle. Some pigment (color) cells of the skin enlarge with age, resulting in the pigmented plaques often seen on the skin of aged persons.

Decreased bone and muscle mass. This process among some older individuals can result in stooped posture, reduced height, loss of muscle power, misshapen joints, and limitations in mobility.

Renal system. The bladder of some persons appears to reduce to less than half its former capacity, and micturition (the desire to urinate) appears delayed until the bladder is near capacity instead of triggering at one-half of capacity. One researcher (Lindeman, 1989) estimates that the average 80-year-old resident has about one-half the glomerular filtration rate of a 30-year-old person.

Hearing and vision. Both hearing and vision appear to become reduced among many aged persons.

5.1.2 Theories of Aging

Most investigators of the causes of aging agree that there is no one theory that currently explains the aging phenomenon fully (Hayflick, 1995; Hefti, 1995; Meites & Quadri, 1995). Reichel, for example, (1983) defines aging as a progressive deterioration in functional capacity occurring after reproductive maturity.

Because no one really knows why people age, there are several theories rather than one generally accepted explanation. Hayflick thinks perhaps the question might more usefully be posed as, Why do we live so long? (Hayflick, 1995). He observes that theorists are increasingly suspecting that the forces that produce age changes are different from those that drive longevity determination (Hayflick, 1995).

There has been an explosion of biogerontologic theory about why we age (Hayflick, 1995). The main criticism of these theories is that changes, such as reduced exercise capacity, may be indicative of certain more fundamental change processes (Hayflick, 1995).

LOOKING FOR ANSWERS

A Limit to the Number of Cell Divisions?

Some theories of aging relate to the genome or genetic apparatus, that is, age-related changes in cell metabolism and function (Hayflick, 1995). Leonard Hayflick, while conducting research at Stanford University, found that normal human fibroblasts (embryonic cells that give rise to connective tissue), when cultured in vitro (in a test tube or other artificial environment), undergo only a limited number of divisions, usually about 50, before they die. His hypothesis is that the life span of a normal human cell is a programmed event under genetic control (Hayflick, 1965). He obtained support for his theory by showing that cells from adult human tissue undergo about 20 divisions before they die. Kane et al. express their doubt about his theory, however (1989).

An Answer in Cancer Research?

Cancer cells appear to be able to continue reproducing indefinitely (Evans et al., 2000; Rimer, 1995). If this is so, what causes noncancerous cells to lose their ability to divide? Some researchers think that the answer to cancer cell divisions may hold information that will reveal the factor that limits the normal human cell's ability to continue dividing.

Somatic Mutation Theory

Some researchers have speculated that a sufficient level of accumulation of mutations in body cells produce the physiologic decrements we identify as aging (Hayflick, 1995).

The Error Theory: A Loss in Genetic Programming?

At the University of California, Bernard Strehler (1962) hypothesized that age-related changes in cell metabolism are a programmed loss of the genetic material found in the DNA molecule (the molecule of heredity in most organisms). Essentially this is based on the theory that there is increasing inaccuracy in the protein synthesis. The idea is that the ends of linear chromosomes the telemere length decreases until cell division ceases (Evans, et al., 2000; Hayflick, 1995).

Random Mutations?

When he was working at the Boston University Medical School, Marott Sinex (1977) proposed that random mutations of cells may produce aging by causing damage to DNA molecules. His theory is that as mutations (changes) accumulate in the body cells, they progressively lose their ability to reproduce and perform their original functions.

Program Theory

Proponents of this approach contend that the events we associate with aging are programmed into the genome, that just as progressive maturation is programmed, so is progressive deterioration is programmed (Hayflick, 1995).

An Autoimmune Explanation?

Several investigators (see H. T. Blumenthal, 1968; Evans et al., 2000) suggest that a progressive failure of the body's immune system (which consists of white blood cells and various antibodies as the first line of defense against diseases), leads to autoimmune responses in older persons. Their idea is that "copying errors" in repeated cell divisions lead to cells that are progressively not recognized by the body, triggering the immune system to attack these cells, thinking foreign cells have invaded (Maddox, 2001).

This is similar to the wear-and-tear theory which postulates that as mutations progress over time unrepaired changes of DNA and similar processes result in aging (Maddox, 2001; Medevedev, 1995).

Entropy and Aging

The second law of thermodynamics postulates that ordered systems move toward disorder. According to this theory, aging is an inevitable expression of the idea that closed systems, such as our bodies, tend to a state of equilibrium in which nothing more happens (Evans et al., 2000).

Longevity-Assurance Genes

In this approach aging is thought to be under the control of hormones and to be genetically based (Hayflick, 1995; Meites & Quadri, 1995).

Stress Theory of Aging: Wear and Tear

Some theorists have suggested that the body simply wears out, or that vital parts wear out, similar to what occurs in machines (Evans et al., 2000; Landfield, 1995; Maddox, 2001; Medvedev, 1995). Hans Selye suggests that the body's response to long-term stress resembles the normal life cycle, leading to the final stage of senescence. In this view, repeated experiences with stress are associated with a speeding up of the aging process (Landfield, 1995). Some researchers have focused on the possible role of adrenal steroids and stress hormones that appear to accelerate aging of the brain (Landfield, 1995).

Neuroendocrine Theory of Aging

Several theorists believe that the brain and the endocrine glands control aging. The concept is that as derangements in normal functioning occurs, tissues and organs are affected in ways that we identify with aging. Some of their thinking is based on the immune-neuroendocrine interactions. Basically, the brain and endocrine glands are believed to affect, for example, the immune system, which leads to impairment of antibody formation (Meites & Quadri, 1995).

Some researchers have focused on the association between caloric restriction and delayed maturing of the neuroendocrine functions, delayed body growth and puberty, lowered blood temperature and cell division, decreased body metabolism, and so on, thus delaying what we think of as the aging process (Maddox, 2001).

Neurotropic Factors and Aging

Neurotropic factors are observed to control the survival of neurons or nerves over time, and some theorists believe that understanding this phenomenon will lead to greater understanding of what we identify as the aging process (Hefti, 1995).

Failure of Collagen?

Collagen is a protein fiber that is distributed in the walls of the blood vessels, the heart, and the connective tissue. With age is there by a reduction in the elasticity of this protein, possibly leading to heart muscle inefficiency and reduced cell permeability that makes cell nutrition more difficult?

Regardless of which, if any, of these explanations of the aging process turns out to be correct, the nursing home administrator must deal with the effects of aging in planning the care of residents/patients in the facility.

5.1.3 Resident Exercise and Fitness

As we will see later, a degradation of function in the cardiovascular system usually interferes with the supply of nutrients and oxygen to the cells (Sullivan, 1995). This, in turn, damages the tissues and organs in the body, leading to the decline of other major organs in the body and other major processes. It is not surprising, then, that a consensus is emerging: Moderate exercise is important to the cardiovascular system of aged persons (Evans et al., 2000; Maddox, 2001). Harris (1989) cites studies by deVries, Frankel, Kraus, Jokl, and others that demonstrate how physical conditioning can improve the cardiovascular and respiratory systems, the musculature, and the body composition of older persons (Harris, 1989). The Paffenbarger study of 16,920 Harvard male alumni attributed 1 to 2 years of increased longevity to men 80 years old who had exercised moderately over the years (Paffenbarger, Wing, & Hsieh, 1986).

This all makes sense. The body systems we have mentioned (and will describe in more detail later) all depend on oxygen and nutrients from the blood (Evans et al, 2000). Exercise increases the blood supplied to the body systems, and improved supplies of oxygen and nutrients lead to improved organ and cell status (Evans et al., 2000).

Claims for the benefits of exercise for older individuals are extensive. Improvement of depression, reduced risk of developing heart disease, improved oxygenation and oxygen transport, greater protection against deterioration of glucose tolerance, improved oxygen transport, and denser bone mass are some of the perceived benefits (Harris, 1989; Maddox, 2001).

A sedentary lifestyle and poor physical fitness are thought to be responsible for some of the typical nursing facility symptoms such as headaches, constipation, joint pain, back aches, insomnia, and fatigue (Harris, 1989).

Keeping the cardiovascular system at its peak through regular exercise, then, is seen to have beneficial effects upon many of the body's systems (Maddox, 2001).

Including of a level of aerobic exercise (i.e., exercise that sustains the heart rate at an elevated level, delivering increased oxygen for specified minimum period of time each week) matched to each resident's capabilities in the plan of care seems appropriate as facility policy (Evans et al., 2000; Maddox, 2001).

In the next sections we explore further some of the possible important relationships between diseases and aging found in the typical nursing facility population. Before turning to an exploration of these relationships, however, the following section is offered, which presents and defines a number of medical and related terms. The section is divided into four vocabulary-building topics: (a) a list of medical and related specialists, (b) therapeutic action of some drugs, (c) abbreviations commonly used in patient charting, and (d) a series of the more common prefixes and suffixes.

5.2 Medical and Related Terms

5.2.1 Medical Specializations

Specialization is typically a 3-year training program taken beyond medical school curriculum, which itself is usually 4 years. By professional custom, physicians usually place only *M.D.* after their names, omitting any reference to certification they may hold as a specialist. The following is not a list of all the prominent specialists, rather, it is a list of those more commonly seen or consulted by residents in the nursing facility.

Cardiologist. A physician who specializes in the diagnosis and treatment of heart diseases.

Chiropodist. See Podiatrist.

Dermatologist. A physician who diagnoses and treats diseases of the skin.

Endocrinologist. A physician who specializes in disorders affecting the endocrine (ductless gland) system. This system includes the pituitary, thyroid, pancreas, and adrenal glands, which secrete hormones into the bloodstream.

Family medicine specialist or practitioner. In 1879, 80% of physicians were general practitioners (GPs), 20% were specialists. With the proliferation of medical knowledge the reverse is true today. The general practice of yesteryear has come full circle, since the late 1980s and is itself a specialty requiring 3 years of internship beyond medical school. In this sense, nearly all physicians are now specialists. They specialize in diagnosing diseases and making referrals to specialists when appropriate and still provide the bulk of care in nursing facilities.

Gastroenterologist. A physician who treats and diagnoses diseases of the digestive tract.

General surgeon. A physician who specializes in operative procedures to treat illnesses or various injuries.

Geriatrician. A physician who concentrates on the treatment of older persons. Gerontology became a specialization only in 1987. (*Note:* There are currently a number of physicians who, during the grandfather period in the late 1980s, became certified gerontologists by taking the written exam only, without undergoing the required 3-year specialization.) Still at issue, and an important question for the nursing home industry, is whether gerontology will be a small subspecialty or will see all of the older population. Current expert opinion is that gerontology will move toward being a small subspecialty because the typical needs of older persons, especially perhaps nursing home residents/patients, will best be met by other specialists, regardless of age. Persons with hip fracture, prostate problems, cardiac problems, will require the care of a specialist (Maddox, 2001). (A **gerontologist,** by contrast, is a professional who studies the problem of the aging population in society and usually is not a medical doctor.)

Internist. A physician who specializes in diagnostic procedures and treatment of nonsurgical cases.

Neurologist. A physician who diagnoses and treats diseases of the brain, nervous system, and spinal cord.

Ophthalmologist. A physician who diagnoses and treats eye diseases and disorders, performs eye surgery, refracts the eyes, and prescribes corrective eye glasses and lenses.

Optician. A technician, not a physician, trained to grind lenses and to fit eyeglasses.

Orthopedist. A physician who specializes in diseases and injuries to bones, muscles, joints, and tendons. An orthopedic surgeon is a physician who specializes in surgical procedures relating to the bones, muscles, joints, and tendons.

Osteopath. A doctor of osteopathy, not an allopathic trained medical doctor, who uses methods of diagnosis and treatment that are similar to those of a medical doctor, but who places special emphasis on the interrelationship of the musculoskeletal to the other body systems.

Physiatrist. A physician who specializes in physical medicine, body movements, and conditioning, much like the focus of a physical therapist, and often associated with sports medicine.

Podiatrist. A trained professional, who is not a medical doctor, who is concerned with care of the feet, including clipping of toenails for diabetics, and who treats ailments such as corns and bunions.

Proctologist. A physician specializing in the diagnosis and treatment of the large intestine, particularly the rectum and anus.

Psychiatrist. A physician who specializes in the diagnosis and treatment of mental disorders.

Psychoanalyst. A psychiatrist who specializes in the use of the psychoanalytic technique of therapy.

Psychologist. A trained professional, not a physician, who studies the function of the mind and behavioral patterns and administers psychological tests.

Pulmonologist. A physician specializing in treatment of the lungs.

Radiologist. A physician specializing in the use of X-ray and similar medical diagnostic machines such as magnetic resonance imaging (MRI), computer automated tomography (CAT) scans, and other medical techniques or modalities.

Rheumatologist. A physician who specializes in the treatment of rheumatic and arthritic diseases.

Urologist. A physician specializing in the diagnosis and treatment of diseases of the kidney, bladder, and reproductive organs.

5.2.2 Medications/Therapeutic Actions of Drugs

(*Note:* The nature and uses of several of the drugs and concepts mentioned but not defined in this section are discussed in the context of individual body systems.)

EXTENT OF DRUG PRESCRIPTIONS IN THE NURSING FACILITY

Medications are among the most common types of treatment prescribed by physicians for the nursing home resident (Jones, 1989). According to one National Nursing Home Survey, 95.5% of nursing home residents receive at least one or more medications (Evans et al., 2000; Hing, 1977; Maddox, 2001). This is not surprising, because admission usually depends on one's being ill and in need of continuing treatment. However, another study revealed that more than half of nursing home residents receive 3 to 7 different medications a day (U.S. Department of Health, Education and Welfare, 1976).

ROUTES USED IN DRUG ADMINISTRATION

Drugs typically function in the body after being absorbed into the blood-stream, usually through the digestive tract, following a pathway similar to that traveled by nutrients from food.

Drugs may be administered several ways in addition to orally (P.O.): intramuscularly (IM) by an injection; directly on the skin (topically); through membranes or other tissue, such as being held under the tongue (sublingually); or as suppositories. Usually medications eventually become inactive in the liver and are removed from the body by the kidney.

Injections and Intravenous Therapy

Injections are provided by facilities for a variety of reasons. Injections rates remained essentially level from 1993 through 1999. In 1993, 11.5% of residents in facilities were receiving injections compared with 12.6% in 1999 (Harrington et al., 2000).

Intravenous therapy rates, on the other hand, rose. Intravenous therapy and blood transfusions are used to provide fluid, medications, nutritional substances, and blood products for residents. The percent of residents receiving these therapies in nursing facilities rose from 1.5% in 1993 to 2.7% in 1999, possibly reflecting an increasingly higher acuity level of residents (Harrington et al., 2000).

FIVE BASIC DRUG ACTIONS

Following are the five basic types of actions that drugs will produce (Poe & Holloway, 1980):

- blocking of nerve impulses
- stimulating of nerve impulses
- working directly on living cells
- working to replace body deficiencies
- any combination of the above

Every person is affected by drugs differently because of individual body chemistries, so every resident/patient must be monitored to determine the appropriateness of different dosages (Evans et al., 2000; Jones, 1989).

As a result of age-related changes in the liver, kidney, and other organs that alter the normal utilization of drugs, older persons are at much greater risk of drug reactions, which are often the result of a buildup or excess amount of drugs in the body. In addition, there may also be an increase in the side effects that are commonly associated with most medications (Jones, 1989).

Policy Implications

Because nursing home residents are more likely to suffer from multiple diseases and use multiple medications, these drug combinations can produce dangerous drug interactions (Maddox, 2001; Roberts & Snyder, 1995). The same residents are also at a much greater risk of suffering from an adverse drug reaction, many of which are the result of chemical incompatibilities among the different medications (Jones, 1989).

For these reasons, the nursing home administrator must ensure that drug regimens in the facility are appropriately monitored by the consulting pharmacist with proper, in-depth periodic reports to the facility management. Special precautions can be mounted to prevent the consequences of illness or disability from drug reactions (Jones, 1989)

Use of PRN. Often physicians rely on what is commonly referred to as PRN (*pro re nata,* meaning "as the thing is necessary") approach. These "prescribe as needed" orders allow licensed nurses to determine when to administer a particular medication. A study of nursing home medication practices by Segal, Thompson, and Floyd (1979) revealed that approximately 46% of medications were prescribed on a PRN basis. These practices, while functional and probably desirable, nevertheless need to be monitored closely.

A policy involving the facility's pharmacy consultant, medical director and nursing staff in a constant monitoring of drug reactions is a major improvement. Increasing concern has been generated concerning polypharmacy (being given too many drugs) among older patients (Evans et al., 2000, p/ 1185) However, closer and more active monitoring seems appropriate, inasmuch as undesirable drug interactions are a major ongoing concern in nursing facility administration.

The five "rights" of medication administration include identifying

1. the right medication
2. the right dose
3. the right time for administration
4. the right route of administration (oral, injection, etc.)
5. the right patient (a picture with the medication administration record [MAR] is always a good idea).

GENERIC AND BRAND NAMES

Familiarity with some of the more commonly prescribed medications by both the generic (chemical) names and brand (manufacturing) names can be useful. In the following discussion the generic names are mentioned first, with the brand names following in parentheses. Brand names are often used among health professionals unless a particular medication, for example, aspirin, is produced by a number of companies. The following are some of the more frequently prescribed medications.

Antianxiety and Antipsychotic (Psychoactive) Medications

Antianxiety and antipsychotic medications act on the central nervous system to enable residents/patients to deal with changes in their own behavior or stressful and anxiety-provoking changes in their environment. The two major classes of this type of drug are tranquilizers and sedatives/hypnotics.

These medications act directly on the major control center—the brain—and should be administered very cautiously. Many of the drug-related fatalities among older persons are associated with these medications (Basen, 1977; Maddox, 2001).

Some of the most commonly prescribed tranquilizers and sedatives/hypnotics used in the nursing home are thioridazine and chlordiazepoxide. Thioridazine (Mellaril) is a major tranquilizer and/or antipsychotic drug prescribed for mild to moderate anxiety relief. This medication has been used for longtime alcoholics to control their illness. Chlordiazepoxide hydrochloride (Librium) is a minor tranquilizer prescribed for relief of anxiety.

The side effects associated with these medications include drowsiness, dizziness, disorientation, and allergic reactions (Evans et al., 2000). An extensive and apparently successful effort has been made over the past few years to reduce the number of antipsychotic drugs used in the typical nursing facility (Ray, 1993; Selma, Palla, Paddig & Brauner, 1994).

Vitamins and Minerals

Vitamins and minerals are the most common classes of medications prescribed for the older nursing home residents, according to the National Nursing Home Survey (Evans et al., 2000; Hing, 1977). Ferrous sulfate, which is an iron supplement, and multivitamins are among the most popular in this category.

A common side effect of iron supplements is irritation of the gastrointestinal tract, which may cause some stomach upset. Too much iron is suspected of contributing to heart attacks. Other frequently prescribed minerals include calcium and potassium supplement.

Analgesics

Analgesics are often administered for pain relief (Sengstaken & King, 1993). Acetylsalicylic acid, or aspirin, may be relatively safe, except for nursing home residents/patients with kidney problems and ulcers. Aspirin may also act as an anti-inflammatory agent for arthritic patients. Such medications serve to reduce the amount of damage to the joints and to lessen the painful side effects associated with the inflammatory process.

Some of the side effects associated with aspirin include stomach upset, ringing in the ears, deafness, dizziness, confusion, and irritability (Gotz & Gotz, 1978).

Acetaminophen (Tylenol) is an analgesic similar to aspirin, but without anti-inflammatory properties, and hence it may serve only as a pain reliever. Some side effects associated with it are redness and itching of the skin and possible liver damage.

Narcotics are another group of much stronger analgesics. Federal regulations require that they be kept under lock and key in a safe place because of their potential for abuse. A dangerous side effect with these drugs is the potential to depress breathing and respiratory functions that are controlled by the central nervous system. Alterations in consciousness or blood pressure may also occur. Some of the more commonly prescribed narcotic analgesics include codeine (Methylmorphine), meperidine (Demerol), morphine sulfate, and oxycodone terephthalate (Percodan).

Laxatives and Gastrointestinal Agents

Gastrointestinal agents are among some of the more commonly prescribed medications for nursing home residents/patients. Laxatives are also referred to as cathartics. This category includes suppositories, such as bisacodyl (Dulcolax), bulk laxatives like plantago seed (Metamucil) and stool softeners such as milk of magnesia (Cooper, 1978).

Often these agents are prescribed with other medications to neutralize their irritating effects on the gastrointestinal tract. Antacids, one of the most commonly indicated for this purpose, unfortunately may also cause side effects such as diarrhea. Milk of magnesia is frequently prescribed for gastrointestinal problems.

CARDIOVASCULAR AGENTS

Various groups of cardiovascular agents work to reduce blood pressure by different actions (this and similar topics are explored at length later in this section).

Methyldopa (Aldomet) is an antihypertensive that works directly on the central nervous system to lower blood pressure. Orthostatic hypotension, or decreased blood pressure on standing, may be associated with this medication and increases the likelihood of residents/patients falling (Gotz & Gotz, 1978).

Diuretics work by forcing the body to excrete excess fluids. Furosemide (Lasix) and hydrochlorothiazide (Esidrix) are commonly prescribed. But they cause the body to excrete potassium, and this may result in muscle weakness, lethargy, and muscle cramping.

Other medications act directly on heart muscle Digoxin (Lanoxin R acts to slow down the heart rate by decreasing the speed of impulses traveling along muscle fibers. Propranolol hydrochloride (Inderal) is another medication that works to block chemicals from increasing the heart rate. Some side effects from these medications include a loss of appetite, nausea, vomiting, confusion, blurred vision, and arrhythmias (irregular heartbeats).

Anti-anginal medications work to alleviate the pain associated with a decreased oxygen supply to the heart muscle. Nitroglycerin (NTG) works as a vasodilator to increase the size of blood vessels so they will carry more oxygen. This medication is administered sublingually (under the tongue).

Antidepressants

Amitriptyline hydrochloride (Elavil) is one of the most commonly prescribed drugs for older residents in a nursing facility (Cooper, 1978). This medication also acts as a tranquilizer. The extent of its use is not surprising, considering that depression is one of the most common forms of illness (see Jones, 1989, pp. 55–56). Depression is also common among residents/patients suffering from other chronic ailments, especially Alzheimer's and Parkinson's diseases (Evans et al., 2000; Kaszniak, 1995; Maddox, 2001)

Some of the side effects associated with antidepressant medications such as Elavil include confusion, drowsiness, decreased blood pressure, constipation, dry mouth, heart flutter, rashes, and retention of urine.

Antiinfectives

Antiinfectives kill or decrease the growth of infectious organisms, complementing the natural body defense mechanisms.

Antibiotics are one of the more notable groups of medications within this class. Among the different types are the penicillins, cephalosporins, and tetracycline. One of the most important side effects associated with these medications are allergic reactions, which are often identified by skin rashes.

Some antibiotics may be used to combat fungal and viral infections. Intravenous (IV) therapy is introduced when dealing with the more resistant organisms.

Miscellaneous Medications

R*espiratory agents:* Expectorants, including ammonium chloride (Robitussin) terpin hydrate, and acetylcysteine (Mucomyst) are used to break up and expel mucus from the respiratory tract. The first two medications are taken orally; the third is usually administered by inhalation in the form of a vapor. Tetracycline and ampicillin can be effective antibiotics for residents/patients with respiratory tract infections due to chronic bronchitis (Evans et al., 2000; Rodman & Smith, 1977).

Optical medications: Mydriatics are often used for residents/patients with glaucoma. Pilocarpine and physostigmine are two medications that are often prescribed. They act to decrease the fluid buildup in the eye resulting from glaucoma. These medications are administered as eyedrops. Some of their more common side effects are headaches, diarrhea, and sweating.

CONTROLLED-DRUGS SCHEDULES

Federal regulations require all drugs and biologicals to be stored in locked compartments. Separately locked, permanently affixed compartments are required for Schedule II drugs listed in the Comprehensive Drug Abuse Prevention and Control Act of 1970.

Formerly, drugs were regulated under the 1914 Harrison Narcotic Act, which placed them into classes A, B, X and M narcotics. Subsequently, each state passed drug acts. Today pharmacists and nursing facilities must meet the individual state drug laws and the federal drug law. Most states have passed a State Uniform Controlled Substances Act, some with six instead of five group classifications.

The federal government has classified drugs into the following five schedules.

Schedule I Drugs: drugs with a high abuse potential and no accepted medical use in the United States, for example, heroin, marijuana, LSD, peyote, mescaline, and certain other opiates and hallucinogenic substances.

Schedule II Drugs: drugs with accepted medical use in the United States, having high abuse and dependency potential, for example, opium, morphine, codeine, methodone, cocaine, amphetamine, secobarbital, methaqualone (Quaalude), and phencyclidine ("angel dust"). These were formerly Class A narcotics.

Schedule III Drugs: Drugs with less abuse potential than schedules I and II drugs. Several compounds are included, for example, Empirin compound with codeine, Tylenol with codeine, and Phenaphen with codeine. These were formerly Class B drugs.

Schedule IV Drugs: drugs with less abuse potential than Schedule III drugs, such as, barbital, Librium, diazepam (Valium), and Dalmane.

Schedule V Drugs: drugs with less abuse potential than Schedule IV drugs. These typically are compounds containing limited qualities of narcotic drugs for antitussive (anti-cough) and antidiarrheal purposes. Examples are Lomotil, Phenergan (expectorant with codeine), and Robitussin A-C syrup. These were formerly Class X (exempt narcotics) under the Harrison Act.

THERAPEUTIC ACTION OF DRUGS

Analgesic—reduces pain, e.g., aspirin.

Antacid—neutralizes the acid in the stomach, e.g., Maalox

Antianemic—used in treatment of anemia, e.g., liver extract.

Antibiotic—destroys microorganisms in the body, e.g., penicillin.

Anticoagulant—depresses (slows) the clotting of blood.

Antidote—used to counteract poisons.

Antiseptic—slows down growth of bacteria, but does not kill all of the bacteria, e.g., hydrogen peroxide.

Antispasmodic—relieves smooth muscle spasm, e.g., Valium (diazepam).

Antitoxin—neutralizes bacterial toxins in infections, e.g., tetanus antitoxin.

Astringent—used to constrict skin and mucous membranes by withdrawing water, e.g., alum.

Carminative—an agent that reduces flatulence (gas) in the stomach or intestinal tract.

Cathartic—laxative, purgative, inducing bowel movements, e.g., cascara sagrada.

Caustic—destroys tissue by local application, e.g., silver nitrate.

Chemotherapeutics—chemicals used to treat illness, e.g., sulfanilamide for streptococcal infection.

Coagulant—stimulates clotting of the blood.

Diaphoretic—used to induce perspiration.

Disinfectant—destroys pathogenic organisms, e.g., Zephiran Z. chloride).

Diuretic-stimulates elimination of urine, often used with medications prescribed to reduce hypertension, e.g., diazide.

Emetic—induces vomiting, e.g., warm salt water.

Emollient—used to soften and soothe tissue, e.g., cold cream, petroleum jelly.

Expectorant—used to induce coughing, an agent that increases bronchi-
al secretion and facilitates its expulsion (coughing), e.g., Robitussin.
Hypertensive—helps raise blood pressure.
Hypnotic—assists patients residents to fall asleep, e.g., Nembutal
Miotic—constricts the pupil of the eye.
Mydriatic—dilates the pupils of the eye.
Sedative—relieves anxiety and emotional tensions, e.g., Seconal
Tonic or stimulant—used to stimulate body activity, e.g., Eldertonic or
Ritalin
Vasoconstrictor—causes blood vessels to narrow or constrict.
Vasodilator—expands or dilates blood vessels.
Vitamins—used in replacement therapy, e.g., vitamin C.

5.2.3 Abbreviations

aa	of each
Abd	abdomen
ac	before meals
Ad lib	as much as desired, at pleasure
A/G	albumin/globulin ratio
AIDS	acquired immune deficiency syndrome
amp	ampule
amt	amount
aq	water
aq dist	distilled water
ASHD	arteriosclerotic heart disease
BE	barium enema
BID	twice a day
BMR	basal metabolic rate
BP or B/P	blood pressure
BRP	bathroom privileges
c	with
Ca	carcinoma
CAD	coronary artery disease
caps	capsules
cath	catheter
CBC	complete blood count
cc	cubic centimeter
cf	compare

CNS	central nervous system
COLD	chronic obstructive lung disease (same as COPD)
comp	compound
COPD	chronic obstructive pulmonary disease
CVA	cerebral vascular accident
d/c	discontinued
Diab	diabetic
Diag or **Dx**	diagnosis
Dicsh or **D/C**	discharge
Diff	differential blood count
Dil	dilute
Disc	discontinue
dx	diagnosis
EEG	electroencephalogram
EKG	
or **ECG**	electrocardiogram
exam	examination
fl or **fld**	fluid
FUO	fever of unknown origin
Fx	fracture
GI	gastrointestinal
gm	gram
gr	grain
gtt(s)	drop(s)
H or **hr**	hour
hs	at bedtime
hypo	hypodermically
inf	infusion
IDDM	insulin dependent diabetes mellitus
IM	intramuscular
IV	intravenous
KUB	kidney-ureter-bladder
l	liter
lab	laboratory
Lat	lateral
lb	pound
liq	liquid
mg	milligram
min	minute
ml	milliliter
mm	millimeter
MN	midnight
MRSA	methicillin-resistant Staphylococcus aureus
N	noon

NIDDM	noninsulin dependent diabetes mellitus
no	number
noct	at night
NPO	nothing by mouth
NV or **N/V**	nausea and vomiting
od	right eye
os	left eye
OT	occupational therapy
ou	each eye
oz	ounce
p	pulse
pc	after meal
PEARL	pupils equal and reactive to light
po	by mouth
prn	as needed
prog	prognosis
PROM	passive range of motion
PT	physical therapy
pt	pint
PX	physical examination
qd	every day
qh	every hour
qhs	each bedtime
qid	four times a day
qn	every night
qod	every other day
qs	sufficient quantity
ROM	range of motion
Rx	prescription
s	without
SOB	shortness of breath
sol	solution
sos	one dose, if necessary
spec	specimen
SS	soap solution
ss	half
stat	immediately
surg	surgery
T	temperature
tab	tablet
TB	tuberculosis
TID	three times a day
tinct or **tr**	tincture
TO	telephone order

TPR	temperature, pulse, and respiration
u	unit
ung	ointment
URI	upper respiratory infection
UTI	urinary tract infection
VO	verbal order
vol	volume
vs or vs	vital signs
WBC	white blood cells
W/C	wheelchair
wt	weight

5.2.4 Prefixes

a-, an- *without,* e.g., anorexia (loss of appetite)

ab- *from, off, away,* e.g., abnormal (not normal)

ad- *toward, to, at*

adeno- *gland,* e.g., adenoma, a benign (noncancerous) epithelial (surface-covering) tumor in which the cells form recognizable glandular structures

ambi- *both,* e.g. ambilateral (relating to both sides)

an- *without,* e.g., anoxia (absence of oxygen supply to the tissues despite adequate perfusion of the tissue by blood, sometimes used to mean hypoxia or reduced oxygen supply, as in anoxic encephalopathy (for degenerative brain disease, meaning a degenerative brain disease characterized by insufficient supply of oxygen)

ana- *up, toward,* e.g., anabolism (building up metabolism)

angio- *relating to a vessel,* e.g., angiofibrosis (hardening of a vessel wall)

ante- *in front of, before,* e.g., ante cibum (before a meal)

arthro- *pertaining to the joints,* e.g., arthropathy (any disease affecting the joints)

auto- *self, same,* e.g., autoanalysis (analysis by a person of his or her own disorder)

bact *relating to bacteria,* e.g., bacteuria (the presence of bacteria in the urine)

bi- *two,* e.g., bilateral (relating to both sides)

bio- *relation to life,* e.g., biopsy (the process of removing tissue from living residents/patients for a diagnostic examination)

brady- *slow,* e.g., bradycardia (a slow heart)

broncho- *relating to the trachea or windpipe,* e.g., bronchoedema (swelling of the mucosa of the bronchial tube)

carcino- *pertaining to cancer,* e.g., carcinogen (any cancer-producing substance) or carcinoma (a malignant neoplasm or cancer)

cardio- *pertaining to the heart,* e.g., cardioplegia (paralysis of the heart) or cardiomyopathy (a generalized term denoting heart disease)

cata- *downward, against,* e.g., catabolism (the breaking down in the body of complex chemical compounds into simpler ones, often accompanied by the liberation of energy)

celio- *pertaining to the abdomen,* e.g., celiectomy (excision of the stomach) or celiocentesis (puncture of the abdominal cavity)

cephalo- *head,* e.g., cephalogram (an X-ray image of the structures of the head)

cervico- *neck or cervix,* e.g., cervicovesical (pertaining to the urinary bladder and the cervix)

chiro- *pertaining to the hand,* e.g., chiroplasty (plastic surgery on the hand)

chole- *pertaining to bile,* e.g., cholecystotomy (incision into the gall bladder)

circum- *around,* e.g., circumcorneal (around or about the cornea of the eye)

com-, con- *with, together,* e.g., complication (a disease or adverse condition associated with another disease or adverse condition)

contra- *against, opposite,* e.g., contraindicated (not recommended, advised against)

counter- *against, opposite,* e.g., counteraction (action of a drug or agent opposed to that of some other drug or agent)

cranio- *pertaining to the head,* e.g., cranioplasty (any plastic operation on the skull)

cysto- *pertaining to the bladder,* e.g., cystitis (inflammation of the urinary bladder) or cystocele (hernia of the bladder)

cyto- *relation to a cell,* e.g., cytolysis (the dissolution of a cell)

de- *down, away from,* e.g., defibrillation (the arrest of fibrillation—irregular or rapid randomized contractions of the cardiac muscle—and restoration to normal rhythm); debridement (removal of foreign material and contaminated or devitalized tissue adjacent to a traumatic or infected lesion until healthy tissue is exposed, to debride a pressure sore); detrusor (a general term for a body part, such as a muscle, that pushes down)

derm- *pertaining to the skin,* e.g., dermatitis (inflammation of the skin)

dextro- *toward or on the right side,* e.g., dextrocardiogram (the part of the electrocardiogram that is derived from the right ventricle of the heart)

di- *double, twice,* e.g., diarthric (relating to two joints)

dia- *through, apart,* e.g., diagastric (through the stomach)

dys- *painful, difficult,* e.g., dysphasia (difficulty in talking) or dyspnea (difficulty in breathing)

ecto- *out, away from,* e.g., ectoderm (the outermost layer of the skin)

em-, en- *in,* e.g., embolic (pushing or growing in)

encephalo- *condition in the brain or head,* e.g., encephalomyolitis (an acute inflammation of the brain and spinal cord) or encephalosclerosis (a hardening of the brain)

endo- *within, inner,* e.g., endocarditis (inflammation of the endocardium or lining membrane of the heart) or endoscope (an instrument for the examination of the interior of a body canal or hollow area)

entero- *relating to the intestines,* e.g., enterocolitis (inflammation of the mucous membrane of both small and large intestines)

epi- *above, upon, over,* e.g., epidermitis (inflammation of the epidermis or the superficial layer of the skin)

eu- *good,* e.g., euphoria (a feeling of well-being, commonly exaggerated and not necessarily well founded) or eupnea (easy, free respiration)

fibro- *pertaining to fiber,* e.g., fibromyalgia (a condition characterized by fatigue, stiffness, and chronic pain of the muscles, tendons, and ligaments)

gastro- *stomach,* e.g., gastrostomy (the establishment of an artificial opening into the stomach, usually for feeding purposes)

glyco- *relationship to sweetness* (sugar), e.g., glycogen (the chief carbohydrate storage material in animals formed by and largely stored in the liver and, to a lesser extent, in the muscles)

gyneco-, gyno- *pertaining to a female,* e.g., gynecology (the science of diseases of women, especially those of the genital tract)

hemato-, hema- *pertaining to the blood,* e.g., hemorrhage (bleeding, a flow of blood) or hematuria (blood in the urine)

hemi- *half,* e.g., hemialgia (pain affecting one entire half of the body) or hemiplegia (paralysis of one side of the body)

hepato- *liver,* e.g., hepatitis (inflammation of the liver)

histo- *relationship to tissue,* e.g., histolysis (disintegration of the tissue)

hydro- *pertaining to water,* e.g., hydrocyst (a cyst or sore with clear, watery contents)

hyper- *excessive,* e.g., hyperesthesia (abnormal acuteness of sensitivity to touch, pain, or other stimuli)

hypno(a)- *relating to sleep,* e.g., hypnotherapy (the treatment of disease by inducing prolonged sleep)

hypo- *deficiency, lack of,* e.g., hypochondria (a false belief that one is suffering from some disease) or hypotension (abnormally low blood pressure)

hystero- *relating to the uterus,* e.g., hysterogram (an X-ray of the uterus)

ileo- *relating to the ileum,* (remote end of the small intestine), e.g., ileocolitis (inflammation of the mucous membrane of both ileum and colon)

infra- *below, beneath,* e.g., infracardiac (beneath the heart, below the level of the heart)

inter- *between,* e.g., intercostal (between the ribs)

intro- *in, into,* e.g., introgastric (leading or passed into the stomach, such as a nasogastric tube for feeding)

kerato- *relating to the cornea or horny tissue,* e.g., keratoconjunctivitis (inflammation of the conjunctiva at the border of the cornea of the eye)

labio- *relating to the lip,* e.g., labiocervical (pertaining to the lip and to the neck)

macro- *large, long,* e.g., macrocyte (a giant red cell)

mast- *relating to the breast,* e.g., mastectomy (amputation of the breast)

mega- *large, oversize,* e.g., megacardia (enlargement of the heart)

meta- *after, beyond, transformation,* e.g., metastasis (the shifting of a disease)

micro- *small,* e.g., microinfarct (a very small infarct, that is death of tissue due to lack of blood supply, due to obstruction of circulation in capillaries or small arteries)

multi- *many,* e.g., multicellular (composed of many cells)

myel- *pertaining to the spinal cord,* e.g., myeloplegia (spinal paralysis)

myo- *relating to muscle,* e.g., myotrophy (muscular atrophy) or myocardial infarction (death of some heart muscle due to lack of blood supply, a heart attack)

necro- *relating to death,* e.g., necrocytosis (death of cells)

neuro- *relating to the nerves,* e.g., a neurogenic bladder (one which is controlled by the nervous system rather than by voluntary control of the person) or neruroleptic (an antipsychotic agent)

nephro- *pertaining to the kidney,* e.g., nephritis (inflammation of the kidney)

odont- *relating to the teeth,* e.g., odontalgia (a toothache)

omo- *pertaining to the shoulder,* e.g., omodynia (pain in the shoulder joint)

opthalmo- *relating to the eye,* e.g., opthalmoplegia (paralysis of the motor nerves of the eye)

opto- *relating to vision,* e.g., optometer (an instrument for determining the refraction of the eye)

ortho- *straight,* e.g., orthostatic (standing upright from a sitting or re-clining position)

osteo- *pertaining to the bones,* e.g., osteoporosis (reduction in the quantity of bone or atrophy of skeletal tissue)

oxy- *sharp, acute,* e.g., oxyesthesia (a condition of increased acuity of sensation)

pachy- *thick,* e.g., pachylosis (a condition of roughness, dryness, and thickening of the skin)

pan- *all,* e.g., pancarditis (diffuse inflammation of the heart)

patho- *disease,* e.g., pathogenesis (the origin or development of a disease)

per- *through,* e.g., perfusion (the act of pouring over or through, especially the passage of a fluid through the vessels of a specific organ)

peri- *around,* e.g., peribronchitis (inflammation of the tissues surrounding the bronchial tubes)

phlebo- *relating to a vein,* e.g., phlebitis (inflammation of a vein)

pneumo- *lung,* e.g., pneumonia (inflammation of the lung)

poly- *many, much,* e.g., polyarthritis (inflammation of several joints)

procto- relating to the anus, e.g., proctoscope (a short tubular instrument with illumination for inspecting the rectum). A sigmoidoscope, a foot-long tube, is used to examine the sigmoid (shaped like the letter M) colon, the left colon from the descending colon to the rectum. A colonoscope is used to examine the entire colon

pseudo- *false,* e.g., pseudodementia (a condition of indifference to one's surroundings without actual mental impairment)

psycho- *pertaining to the mind,* e.g., psychotherapy (counseling help)

pyo- *signifying pus,* e.g., pyoderma (any infection of or on the skin that contains pus, i.e., a collection of white blood cells and other materials generated by the immune response)

rachi- *spine,* e.g., rachiocampsis (curvature of the spine)

rhino- *nose,* e.g., rhinoplasty (a repair of the nose)

sub- *under,* e.g., subcutaneous (under the skin)

syn- loss, e.g., syncope (to faint, a temporary loss of consciousness due to generalized cerebral ischemia, i.e., too little blood getting to the brain)

tachy- *rapid,* e.g., tachycardia (rapid beating of the heart)

thermo- *heat,* e.g., thermophobia (morbid fear of heat)

uni- *one,* e.g., unicellular (composed of one cell)

uro- *relating to the urine,* e.g., urosepsis (septic poisoning from retained and absorbed urinary substances)

vaso- *vessel,* e.g., vasoconstriction (narrowing of the blood vessels) or vasodilation (widening of the blood vessels)

5.2.5 Suffixes

-ac *pertaining to,* e.g., cardiac (pertaining to the heart)

-algia *pain,* e.g., neuralgia (nerve pain)

-cele *hernia,* e.g., protrusion of a portion of an organ or tissue through the wall that normally contains it

-centesis *surgical puncture,* e.g., paracentesis (a puncture of the body cavity for removing fluid)

-clasis *breaking,* e.g., thromboclasis (the breaking up of a blood clot)

-clysis *washing, irrigation,* e.g., enteroclysis (enema of the intestines)

-cyte *cell,* e.g., hematocyte (any blood cell)

-ectasia *dilation, stretching,* e.g., gastrectasia (dilation of the stomach)

-ectomy *excision (cutting out) of,* e.g., tonsillectomy (cutting out of the tonsils)

-emesis *vomiting,* e.g., hyperemesis (excessive vomiting)

-emia *denoting a condition of the blood,* e.g., glycemia (sugar in the blood)

-genesis condition of producing, e.g., carcinogenesis (the origin or production of cancer)

-itis *inflammation,* e.g., dermatitis (inflammation of the skin)

-lith *stone,* e.g., nephrolith (kidney stone)

-lysis *breakdown,* e.g., hemolysis (the destruction of red blood cells)

-malasia *softening,* e.g., osteomalasia (a disease characterized by gradual softening and bending of the bones)

-megaly *enlargement,* e.g., cardiomegaly (enlargement of the heart)

-odynia *painful condition,* e.g., cardiodynia (pain in the heart)

-oma *tumor,* e.g., carcinoma (a malignant tumor)

-opsy *vision,* e.g., biopsy (excision of a small piece of living tissue from a patient for microscopic examination)

-orexia *appetite, desire,* e.g., anorexia (loss of appetite)

-orrhaphy *suture,* e.g., gastrorrhaphy (the suture of a perforation of the stomach)

-orrhea *flow, discharge,* e.g., gastrorrhea (excessive secretion of gastric juice or mucus by the stomach)

-ostomy *to make a new opening,* e.g., colostomy (the establishment of an artificial anus by an opening into the colon)

-otomy *incision, to cut into,* e.g., nephrotomy (an incision into the kidney)

-path *morbid or diseased,* e.g., a sociopath (a person who feels no remorse or guilt about behaving in socially unaccepted ways and feeling no guilt or remorse)

-pathy *disease,* e.g., neuropathy (any nerve disease) or angiocardiopathy (disease of the heart or blood vessels) or cardiomyopathy a disease of the heart; diabetic neruropathy is an often heard term in the nursing facility

-penia *deficiency,* e.g., leukopenia (any situation in which the total number of leukocytes-white blood cells-in the circulating blood is less than normal)

-pepsia *digestion,* e.g., dyspepsia (indigestion or upset stomach)

-pexy *fixation, to put into place,* e.g., nephropexy (surgical attachment of a floating kidney)

-phobia *fear,* e.g., claustrophobia (fear of being closed in a small space)

-plasty *surgical repair,* e.g., thoracoplasty (reparative or plastic surgery to the chest)

-pnea *breath,* e.g., polypnea (very rapid breathing)

-rhythmia *rhythmical,* e.g., arrhythmia (any variation from the normal rhythm of the heart)

-sclerosis *hardening,* e.g., arteriosclerosis (hardening of the arteries)

-spasm *sudden violent involuntary contraction of muscles,* e.g., myospasm (spasm of a muscle)

-stasis *arrest, control,* e.g., cholestasia (an arrest in the flow of bile from the liver)

-taxis *order, arrangement,* e.g., thermotaxis (regulation of the temperature of the body

-tripsy *cru*shing, e.g., lithotripsy (the crushing of a stone in the kidney by a machine called a lithotripter that uses sound waves to break stones into minute particles, which can then be passed in the urine)

-trophy *development, nourishment,* e.g., hypertrophy (an overgrowth or increase in the bulk of a body part or organ)

-uria *urine,* e.g., albuminuria (the presence of protein in urine, chiefly albumin, which is any protein that is soluble in water)

5.3 The Aging Process As It Relates to Diseases Common to the Nursing Home Population

It is useful for the administrator to be familiar with the rudiments of biological processes and human anatomy and to be able to recognize the parts of the body that are most affected by the aging process. In this way the administrator will be better able to appreciate the special problems with which the facility must cope.

All physical processes in the body may undergo some changes as a result of aging, including a slowing down, a decrease in the overall energy reserve, breakdown of some of the body functions, and an alteration of some individual cell structures, which ultimately affects the functioning of some body tissues and organs as well.

The systems referred to are groups of structures that perform a specialized function for the body. Below is a list of ten systems of the body processes and structures as they are most commonly categorized. They are presented to reflect also the prevalence of diseases affecting them in the nursing home population.

It is important to remember that these systems are highly interrelated and that most nursing home residents typically suffer from multiple chronic diseases that may affect combinations of body systems (Kane et al., 1989).

1. *Blood circulation*—the basic processes and structures that enable the body to transport oxygen to the cells and tissues.
2. *Breathing*—the process by which the body obtains oxygen from the environment and distributes it throughout the body.
3. *Nervous system*—responsible for controlling all of the body functions and ensuring that they are functioning properly; these are the regulatory activities.
4. *Digestion*—the process by which the body breaks down food into a form in which the nutrients may be used by the individual cells.
5. *Nutritional needs*—needs of the body for nutrients (Evans et al., 2000).
6. *External and internal defense mechanisms*—the skin and an internal immune system, which play important roles in protecting the body from any harmful invasions.
7. *Musculoskeletal system*—the bones, muscles, tendons, and joints used in movement (Tonna).
8. *Excretory system*—the way in which the body removes fluid and chemical waste products.
9. *Reproductive system*—sexuality in older persons.
10. *Emotional and mental well-being*—the psychological status.

5.3.1 Blood Circulation

The circulatory system, also called the cardiovascular system, may be thought of as an elaborate pumping mechanism (Rosendorff, 1983). It is powered by the heart, which pumps the blood throughout the body within a network of blood vessels (arteries and veins).

COMPONENTS OF THE CIRCULATORY SYSTEM

Arteries

Arteries are the vessels that carry blood rich in nutrients away from the heart to the rest of the body cells.

Nutrients obtained from food are processed in the digestive tract. Combined with oxygen, nutrients permit individual cells to perform the chemical reactions that produce energy.

Oxygen is a colorless, odorless, gaseous chemical element that is found in the air. Oxygen is most plentiful in the arteries, which divide into smaller and smaller branches until they become capillaries. These capillaries are the smallest blood vessels and form a network connecting the smallest arteries to the smallest veins (see Figure 5-1). It is here at the capillaries that the function of oxygenation occurs.

Oxygenation is the transfer of oxygen from the blood cells at the capillary level into the necessary tissues in exchange for carbon dioxide. Carbon dioxide is also a gas. It is produced as a waste product of the chemical reactions in the cells.

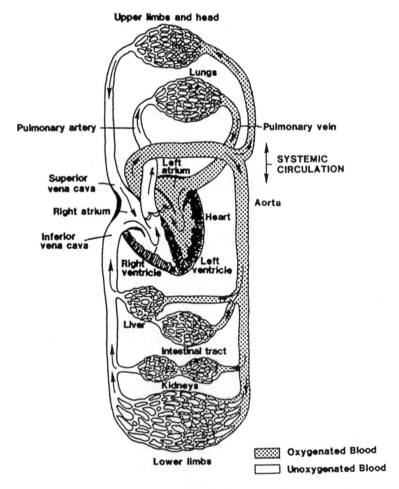

FIGURE 5-1. Representation of the circulatory and oxygenation process.

Veins

The blood cells carry carbon dioxide through the vein network and back to the heart. Veins return blood that is carrying carbon dioxide back to the heart through the superior (from upper body) and inferior (from lower body) vena cava (see Figure 5-1).

The blood then enters the right side of the heart. When a sufficient amount of blood has collected, the right ventricle of the heart contracts, actually squeezing its contents into the artery that leads to the lungs (pulmonary artery).

Lungs

Within the lungs the carbon dioxide that has been collected by the veins is discarded and exchanged for oxygen. The carbon dioxide is then exhaled into the air as the breath is expelled. It has followed the reverse of the oxygen pathway until it is removed from the body. This is a simplification of the respiratory process (breathing), which will be discussed further in the next section.

The newly oxygenated blood returns to the heart through the pulmonary vein. The blood is then channeled into the left side of the heart. When enough blood has collected, this blood is then pumped forcefully out of the heart into the aorta. The aorta is the largest artery from which all the smaller arteries branch off, carrying blood that is rich in oxygen throughout the rest of the body again. This process occurs with every heartbeat (Pierce, 1995).

The Heart

The heart itself is a complex organ. It is a muscle composed of various types of cells to facilitate the pumping process. The heart requires oxygen to function and is supplied by a network of coronary arteries that stem from the aorta (see Figure 5-2).

The inner structure of the heart is also very complex, with four distinct chambers and a valve network that regulates blood flow.

CELL CHANGES

Any substantial change in these structures or the circulatory process itself can eventually affect all the body cells. The significance, then, of the oxygenation process is that when the health of cells has deteriorated, it is usually due to a change in the cardiovascular system that interferes with the supply of nutrients to the cells and with the supply of oxygen.

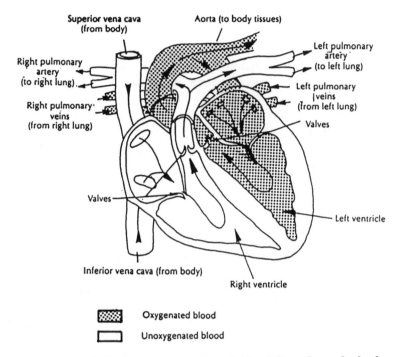

FIGURE 5-2. Schematic representation of blood flow through the heart.

This in turn damages the tissues and organs in the body, leading to the decline of other major processes.

AGING EFFECTS

The extent to which the aging process plays a role in this deterioration is still being argued. It is known that the cardiovascular system (heart and blood vessels) is not designed to last indefinitely. Many of the cells are not capable of dividing and remain part of the system for long periods of time.

Decreased Elasticity

A specific age-related change in the heart may include a lessening of the force of contraction (pumping) due to the decreased elasticity of muscle. Elasticity is the ability of the heart muscle to stretch and return to normal size spontaneously. When this property has been decreased in the heart muscle, the heart becomes stretched. This loss of elasticity reduces the force of contractions by the heart, which ultimately diminishes the amount of blood pumped by the heart (also termed cardiac output).

Decreased Cardiac Output

The reduced cardiac output is also due to an increased resistance to blood flow within the blood vessels and a loss in the heart's ability to compensate by beating faster. This added resistance to blood flow within the blood vessels may be a direct result of arteriosclerosis (hardening of the arteries) or more specifically atherosclerosis (one type of arteriosclerosis (Golden, 1995; Maddox, 2001).

A change in any one of these components will affect the other two. If the amount of blood circulated is reduced, the organs and tissues will receive fewer nutrients and less oxygen, resulting in some cells dying (if deprived for more than 3 to 5 minutes).

It is estimated that in older individuals the blood flow to the kidneys is reduced by as much as 50%, and to the brain by as much as 20%, due to these same processes (Kenney, 1982). These changes can explain changes in other systems associated with age.

Blood Pressure Changes

There is much debate among scientists about the role of the aging process and its effect on blood pressure. In many older persons the blood pressure does increase (O'Brien & Bulpitt, 1995). This increased pressure may be attributed to the stiffness of the large arteries (arteriosclerosis) and *peripheral vascular resistance* (the resistance in the blood vessels throughout the body) that are commonly associated with the aging process. Other studies of individuals in isolated areas reveal no changes in blood pressure levels for older persons. Some investigators feel there is a strong association of social and environmental factors contributing to the presence of high blood pressure in any individual (*hypertension*) ("Best Drugs," 1995; Kane et al., 1989).

Blood vessel changes due to this progressive stiffening indicate that they become like rigid tubes (Finch & Haflick, 1977). This promotes the resistance to blood flow throughout the body (peripheral vascular resistance) and may exacerbate an already adversely affected heart function and increased blood pressure.

The vein walls tend to weaken with increased deposits of fats, cholesterol, fibrin, platelets, cellular debris, and calcium over time. The capillary walls become thickened, thus decreasing their ability to exchange oxygen with the cells. This thickening also contributes to the overall decrease in perfusion of (flow of nutrients into) the tissues and organs.

SIX COMMON CARDIOVASCULAR DISEASES

Cardiovascular disease is the major cause of death in the older population. Some problem associated with heart disease is the primary diagnosis of approximately 40% of long-term nursing home residents. The
distinction between changes related to the aging process and those related to disease is a fine one. This dilemma becomes clear with the discussion of arteriosclerosis.

Arteriosclerosis

Usually, arteries are smooth inside and can stretch to permit the passage
of more blood and oxygen when needed. With arteriosclerosis, the blood
vessels are not as responsive as they previously were. Everyone has
arteriosclerosis to some degree. Almost half of all long-term nursing
home residents manifest disease changes due to chronic arteriosclerosis.
Two forms of this condition (atherosclerosis and aortic stenosis) account
for much of the heart disease in older individuals.

Aortic Stenosis. The term describes a narrowing of the aorta, which is
the major artery leading from the heart that channels the oxygenated blood
supply to the rest of the body. Stenosis, or narrowing of the vessel, increases
the workload specifically for the left ventricle of the heart, because it now
has to pump harder to overcome the obstructive resistance to blood flow.

The increased workload eventually is felt by the entire heart, and
when combined with the normal changes attributed to the aging process,
this disease places considerable stress on the cardiovascular system. It
can result in congestive heart failure, which will be discussed at the end
of this section.

For many residents/patients, the cause of the disease is either the
result of scarring from a childhood case of rheumatic fever or calcified
deposits lining the blood vessels.

Some of the **symptoms** of aortic stenosis are difficulty in breathing,
dizziness, high blood pressure, chest pain, and symptoms associated
with congestive heart failure.

Treatment can consist of surgical correction, rest to decrease the
workload on the heart, and medication therapy.

Atherosclerosis. In this, the most common form of arteriosclerosis,
there is a progressive buildup of fat deposits on the inner lining of blood
vessel walls. The disease does not usually manifest itself until the blood
vessel becomes completely obstructed or shows a marked decreased ability
to facilitate blood flow. The symptoms can be found affecting the body
anywhere that an initial pathology (a disease-related change in a tissue

or organ) may be present; this usually includes the main arteries. In 1980, atherosclerosis caused twice the number of deaths as cancer in older groups.

Cerebrovascular Disease

This disease manifests itself through restricted blood flow to the brain, caused by occlusions within the carotid arteries that supply blood to the brain. It is one of the most important causes of strokes (Maddox, 2001).

Long-term nursing home residents who may be predisposed to cardiovascular disease are those with high blood pressure, previous history of heart disease, and those who are overweight (Birchenall & Streight, 1982). The specific symptoms of the disease depend on the affected area in the brain. *Transient ischemic attacks* (also termed "mini-strokes") are caused by a temporarily diminished blood supply to the brain.

Signs of cerebrovascular disease can be slurred speech, blurred vision, dizziness, numb hands and fingers, and mental confusion. Some of these symptoms could be easily attributed to the aging process rather than to this underlying disease pathology.

A much more severe consequence of cerebrovascular disease is *stroke,* or cerebrovascular accident (CVA). This occurs when the lack of oxygen for a much larger area of the brain causes permanent damage. Again, the resulting damage will depend on the area of the brain affected and may range from temporary loss of taste or smell to paralysis of many of the body parts.

Peripheral Vascular Disease

This actually describes a group of diseases that affect the veins, arteries, and other blood vessels of the extremities (Birchenall & Strieght, 1982). The symptoms are a result of decreased blood flow to the affected area. The most frequent symptom is *intermittent claudication,* which is a complex of **symptoms** (Evans et al., 2000) including the following:

- pain on movement of an extremity
- pain that is chronic in a localized area
- cold, numb feet
- changes in skin integrity, such as ulcers or infections that are slow to heal

Coronary Artery Disease

Also known as chronic ischemic heart disease, here the heart muscle itself suffers from a lack of oxygen due to blockages in the coronary arteries that usually supply it (Evans et al., 2000).

The popular coronary artery bypass graft surgery is a common treatment for persons with severe blockages who do not respond to medical therapy. Because this is major surgery, some nursing facility residents/patients would not be considered good surgical risks for such treatment. This may be increasingly true inasmuch as a growing number of researchers are beginning to believe that medical treatment may be as effective as surgery.

Symptoms can include chest pain (commonly called angina), which results from a lack of oxygen to certain areas of the heart muscle. Pain may be located anywhere in the chest, especially in the left arm or neck. This symptom is commonly found in residents/patients over 60 years of age (Kleiger, 1976).

Myocardial infarction (MI, literally meaning heart muscle death) results when a large enough area of the heart muscle does not receive oxygen for a period of time (Evans et al., 2000). With a massive myocardial infarction, the heart can no longer continue to act as a pump and may completely stop beating. There is a greater chance that residents/patients over 60 years old will die from a heart attack than will younger patients (Evans et al., 2000; Kleiger, 1976).

The phases in coronary artery disease range from diffuse, incomplete blockages throughout the arteries, to one or more large blockages that occlude more of the blood flow.

Symptoms can range from none at all to various types of angina or, most serious, to a complete cessation of heart activity that occurs after MI or complete heart block (Evans et al., 2000).

Treatment varies. Initially, patients without severe manifestations of the disease can be treated conservatively with restrictions on sodium and fat in their diet. Medications commonly used in the nursing facility are nitroglycerin and propranolol.

Nitroglycerin, the most common medication prescribed for persons with angina, is administered sublingually, under the tongue. This drug lowers the blood pressure by dilating the blood vessels, including the coronary arteries, to decrease resistance to blood flow.

Propranolol hydrochloride (Inderol) is referred to as a beta blocker because of its action in blocking body chemicals that increase the heart rate. The medication slows the heart down, thereby decreasing blood pressure and lowering the amount of oxygen required by the heart muscle.

There are also a variety of antiarrhythmic medications available, which are prescribed in accordance with the particular type of arrhythmia diagnosed.

A common result of prolonged or diffuse coronary artery disease is the inability of the heart to initiate contractions independently. When this occurs, another type of treatment is often prescribed: a permanent pacemaker. The pacemaker is a mechanical device implanted under the skin with its wires attached to the heart muscle to provide a continuous flow of electrical impulses that stimulate the heart to contract with a steady rhythm and can now be monitored by phone lines.

High Blood Pressure

High blood pressure, also called hypertension, is usually considered to be present when the blood pressure measurement is consistently greater than 160/95.

These numbers are a measurement of the amount of pressure the blood exerts on the walls of the arteries. The first number measures the maximum pressure (systolic) exerted when the heart is fully contracted near the end of the stroke output of the left ventricle. The second number measures the minimum (diastolic) pressure when the heart ventricles are in the period of dilation or fully relaxed. This must be monitored for each individual to account for height and weight variations (Evans et al., 2000).

There are two types of high blood pressure: essential hypertension and secondary hypertension. The cause of essential hypertension is unknown, and therefore the disease is without a complete cure, but it can be successfully controlled by medication. Secondary hypertension in older persons results from other underlying diseases, including anemia, fever, endocrine disease or hormonal disruption, arteriosclerosis, or kidney disease (Evans et al., 2000; Rubin, 1981). These diseases place a greater demand on the heart and may cause the blood pressure to increase during the disease episode or permanently.

The effects of continued high blood pressure, regardless of the cause, may be harmful to various organs within the body, especially the heart, brain, kidney, and eyes. When a person has high blood pressure, the heart must automatically pump harder to circulate the blood throughout the body. Eventually it begins to fail from being overworked for such long periods of time. This in turn reduces the blood flow to the vital organs, damaging their functioning as well.

Some **signs** of hypertension are prolonged, elevated blood pressure greater than 160/95, or the individual's norm, and prolonged presence of risk factors such as overweight, smoking, high salt intake. Using the 160/95 definition, 40% to 50% of individuals over age 65 are hypertensive and should be actively treated (Kane et al., 1989). More recently, the threshold of concern for beginning treatment has been lowered to 140/90 (Maddox, 2001).

Treatment typically includes prescribing weight loss and diet therapy, including restricted salt intake. The goal of medication therapy is to use as few drugs as possible. Some of the most common medications used in a nursing facility include diuretics, nitroglycerin, and propranolol.

Diuretics are frequently used to get rid of the excess fluids in the body in order to decrease the heart's workload by decreasing the blood volume that it must pump. Vasodilators such as nitroglycerin are used to dilate blood vessels and therefore decrease the amount of resistance against which the heart must work. Cardiac drugs such as propranolol may also be used to relieve the workload of the heart by decreasing its rate of contractions or pumping.

Congestive Heart Failure

This is not a disease but actually a complex set of many symptoms associated with an impaired performance of the heart (Evans et al., 2000). A progressively weakening heart results in an increasing inability of the heart to pump enough oxygen to the various tissues of the body. This failure results in a congestion of blood that backs up in the circulatory system, which causes fluids to leak out of the bloodstream into the various tissues and organs, most notably the lungs. Taken together, these constitute the disease process called congestive heart failure (CHF) (Evans et al., 2000) (See Figure 5-3).

The cause of congestive heart failure may be a variety of diseases or conditions, most notably arteriosclerosis, coronary artery disease, uncontrolled high blood pressure or a problem with one of the heart valves, heart attack, alcoholism, or chronic exposure to agents harmful to the body tissues (Evans et al., 2000). The lifetime prevalence of alcoholism of older hospitalized persons has been reported as 20.4% for those aged 60—69, declining to 13.7% among patients aged 70—79 and to 0% for those aged 80 and older (Maddox, 2001).

The symptoms usually are seen in other organs and can be classified according to whether the heart failure primarily affects the left or right side of the heart.

Right-sided failure of the heart produces the following **symptoms**:

- edema: a build-up of fluids outside of the blood vessels that forces fluid into the tissues; occurs mostly in the ankles
- gradual loss of energy
- anorexia (loss of appetite for food)
- constipation
- weight gain (because the kidneys cause the body to retain too much sodium and water)
- grayish or blue color of the skin due to decreased blood flow

Left-sided failure of the heart is indicated by different **symptoms**:

- frequent coughing or wheezing
- shortness of breath (dyspnea) a result of the blood backing up into the lungs thus decreasing the amount of space in the lungs available

Congested Heart

Congestive heart failure occurs when a healthy heart (*right, top*) loses its ability to contract fully. As a result, too much blood remains in the heart after each pump cycle, and the heart cannot supply the body with an adequate amount of oxygenated blood (*bottom*).

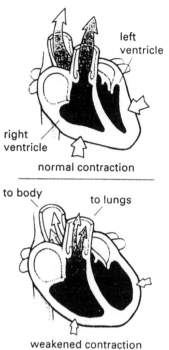

FIGURE 5-3. Congested heart.
From *Johns Hopkins Medical letter,* 1995, 7(10), p. 4. Reprinted with permission.

to hold air; is one of the definitive signs of CHF usually occurring after exercise (Anderson, 1976; Evans et al., 2000)

- confusion and loss of memory are severe symptoms that suggest the disease has progressed far enough to damage the brain tissue

Treatment generally consists of rest; monitoring weight to guard against sudden changes; diet therapy, including reducing salt intake and encouraging potassium intake with foods like bananas and oranges; and oxygen therapy to improve the oxygen content of red blood cells, because there is less and less exchange area available in the lungs (Moss, 1989).

Technological advances are being made in providing oxygen to residents/patients. Machines called oxygen concentrators are available, obviating the constant need for oxygen tanks. The advantage is an ability to use ambient air in the resident/patient's room to produce the required oxygen. The potential disadvantage is that, unlike the bulky and unsightly tanks, the oxygen concentrator must have a continuous supply of electricity.

Medications can include Digoxin (Lanoxin) which acts directly on the heart muscle to increase the force of contraction. This is an extremely powerful medication that may cause severe side effects in older persons when the level of the medication becomes too high in the blood. Confusion or severe behavioral changes may indicate this is occurring (Gambert, 1983; Kane et al., 1989).

To avoid fluid buildup, *diuretics* are also often prescribed to aid the body in eliminating toxic wastes and fluids that have accumulated (Crow, 1984). Some of the more powerful diuretics deplete the body's supply of important electrolytes, such as sodium and potassium. Low levels of potassium can be particularly dangerous for the older resident/patient, who is especially vulnerable to such imbalances. Potassium supplements are frequently prescribed, in addition to dietary supplements, to increase the blood level of this naturally occurring mineral.

5.3.2 Respiratory System

The chief function of the respiratory process is to provide the body with oxygen while removing excess carbon dioxide. These processes occur during breathing, when air enters and exits the body through the nose and mouth. The air that enters the body is rich in oxygen, the gas necessary for many of the cells' basic chemical functions. The respiratory and circulatory systems are very closely related, because both are involved with the oxygenation process.

THE OXYGENATION PROCESS

The circulatory system can be likened to a train, carrying the oxygen in each "car" or blood cell. The lungs, then, are the depots where the blood cells pick up oxygen and deposit carbon dioxide. The structures in the body that help the respiratory system do its work include the mouth, nose, pharynx, trachea, bronchi, bronchioles, lungs, alveoli, diaphragm, and various respiratory muscles. The respiratory process involves all of these structures to promote the inhalation and exhalation of air that transports gases to the blood cells and diffuses oxygen into the body (Rosendorff, 1983).

After the air is inhaled through the nose or mouth, it travels through the trachea which leads to the bronchi of the lungs. There, the two bronchi, the main airways into the lungs, divide and subdivide numerous times before ultimately forming the bronchioles (see Figure 5-4). The

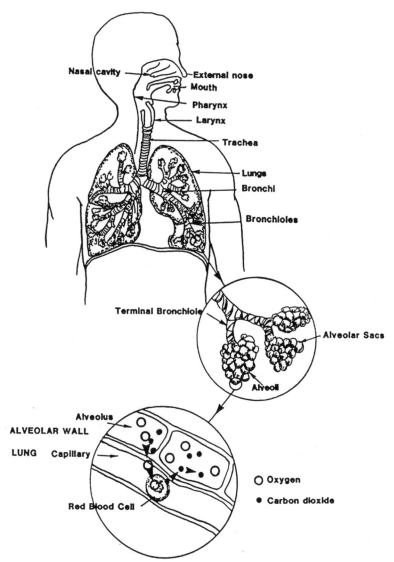

OXYGEN–CARBON–DIOXIDE EXCHANGE AT ALVEOLAR WALL WHERE
PERMEATION OF OXYGEN AND CARBON DIOXIDE CELLS OCCURS

FIGURE 5-4. The respiratory tract. Oxygen–carbon dioxide exchange at alveolar wall where permeation of oxygen and carbon dioxide cells occurs.

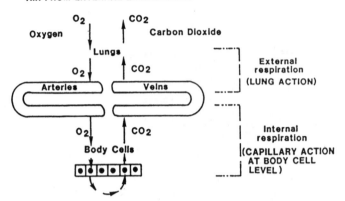

FIGURE 5-5. Diagram of events occurring simultaneously during respiration.

bronchioles are the smallest airways in the lungs and eventually terminate in the numerous alveoli that are the basic respiratory units (see Figure 5-5).

Alveoli are the many air-filled sacs that are the site of the actual oxygen–carbon dioxide exchange. In this transaction, oxygen is absorbed by the blood, and carbon dioxide is released into the air as the breath is exhaled. Much of the volume within the lungs is taken up by blood undergoing this stage of the oxygenation process.

Because the respiratory and cardiovascular systems are closely related, any damage to one of these systems is likely to directly affect the other (Kart, Metress, & Metress, 1978). A number of other structures are essential for breathing, including the diaphragm and associated respiratory muscles of the chest. These structures aid the lungs in expanding and contracting with each inhalation and exhalation.

AGE-ASSOCIATED CHANGES

Changes associated with the aging process do occur. However, in the older person without any significant disease, the overall result of these changes should not be incapacitating or prevent the person from carrying on the activities of daily living (Kart et al., 1978).

One of the reasons for this is that the lung, unlike the heart, has a remarkable ability to repair itself after infection or damage. These repairs usually leave only minor traces that could later be mistaken for degenerative changes (Woodruff & Birren, 1975). A list of changes due to aging that do affect the respiratory system includes the following (Kenney, 1982):

- decreasing size (and therefore capacity) of the alveoli
- loss of elasticity of lung tissue
- stiffening of the ribs (requiring muscles to work harder to pump air in and out of the lungs)
- changes in the shape of the chest
- decreased resistance to infection

The decreased capacity of the alveoli is not in itself enough to cause any dramatic changes in the breathing process. However, this does reduce the efficiency of the breathing mechanism and may lead to disability and respiratory problems over time (Weg, 1983).

Older individuals are more prone to infections than the rest of the population (which is explored further in this section). When these additional factors are coupled with the fact that the lungs receive foreign materials continuously from the outside air, it is not surprising that many older persons suffer from some form of lung disease.

INFLUENCE OF THE ENVIRONMENT ON THE LUNGS

Because the lungs are in almost direct contact with the air outside, the environment may play a more important role in the development of disease in the lungs than in any other body system. Environmental exposure to a lung irritant over a prolonged period of time often produces the type of changes that result in respiratory disease. Some examples are miners' exposure to coal dust, welders' to asbestos, and chronic cigarette smokers' to tar and nicotine. Lung infection is one of the more common causes of death among older persons (Garagusi, 1989).

CHRONIC RESPIRATORY DISEASE

Approximately 6% of long-term nursing home residents/patients suffer from some type of chronic respiratory disease. The most common classification of lung disease is chronic obstructive lung disease (COLD) or chronic obstructive pulmonary disease (COPD). The COPD diagnosis includes chronic bronchitis, asthma, and emphysema (Shashaty, 1989). There is no cure for these diseases, but there are a variety of treatments available ("Keeping Active," 1994). New diagnostic instruments are becoming available such as a pulse oximeter, which uses infrared light through the finger to read the oxygen level within 30 seconds. Spirometers are used to detect the amount of lung volume the individual can exhale, then the results are compared with predicted curves.

The main complication brought on by COPD is that the body is unable to rid itself of the air containing carbon dioxide. This may be because of a disruption of the alveoli or because the bronchial tubes are not expanding and permitting the gases to escape during respiration.

Chronic bronchitis and emphysema are two diseases of this type that are most commonly seen in the long-term nursing facility resident/patient. The signs, symptoms, and treatment of the respiratory diseases mentioned are very similar because they all affect the lungs. The symptoms listed following the discussion of the next two diseases will apply to all the diseases in the remainder of this section.

Chronic Bronchitis

As the name suggests, chronic bronchitis is caused by a continuing irritation of the bronchi (the two airways into the lungs). The inside of these airways swell and become clogged with mucus secretions, making it more difficult to breathe. This may be due to something irritating from the environment or a recurrent infection. Chronic smokers are the ones most likely to develop bronchitis. This disease is the most common respiratory condition found in older persons and is defined as a chronic productive cough in more than 3 months of two successive years, unexplained by another diagnosis (Shashaty, 1989).

Asthma is characterized by bronchial reactions to internal or external stimulants. It is generalized reversible airways obstruction. Usually a bronchodialator is administered orally, by inhalation or both (Shashaty, 1989).

Emphysema

Emphysema results in a loss of elasticity in all of the lung tissue. As a consequence, the lung is less able to hold as much air, but the alveoli tend to have air trapped inside causing carbon dioxide to build up. The increasing amount of carbon dioxide only worsens the respiratory condition because the body is triggered to obtain more and more oxygen to compensate for this imbalance. Continuous oxygen therapy may be supplied from large oxygen tanks, liquid oxygen reservoirs, or an oxygen concentrator. Oxygen therapy reduces lung hypertension and promotes oxygenation of the other body systems (Shashaty, 1989).

The causes of emphysema are similar to those of bronchitis, the most common one being a recurrent infection or chronic irritant to the lung. Emphysema is much more serious than bronchitis, and usually residents/patients with this disease die from heart failure as a result of prolonged stress on the cardiovascular system.

Symptoms common to most lung diseases are chronic cough, increased production of thick white mucus, and some shortness of breath. These symptoms are a result of the body's attempting to rid itself of whatever is irritating the respiratory tract. Irritation of the inner lining of the respiratory tract results in the increased production of mucus, which is intended to coat the cause of the irritation and assist its excretion from the body.

A cough is another way the body has of rejecting whatever is causing the irritation. When this irritation is chronic, these mechanisms are continually being triggered.

These symptoms can be found in more severe forms of lung disease:

- stress on the entire cardiovascular system with related symptoms
- enlarged heart
- heart failure (with emphysema)
- thick mucus plugs blocking the smaller airways within the lung
- alveoli that have become overinflated and eventually burst, decreasing the amount of space available for oxygen exchange
- barrel-shaped chest
- poor appetite
- weight loss
- dizziness

Treatments include medications to minimize airway irritation and obstruction, such as bronchodilators (to relax the breathing tubes, widening them and thus improving air flow) and expectorants, to thin the mucus so that coughing is more productive.

Pneumonia

Pneumonia is an infection in the lungs caused by either a virus or bacteria. Residents/patients with chronic obstructive lung disease are much more susceptible to this infection because bacteria grow in stagnant areas like those where the mucus is collecting. This infection further complicates the older person's ability to breathe and causes disruptions in other systems.

The **signs and symptoms** are very similar to those already described and may include a fever or very weak condition resulting from the infection. **Treatment** generally includes some type of antibiotic therapy when bacteria are the cause of this infection. A study of 124 nursing home patients with nursing home–acquired pneumonia, some of whom were treated in the nursing home and some in the hospital, revealed that the majority of episodes were successfully treated with oral antibiotics (Delague, Guay, Straub, & Luxemberg, 1995; Evans et al., 2000).

Chronic Tuberculosis

Tuberculosis is an infectious disease more commonly found among nursing home residents/patients because of their higher risk of infection, resulting from multiple chronic diseases (L. F. Cohen, 1995b; Maddox, 2001).

Tuberculosis may infect a young person, but oftentimes a healthy immune system wards off the disease, which goes into a dormant state. As a person ages, this immunity may break down with an infection, and the dormant disease may become active (Evans et al., 2000; "Tuberculosis," 1995).

Symptoms and signs are similar to those listed for COLD, except that the secretions contain the tuberculosis bacteria. The disease is termed infectious because it may easily be transmitted through the secretions or when a patient coughs.

One of the most important **treatments** then, is to isolate the person as long as he or she is coughing and producing sputum. To prevent the spread of infection, staff and visitors generally are required to wear masks and gloves when in contact with the resident/patient or when in his or her room.

Lung Cancer

Lung cancer is a chronic lung disease and is among the leading causes of death for American men. It is also the most prevalent from of cancer found among nursing facility residents/patients. Because the disease affects the lungs, **symptoms** are similar to those of COLD.

Generally, the nursing home resident/patient is receiving palliative **treatment** (just enough therapy to be comfortable) (Evans et al., 2000; Maddox, 2001). **Other types of treatment** include radiation, chemotherapy, or surgery, depending on the size and location of the tumor (Evans et al., 2000). With improved understanding of this disease process, new drug regimens and improved radiation treatments, lung cancer is becoming treatable (Evans et al., 2000; "Lung Cancer Is Always Treatable," 1995).

Respiratory Therapy Rates

Respiratory treatment is provided by respirators/ventilators, oxygen, inhalation therapy, and other treatment. In 1993, 6% of facility residents received treatment compared to 9% in 1999. Rates varied: Wyoming reported 20% of residents receiving respiratory treatment compared to 6% in Hawaii (Harrington et al., 2000).

5.3.3 Nervous System

One of the body's most important mechanisms is the nervous system, which acts as its control enter by coordinating functions and maintaining order. The brain can be thought of as a computer system with the nerves and spinal cord transferring input and output messages to and from each part of the body (Brody, 1995a).

Some specific nervous systems functions for control of the body include responding to events outside the body through the five senses, performing voluntary activities such as walking, and storing memories, ideas, and emotions so they may be used at a later time for various thought processes. The nervous system also perform automatic responses such as breathing, maintaining heart rate, and controlling temperature.

COMPONENTS OF THE CENTRAL NERVOUS SYSTEM

The central nervous is composed of the brain, spinal cord, and nerves (Brody, 1995b). The brain is considered by some to be the most important organ in the body because it is accorded a high level of priority among body functions. When the body is undergoing a great deal of stress, other organs will reduce nutrient intake so that more nutrients can be directed to the brain.

The brain is protected by the skull and surrounded inside by a protective layer of cerebrospinal fluid. This organ is very specialized, with different areas responsible for different body functions.

The cranial nerves connect the brain with the areas of the body responsible for sensory perception (identifying what is outside the body through the senses, including taste, smell, and hearing). The base of the brain is called the medulla. It is primarily responsible for controlling motor activity or movement. It is this area that connects the brain to the spinal cord.

The spinal cord looks like a tree trunk, with the nerves representing the branches of the tree and eventually leading to the blood vessels, muscles, and organs throughout the body.

The brain itself is made up of many specialized cells that are unique to the individual areas of the brain in which they are found. Because the brain cells perform complex processes, they need large amounts of oxygen to function continually. A lack of oxygen to the brain causes the cells and their tissues to die within minutes.

The nerves are composed of many individual fibers that are encased in a fatty substance called myelin for the same reason that electrical wires are covered with a plastic coating: to prevent them from "shorting out." These individual fibers are composed of neurons, which are the nerve cells. Unlike the heart cells, nerve cells can be replaced or regenerate themselves, although at a very slow rate.

The nerve fibers form an intricate network that is responsible for carrying a variety of messages to the brain. These messages are carried in the form of electrical impulses that stimulate the appropriate area of the brain, triggering either an involuntary response reaction (reflex) or a thought process (cognitive).

The nerve fibers form a complex series of pathways that impulses travel along to reach the brain. It is important to remember that the left side of the brain controls the functions on the right side of the body, and the right side of the brain controls functions on the left side of the body.

POSSIBLE EFFECTS OF AGING

The effects of aging on the nervous system are most commonly believed to be the result of a change in the system that reduces the oxygen supply to the brain cells. This can lead to permanent alterations to those cells that are so sensitive to the level of the oxygen supply (Chui, 1995ap. 174; Hefti, 1995; Woodruff & Birren, 1975).

Apparently the weight of the brain decreases with age, possibly because of some loss of brain cells and nerve fibers (Kenney, 1982). Researchers, using refined instruments, have been able to detect changes in the neurological system of older persons when observing the speed with which impulses are transmitted to the brain. But this change is not directly associated with a slowing down of functioning in the thought process. It is probably a myth that older people's thought or cognitive process is much slower than other age groups.

PERCEPTUAL CHANGES

One of the perceptual changes commonly attributed to the aging process is a decreased sensitivity to touch (Kenney, 1982).

Some of the visual changes associated with age include loss of range of vision for near objects, decreased flexibility of the lens of the eye, and reduced clarity of vision, or the "dusty windshield" effect of the lens of the eye, accompanied by a loss in ability to distinguish pastels (Evans et al., 2000).

There may be a change in the central processing of sound in the inner ear. This has not been proved as yet, so residents/patients who are hard of hearing are not necessarily that way just because of age. There does appear to be a loss of ability to hear high-pitched sounds; speaking to residents/patients in deep tones can help compensate for this loss.

In many older individuals, the taste buds appear to have degenerated, and the amount of saliva produced also appears to be diminished, producing a change is the capacity to taste different flavors (Evans et al., 2000). An abuse of salt may be the result of a patient's efforts to improve or increase taste sensations. Ability to taste sweets is apparently unaffected, which may explain the preference of many older residents/patients for eating dessert first.

There may also be an age-related decrease in neurons responsible for smell, resulting in the loss of smell for different odors.

Some older people also appear to dream less and have increased periods of wakefulness throughout the night (Libow, 1981).

Diseases associated with the nervous system include those that affect sensory components, impair mobility and communication processes, and affect the ability to distinguish reality from fantasy (Steffl, 1984).

THE EYE

The eye is a complicated structure, held in place by muscles. The retina is the innermost layer of the eye and contains receptor cells that actually generate electrical nerve impulses when hit by light. These impulses are carried to the brain along the nerve fibers that leave the retina and form the optic nerve. This nerve leads to the area of the brain responsible for vision. The retina is protected by the lens covering the eye.

The lens can be thought of as a layer of skin, except that all of the old cells on the lens cannot be discarded like old layers of skin, and they are continually compacted within the eye (Corso, 1981). The aqueous humor is a substance that bathes the eye and protects it as well.

Presence of Eye Problems

Approximately 33% of all long-term nursing home residents experience some form of visual impairment, and 5.5% of these patients are blind. About 61% were found to wear some type of eyeglasses to correct their vision.

The aging process may result in an overproduction of aqueous humor, resulting in a large amount within the eye. When this happens, glaucoma may result.

Glaucoma. Glaucoma is a chronic condition that is actually a complex of many different symptoms. This condition is not a direct result of the aging process, but the incidence of the disease is definitely greater among older individuals (Corso, 1981; Kane et al., 1989).

There are four different types of glaucoma: chronic, acute, secondary, and congenital. In each of these, the primary problem is that fluids within the eye undergo increasing pressure changes. These fluids are continually being formed, but not draining from the eye chamber because of some disruption in the drainage system (Kasper, 1989). As a result, the eyeball itself becomes very hard. This also causes an extremely painful pressure in the eye, which can lead to a range of other conditions.

Symptoms of glaucoma can induce acute pain in the eye, elevated blood pressure, blurred vision, and halos around lights. Untreated glaucoma can lead to blindness.

Treatment usually varies with the form or state of disease, but initially medical therapy is used to promote the drainage of excess fluids from the eye. As a rule, medications are the critical variable in preventing blindness from glaucoma (Steffl, 1984).

Mydriatics are a kind of medication that usually come in the form of eyedrops that act to dilate the pupil of the eye, helping to drain off some of the excess fluid.

Cataracts. A cataract is a cloudiness that affects the transparency of the lens to the extent that light cannot get through to the retina. The retina is the area of the eye that transforms light into the objects seen. Usually cataracts form in both eyes.

The major **symptom** of cataracts is increasingly blurred vision, with perceptions of shadows. **Treatment** usually consists of eyeglasses or contact lenses. The lens of the eye can be surgically removed and replaced with a new manufactured one (lens implant).

Importance of Vision Among Residents/Patients

When older persons with visual impairments are helped to see better through intervention, they adapt better to the area around them. Interventions do not need to be complex. They can include providing large-type books, magazines, and newspapers; painting color-coded boundaries and walkways throughout the facility for easy identification (e.g., a painted baseboard in the hallway that helps distinguish spatial location); and using large letters and numbers in all visual displays such as doors, elevators, and clocks.

HEARING

The structures of the outer ear include those portions of the ear external to the eardrum (tympanic membrane). The middle ear contains three small bones that conduct the sound waves; they are called the incus (the anvil), the malleus(hammer), and the stapes (stirrup).

The inner ear contains the cochlea, which transmits sound waves to nerve impulses that travel down the auditory nerve (the eighth cranial nerve) to the auditory center of the brain.

Hearing Impairments

Presbycusis is the term used to describe any hearing impairment in old age (Kane, Ouslander, and Abrass, 1989). Approximately 26% of long-term nursing home residents/patients suffer some hearing impairment, and it has been estimated that 5% of the residents/patients are deaf. However, only 6% of them use hearing aids (which, in any case, are not always helpful) (Kennie & Warshaw, 1989).

Hearing impairments can also be due to a buildup of wax in the ear or to what is known as a conductive or sensorineural hearing loss. Conductive disorders and ear wax are the only ones that may be treated effectively. Usually surgery or hearing aids are prescribed for those with a conductive loss. The sensorineural disturbances result from a disruption in the structure of the inner ear or the nerve pathway to the brain stem.

Symptoms of hearing impairment can include tinnitus (an intermittent, sometimes constant, ringing in the ears), progressive hearing loss, and increased inability to hear high-frequency sounds, including shouting, warning bells, or buzzers (Yoder, 1989).

Treatment can include a hearing aid when appropriate, sign language, lip-reading, speech reading, slow, well-enunciated communication, facing the resident/patient whenever speaking to him or her, and providing appropriate warning signals to communicate the presence of fires or other dangerous occurrences within the facility.

MOBILITY AND COMMUNICATION

Cerebrovascular Accident

A cerebrovascular accident (CVA), also known as a stroke, can be one of the most debilitating conditions that an older person faces (Evans et al., 2000). It is believed that 16% of long-term nursing home residents have suffered some form of stroke.

The cause of stroke is lack of oxygen to the brain. For treatment purposes, it is important to distinguish among the three types and causes of stroke. Cerebral thrombosis is blockage by a thrombus (clot) that has built up on the wall of a brain artery and accounts for about 40% to 50% of strokes. Cerebral embolism is blockage by an embolus (usually a clot) swept up from below into an artery in the brain and accounts for 30% to 35% of strokes. The third mechanism of stroke occurs when there is rupture of a blood vessel and bleeding within or over the surface of the brain, which accounts for 20% to 25% of cases (Grob, 1989). New evidence suggests that getting a stroke victim to the hospital as rapidly as possible may permit minimizing the damage by quick treatment once it is determined whether the stroke is due to a clot that can be dissolved by a blood thinner or to hemorrhage (a burst artery), which requires different treatment.

Warning **signs** can include headache, dizziness or confusion, visual disturbance, slurred speech, or loss of speech or difficulty swallowing.

Degrees of Disability

The degree of disability resulting from a stroke may range from only a slight impairment to complete immobility and loss of voluntary muscle control (Van Vliet, 1995b). **Symptoms** following a stroke are usually specifically related to the area of the brain affected and may include the following:

- muscle weakness on one side of the body (hemiplegia)
- difficulty standing or walking
- poor balance
- pain in arms and legs
- fatigue
- poor vision
- confusion
- difficulty in spatial judgment, distortion
- complete loss of muscle control (quadriplegia)
- paralysis of the body below the upper extremities (paraplegia)
- difficulty speaking (aphasia)

Aphasia. Aphasia is the term used to describe an inability to interpret and formulate language (Maddox, 2001; Van Vilet, 1995a). Specifically, such problems may be seen as a slowdown in the ability to retrieve vocabulary and inappropriate use of grammar or words, as well as problems in understanding what is being said.

Usually this occurs because the area of the brain responsible for speech is damaged during the stroke. There are many different types of aphasia, with the most severe resulting in an individual's being unable to understand what others are saying (receptive aphasia).

Other types of aphasia result in an inability to express in words what the individual really wants to communicate (expressive aphasia). At other times, inappropriate words or vulgar language is used as if the individual had no control of what he or she says.

Dysarthria. Dysarthria (imperfect articulation of speech) is a speech rather than a language abnormality that may accompany paralysis, weakness, or lack of coordination (Yoder, 1989). This deficit can be a frustrating experience for the resident/patient whose other mental capacities are intact. This frustration often leads to emotional upset. The most important need that residents/patients have at this time is the ability to communicate. The incidence of these disorders may exceed 50% of the long-term population in a nursing facility (Corso, 1985).

Individually designed rehabilitative therapy is the most usual form of **treatment.** The ability of a person to recover from a stroke is best correlated with the cause. Lower brain stem damage from a stroke has a more favorable prognosis than an assault on the upper part of the brain (Adams, 1981).

Rehabilitation therapy usually focuses on standing, ambulating, taking initial steps, and walking with a cane or other appliance. Physical and occupational therapists are integral member of the rehabilitation team for these residents/patients.

Parkinson's Disease. Parkinson's disease is actually a group of symptoms that can progressively lead to complete disability in those severely affected. Scientists believe that selected groups of neurons (nerve cells) in the brain are lost as a result of this disease, but the cause of this loss remains a mystery (Maddox, 2001).

Symptoms of Parkinson's disease can include tremor, or trembling, of any of the limbs while at rest, rigidity or muscle stiffness, and bradykinesia (a slowness in body movements). Additional symptoms may include the following:

- stooped posture while standing
- walking with short, shuffling steps, garbled speech
- illegible handwriting
- sad, lifeless facial expression
- facial droop
- mood swings
- dementia (an impairment in intellectual ability)

There is no cure for Parkinson's disease, so the **treatment** is determined by the specific symptoms and degree of physical impairment in functioning in (Cohan, 1989).

Often residents/patients with Parkinson's disease suffer from mental disturbances similar to those seen in patients with Alzheimer's disease, and physicians are finding it difficult to distinguish one from the other. Alzheimer's patients have the additional diagnosis of dementia (Evans et al., 2000; Ripich, Wykle, & Niles, 1995).

Dementia

Dementia is a broad, nonspecific term denoting cognitive loss (Reichel & Rabins, 1989). The diagnosis and understanding of mental deterioration among some elderly is still in its early stages.

Riechel and Rabins (1989) identify three major causes of senile dementia: About 60% is due to Alzheimer's type, 25% to infarction of brain tissue due to cerebrovascular disease, and 15% to several other diseases such as paresis, Huntington's chorea, Pick's disease, Parkinsonism, AIDS (F. L.Cohen, 1995a), Wilson's disease, and several others (Evans et al., 2000; Maddox, 2001).

More than one half of long-term nursing home residents/patients may have some form of demented illness (Gwyther, 1983). Dementia is usually thought of as senility in an older person and may include behavior such as forgetfulness, a deterioration in personality, and a decrease in intellectual functioning (Reisberg, 1995).

A common misperception is that these behaviors are all a normal result of the aging process. But none of these senile behaviors are considered to be normal aging effects and are instead due to some type of disease or disruption (Kane, Ouslander, and Abrass, 1989).

Hardening of the arteries due to arteriosclerosis is a disease that may lead to dementia in the older person. In this situation, the arteries do not allow enough oxygen to pass through to the brain, with the result that areas of the brain die. This condition is also refereed to as multi-infarct dementia and may affect 25% of older nursing home residents/patients (Chui, 1995b). The only way physicians currently have of distinguishing between multi-infarct dementia and Alzheimer's (Albert, 1995) disease is to perform a computer automated tomograph (CAT scan). The treatment, however, is no different for either diagnosis.

Rates of Dementia & Other Psychological Diagnoses. Figure 5-6, shows a slight increase in average percent of residents reported with dementia, rising from 37% in 1993 to 41% in 1999. The percent varied from 32% in Illinois to 55% in Maine in 1999.

The percent of residents with other psychiatric conditions (other than organic mental syndromes) such as schizophrenia, mood disorders, and other problems is also reported in Figure 5-6. Other psychiatric conditions varied from 11% of residents in 1993 to 14% of residents in 1999. The percentage of conditions varied from 4% in Hawaii to 21% in Louisiana and Ohio in 1999.

Alzheimer's Disease. Alzheimer's disease is the most common form of dementia seen in persons over 60 years old; its incidence increased dramatically after that age (Maddox, 2001). The Alzheimer's patient displays an intellectual impairment that is irreversible. The disease progression varies from one person to another and can extend from a year to over a decade (Schneck et al., 1982). Alzheimer's type of dementia is also known as primary degenerative dementia, a disorder that involves alteration in the structure, number, and functions of neurons in some areas of the brain's cerebral cortex (Evans et al., 2000; Kane et al., 1989; Maddox, 2001).

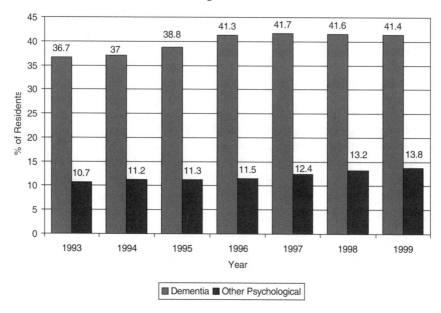

FIGURE 5-6. Percentage of residents in U.S. nursing facilities witih dementia and other psychological diagnoses, 1993–1999.
Nursing Facilities, Staffing, Residents and Facility Deficiencies, 1993–1999, Department of Social & Behavioral Sciences, University of California San Francisco.

Three distinct phases of Alzheimer's disease have been identified: Stage I or early stage is marked by forgetfulness; Stage II or mild stage is characterized by confusion; and Stage III or terminal stage dementia is present (Gwyther & Mason, 1983; Schneck et al., 1982).

The **signs and symptoms** of the disease vary with each stage, but some, including memory loss and behavioral changes, progress in severity until they become profound in the final stage. The following list of signs and symptoms reveals the progressive nature of the disease.

Stage I

- memory loss
- time disorientation
- anxiety
- irritability
- behavior and personality change
- agitation
- inability to concentrate for long periods of time

Stage II

- excessive hunger
- aphasia
- temper tantrums
- restlessness
- muscle twitching
- aimless wandering, sometimes getting lost
- inability to read, write, or do arithmetic calculations
- obsession behavior (e.g., constant washing and rewashing of hands)
- repetitive movements (e.g., tapping, chewing, lip smacking)

Stage III (usually the shortest stage)

- bedridden
- unable to perform purposeful movement (walk)
- poor appetite
- poor articulation
- incontinence
- emaciation
- frequent seizures

The goal of **treatment** is to achieve the highest quality of life while maintaining physical function (Evans et al., 2000). Several nursing home chains as well as individual facilities have installed special Alzheimer's units, usually characterized by enclosed outdoor areas and indoor gates of various types (e.g., coded key pads on doors) to control wandering. Typically, it is the Stage II resident/patient who is the primary type of resident in these units due to the special management needs created by this stage of the disease process. A major recent trend is for assisted living facilities to offer stand-alone Alzheimer's units. It is estimated that 30% to 50% of assisted living facility residents have dementia. About 18% of assisted living facilities offered Alzheimer's special care units in 1999 (Maddox, 2001). This is an area of special concern since staff in these assisted living units have less training than staff in a nursing facility and nearly all such units are locked units, raising serious unlawful-restraint issues in the U.S.

Medications are palliative, often tranquilizers to relax the resident/patient and relieve any agitation or violence. Antidepressants are also used to improve the overall mood.

BREAKING NEW GROUND

Research into treatments appears promising, but no breakthroughs have been achieved. It seems likely that as more is learned, new disease patterns will be identified within the current broad categories of Alzheimer's type, or infarction of the brain tissue due to cerebrovascular disease, or other. Researchers at Harvard Medical School studied 3,623 older Bostonians and found Alzheimer's present in 3% of those aged 65 to 74, 19% of the 75–84-year-olds, and 47% of those 85 or older.

Cognitive losses are being identified more successfully and, it is hoped, will become more treatable. Persons 85 and older make up the fastest growing segment of the United States population. The nursing facility is usually the institution of choice to care for persons of that age who are diagnosed with dementia.

Articles and research reports concerning Alzheimer's disease abound (see, for example, Bennett and Knopman, 1994; Karcher, 1993; Leon & Siegenthaler, 1994; McCaddon & Kelly, 1994; Sterritt & Pokorny, 1994; "Stopgap Benefits," 1995; Swanson, Maas, & Buckwalter, 1993; Zinn & Mor, 1994).

5.3.4 Digestive System

Digestion is the process by which the body breaks down food into needed nutrients. These nutrients are further broken down into particles small enough to pass through tissues and enter the bloodstream for delivery to the appropriate tissues and organs. After absorbing necessary nutrients, the leftover materials or waste products are discarded from the body.

The digestive system is commonly referred to as the gastrointestinal or alimentary tract in reference to the various organs that participate in the digestive process (see Figure 5-7) (Bruns, 1995). A diagrammatic representation of the path of food through the digestive system is presented in Figure 5-8.

MOUTH

Digestion begins when food enters the mouth. Chewing the food is an important step in preparing it for digestion. Saliva, produced by salivary glands in the mouth, contains enzymes that begin breaking down food substances while they are still in the mouth.

ESOPHAGUS

After food is swallowed, it enters the esophagus. The esophagus is the tube (made of smooth muscle) connecting the mouth to the stomach.

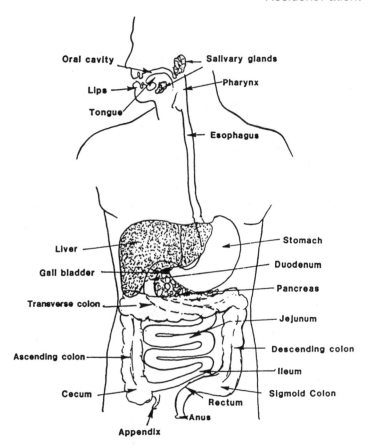

FIGURE 5-7. Organs involved in the digestive processes.

When food is swallowed, the gastric (stomach) sphincter relaxes to allow food into the stomach. Swallowing initiates a wave like movement of the esophagus (called peristalsis) that propels food toward the stomach.

STOMACH

The next phase of digestion begins in the stomach. The stomach has sphincters (muscles) at both ends that close when the stomach is full, enabling the stomach acids sufficient time to bread down the food.

The digestive process in the stomach is controlled by the brain through the nerves, which constantly carry impulses directing the digestion process.

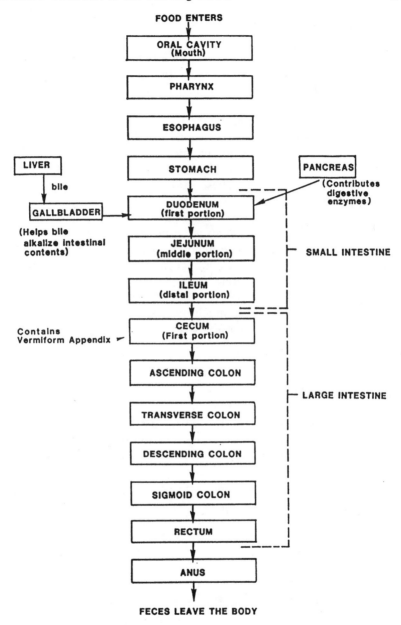

FIGURE 5-8. Diagrammatic representation of the path of food through the digestive system.

INTESTINES

The intestines may be thought of as a long tube. The intestines are also referred to as the bowels or lower gastrointestinal tract (lower GI). Despite its name, the small intestine is actually much longer than the large intestine.

When the digestive contents enter the small intestine (duodenum), further chemical digestive actions occur. The food is in liquid form at this stage and contains powerful enzymes that break down certain substances. The intestines are also filled with bacteria that help to digest some of the food substances. These same bacteria are very harmful to any other part of the body if allowed to escape.

Like the stomach, the intestines also have nerves that carry impulses to and from the brain. These nerves are especially important in stimulating the bowel to move the waste materials along the intestinal tract. As in the esophagus, the intestines contract in snakelike movements (peristalsis), propelling the food along the digestive tract.

If for some reason the brain does not send the appropriate impulses to the intestines, the waste moves much more slowly though these organs. Unlike the esophagus, the intestines do not have the added force of gravity to assist in this process.

LARGE INTESTINE

The large intestine is a continuation of the small intestine and plays its own role in the digestive process. One function of the large intestine is to store the waste so that the body can absorb excess fluids and nutrients before elimination.

By the time waste materials are excreted form the body, they are in a solid form, referred to as feces or stool. It is important to note that usually patients have voluntary control over when they choose to eliminate these waste materials because the sphincters at the very end of the digestive tract are within the realm of voluntary control.

POSSIBLE EFFECTS OF AGING

Mouth

The amount of saliva secreted by the salivary glands may decrease. The saliva also may become thicker, until it is almost like mucus (MacHudis, 1983), and the loss of teeth may also cause digestive complications (Libow, 1981).

Esophagus

In some older persons, food may not travel as quickly through the esophagus. Causes for this appear to be a reduction in the effectiveness of the swallowing mechanism that helps foods move toward the stomach, and the gastric sphincter failing to close as quickly as before (Kenney, 1982).

Stomach

The lining of the stomach can decrease in thickness with age. This decreased thickness of the lining may allow the size of the stomach to increase. The amount of acid produced by the stomach may decrease (Kenney, 1982; Sklar, 1983).

DIGESTIVE DISEASES

The digestive tract is an area of the body about which older nursing-home residents/patients often complain. Physicians use the general diagnosis "gastrointestinal distress" to describe a range of diseases affecting this system.

Esophagus

The esophagus may be a common site of discomfort for the older resident/patient. Esophagitis (inflammation or irritation of the esophagus) is another name for heartburn, a frequent problem for older individuals. Often this sharp, burning pain may be confused with chest pain and may become worse when the person lies flat, allowing stomach contents to reenter the esophagus.

Dysphagia is difficulty in swallowing or transferring food from the mouth to the esophagus (Evans et al., 2000; Gibbons & Levey, 1989; Logemann, 1995). Persons with neurological damage may be subject to this problem. Persons who have recently suffered a stroke can be at increased risk because without this function they may aspirate (inhale particles of) food into their lungs.

Stomach

Peptic ulcers may occur anywhere in the gastrointestinal tract. Two of the most common types are gastric ulcers that affect the midstomach and duodenal ulcers that involve the lower stomach (Evans et al., 2000).

An ulcer is a wearing away of the inner lining of the stomach wall and is due to a chronic buildup of excessive levels of acid. Excessive stress, inactivity, prolonged bed rest, severe trauma, and irritating drugs may all serve to cause or exacerbate this condition. On examination at death, 35% of persons under 50 years of age had gastric ulcers whereas 80% of those over 80 years of age (i.e., the typical nursing facility resident/patient) had gastric ulcers (Gibbons & Levy, 1989).

Medical views on what causes stomach ulcers and their treatment has changed in recent years. Currently, *H. pylori,* a gram-negative spiral bacterium that colonizes the mucus layer overlaying the gastric mucosa, has become known as a transmitted disease, which causes stomach ulcers, contrary to earlier beliefs (Evans et al., 2000). Standard treatment is a triple-antibiotic regimen for 14 days in conjunction with a 6-week course of acid suppression therapy (Evans et al., 2000).

Ulcer symptoms can include sharp burning abdominal pain 1 to 4 hours after eating, nausea, weight loss, blood in vomitus, and blood in stools.

The goal of treatment is to prevent any complications arising from the initial ulceration, thus allowing it to heal. Medications, including antacids, are prescribed to relieve the condition. Long-term treatment for peptic ulcers remains controversial. The preferred approach appears to be to treat for 12 months; others prefer intermittent courses of treatment (Gibbons & Levy, 1989).

Intestines

Constipation is an irregularity in or lack of elimination of waste materials from the body (Kennie & Warshaw, 1989). Twenty-four percent of all long-term nursing home residents/patients have reported this as a problem, and in one study more than 34% of older residents/patients used laxatives at least once a week (Hing, 1977; p. 23; Meza, Peggs, & O'Brien, 1984). "Normal" bowel habits studied in 1,500 older residents/patients indicated that 99% reported anywhere from 3 bowel movements a day to 3 per week (Gibbons & Levy, 1989).

Constipation may initially be a decrease in the number of stools passed, progressing to a complete lack of stool or bowel movements. When the person has not been able to pass stool for a long period of time, an impaction (blockage) has probably occurred. The waste in the large intestine has accumulated in one area and become hard because much of the fluid content has been reabsorbed by the body.

Treatment of constipation can include laxative medications, which are commonly prescribed for nursing home residents/patients. Bulk laxatives, osmotic laxatives, suppositories, and enemas are the different forms of medications that may be prescribed. Increased activity is one of the best treatments.

Hemorrhoids are another painful disturbance that can affect the elimination of waste materials from the body. A hemorrhoid is a vein in either the rectum (internal) or around the anus (external) that becomes enlarged. The external type are usually more painful. Hemorrhoids may either be the cause or result of chronic constipation.

Incontinence is the inability to control the timing of elimination. Some of the causes of this dysfunction may be a neurological disturbance due to disease or trauma to the brain and spinal cord, anal surgery, chronic diarrhea, or mental disturbance. Urinary incontinence is often caused by impaction. Urinary incontinence is a multibillion-dollar health issue that affects almost 60% of nursing home residents Bacteriuria is also prevalent in this group and the two conditions are commonly found together (Ouslander et al., 1995). A number of researchers feel that urinary incontinence is generally manageable (Palmer, Bennett, Marks, McCormick & Engel, 1995). Incontinence care, however, is a major disruptor of the ability of nursing home residents to "get a good night's sleep" (Engel, 1995; Schnelle, Ouslander, Simmons, Alessi, & Gravel, 1993).

Tube feeding. Tube feedings are used to provide nutritional substances to residents into the gastrointestinal system. In 1993, 6% were receiving tube feeding compared with 7% in 1999 (Harrington et al., 2000).

5.3.5 Nutrition

Food provides the body with the nutrients necessary to cell functioning. Adequate nutrition can be of value in the maintenance of fitness and independence as well as prevention of disease (Franz, 1980; Maddox, 2001).

In the earlier section on digestion, the digestive process was described as the time when foods are initially broken down into nutrients so they can be absorbed by the body. The next phase of nutrition is the metabolic process whereby the remainder of the nutrients are absorbed, helping to produce energy and/or control the various body functions.

Metabolism is the transformation process in which nutrients undergo various chemical reactions throughout the body, producing energy while also helping cells perform necessary functions. Calories are the units of measurement for determining the amount of energy that is contained in foods or used by the body. A list of some the nutrients considered essential to the body follows. All of them occur naturally in foods and can be obtained from a well-balanced diet.

Protein is a nutrient that can be broken down into components called amino acids. It is necessary for growth, repair of damaged tissues, transporting nutrients and chemicals throughout the body, and producing various hormones and enzymes.

Carbohydrates can be broken down quickly into readily available fuel for the body. Two common sources are starches and sugars (Halter, 1995). The brain is especially sensitive to any decreased levels of carbohydrates in the body and may be permanently damaged whenever the level is reduced for a period of time.

Fats are considered to be the body's source of energy reserve. Fat forms a protective padding around the major organs, prevents heat loss from the body, and carries vitamins A, D, E and K, helping with their absorption.

Minerals Needed by the Body Include

- *Calcium*—used to build bones and teeth, giving them their hard structure; also helps to clot blood
- *Iron*—important in building healthy red blood cells that are able to carry oxygen
- *Sodium*—acts as a buffering mechanism, helps dissolve substances in the bloodstream, monitors the amount of fluid in the body
- *Potassium*—contained in fluids and tissues; important in muscle contraction, maintains the body fluid balance, and also acts as a buffering mechanism in the bloodstream.

Vitamins act to control certain body functions and regulate the body's utilization of other foods (Maddox, 2001).

FLUIDS

Internally, the body is bathed in fluids that help to eliminate wastes and assist the cells with chemical reactions. Fluids help maintain the integrity of the body by protecting the skin and distributing nutrients to promote healing.

Some Major Body Fluids Include

- *Plasma*—carries red blood cells and essential nutrients throughout the body
- *Cerebrospinal fluid*—protects the brain and spinal cord
- *Lymphatic fluid*—carries white blood cells and fluids from the tissues

In all phases of life, adequate nutrition sustains the building-up processes of the body and impedes the wearing-out processes (Albanese,

1980). However, older residents/patients who have multiple chronic diseases may need even more nutrients than the healthy adults.

POSSIBLE EFFECTS OF AGING

Older persons are believed by some researches to require fewer calories because of reduction in body weight, a decrease in the metabolic rate and often a decline in physical activity (Albanese, 1980; Franz, 1981; Weindruch, 1995). However, at the same time that it may be desirable to reduce the amount of carbohydrates and fats, the older person has an increased demand for nutrients in order to resist the effects of disease. Thus, the appropriate diet for an older person is complex.

Osteoporosis, a softening of the bones, is a concern among numerous older persons. It has been observed frequently in women over 40 (U.S. Barzel, 1995). A lack of sufficient calcium may contribute to a softening of the bones, making some nursing facility residents/patients especially susceptible to bone breakage in falls or other accidents (Maddox, 2001).

Dehydration may occur more easily among older persons if they reduce their fluid intake. A smaller proportion of fat under the skin may permit body fluids to evaporate more readily than previously. Dehydration can occur quickly when an older person has a fever (Beattie & Louie, 1989; Evans et al., 2000) and often has no presenting symptoms or signs (Evans et al., 2000). Rapid weight loss (3%) may indicate dehydration.

Aging may affect other structures that aid in digestion. The loss of teeth can result in changes in the types of foods eaten. Weight loss generally causes problems with fitting of dentures; refitting is often necessary.

A loss in the overall number of cells and muscle mass may decrease body weight. In this situation the body may no longer need as many calories to provide sufficient energy.

As with any person, consuming more calories than needed while remaining relatively inactive can lead to obesity—more and more fat being stored in the tissues as reserve energy. Obesity has been referred to as a frequent form of malnutrition in older persons (Foley, 1981; Kane et al., 1989).

PRESCRIBED DIETS

Although the majority of nursing facility residents/patients will eat normal diets, some residents will have special nutritional needs. Chronic disease and the effects of institutionalization on appetite pose a challenge (E. Kahana, 1995b).

Physicians often prescribe special therapeutic diets for this group.

- *Soft diet*—for residents/patients who need a diet that is low in fiber, soft in texture, and mild in flavor
- *Mechanical soft diet*—same as above, except texture is either chopped, pureed, or ground to make foods easier to ingest
- *Strict full-liquid diet*—consists of foods and liquids that are liquid at body temperature, but can include cold ice cream and hot soup
- *High-fiber diet*—to provide bulk; similar to regular diet, but with foods that are difficult to digest, e.g., fruits, vegetables, whole-grain breads and cereals, nuts, and bran
- *High-calorie high-protein diet*—may include milk shakes, meats, and similar foods to provide additional sources of protein

When residents/patients cannot eat as usual, nasogastric, esophagostomy, or gastrostomy tube feeding may be prescribed by the physician (Evans et al., 2000).

Nasogastric tubes are inserted through the nose and enter the stomach. Esophagostic tubes pass through the neck into the esophagus. Gastrostomy tubes are surgically inserted directly into the stomach.

Gastrostomy tubes may be preferred for patient/residents who need long-term tube feeding, for example, a cancer patient, because they can be more comfortable and there is no chance for fluids to flow into the lungs (aspiration, i.e., when the tube is mistakenly inserted into the trachea instead of the stomach cavity). This often leads to aspiration pneumonia. These tubes also will not irritate the lining of the upper gastrointestinal tract as may nasogastric tubes.

Enteral feeding is a recent innovation using products like Osmolite or Ensure. In this case the feeding tube is inserted nasogastrically, but continues into the duodenum (past the stomach into the opening of the small intestine). A pump feeding tube similar to an IV arrangement delivers the nutrients to enter the duodenum. The obvious advantage is to reduce the possibility of aspiration because the nutrients are introduced into the small intestine itself. The disadvantage is that a permanently inserted tube between the stomach and duodenum must be reinserted with the use of an X-ray machine, usually in a hospital setting, in difficult cases.

ANEMIA AND DIABETES: TWO METABOLIC DISEASE PROCESSES

Two of the most common diseases that disrupt the metabolism of important nutrients are anemia and diabetes (Evans et al., 2000; Sinclair, 1995).

Anemia is a condition in which hemoglobin is deficient, resulting in the body's not getting enough oxygen. The red blood cells contain a substance called hemoglobin, which carries the oxygen. *Diabetes* occurs when the body is unable to metabolize glucose (sugar) because of a problem with the hormone insulin that is produced by a ductless gland, the pancreas (Maddox, 2001).

Anemia

Various types of anemia are found in the nursing facility. It is thought to be due to disease, not old age (Freedman, 1982; Kane et al., 1989), and therapy for each type of anemia is varied. About 5% of long-term nursing home residents probably suffer from some form of chronic anemia.

Anemia is the result of a significant decrease in the number of red blood cells. Having multiple chronic diseases can lead to anemia. Symptoms of anemia are similar to those for heart disease because they also result in a problem with oxygenation (Kravitz, 1989). When anemia is combined with other diseases, such as peripheral vascular disease or coronary artery disease, it may be very serious as well as painful for the resident/patient.

Diabetes

Diabetes affects about 15% of all long-term nursing facility residents/patients. It results from an inability to convert carbohydrates into forms the body can utilize.

Usually, the pancreas produces the hormone insulin, which helps the cells convert sugar (or glucose) into a form for energy for use or storage. Diabetics either produce insufficient amounts of this hormone or have some difficulty utilizing it. The result is large amounts of sugar continually circulating in the bloodstream, causing the condition known as hyperglycemia (high blood sugar).

Chronic hyperglycemia can damage many of the body tissues and can cause complications and disabilities in other systems in the body. In its more extreme form, diabetes is a factor in blindness and amputation for older patients.

There are two different classifications of diabetes: insulin dependent and noninsulin dependent. Individuals with insulin-dependent diabetes mellitus (IDDM) have generally had the disease since childhood and require daily doses (or the equivalent) for the control of the disease. Almost all of the long-term nursing home population fall into this category (Bazzare, 1983). Noninsulin-dependent diabetes mellitus (NIDDM) is usually diagnosed in adults, who are generally able to control the disease by dietary restrictions and the use of oral hypoglycemics (Bazzare, 1983; Beattie & Louie, 1989).

Much of the treatment provided to nursing home residents involves monitoring the blood sugar level. It is often unclear who is truly a diabetic. Glucose tolerance progressively deteriorates with each decade of life. One researcher formulated a percentile system demonstrating decreasing glucose tolerance with age (Andres, 1989). Thus, the physician practicing in a nursing facility must guard against treating a laboratory value that represents an altered physiologic state as a true case of diabetes (Reichel, 1983).

5.3.6 External and Internal Defense Mechanisms

The body is equipped with two different special defense mechanisms to protect it from harmful disruptions in the environment.

THE BARRIER, SYSTEM OF DEFENSE

The first type acts as a barrier preventing harmful substances from entering the body. The largest organ, the skin, is one such barrier (Orentreich, 1995). While protecting the body from harmful organisms, the skin also seals in essential body fluids and regulates the body temperature (Frantz & Gardner, 1994) . The respiratory, intestinal, and urinary tracts also have barrier-like components to protect the body from foreign materials that may enter through their systems.

In the respiratory tract, thousands of cilia (small hairlike elements) line the passageways and help propel outward any foreign materials that may be inhaled from the air. Coughing expels these particles from the body and back into the environment.

Two additional protections are the acid composition of gastric juices and urine, which also act to protect the digestive system and the urinary tract from the entrance of harmful organisms.

THE CHEMICAL DEFENSE SYSTEM

The immune system is often referred to as the second line of defense; it protects the internal structures of the body. Whenever foreign material or an antigen enters the body, the components of the immune system recognize this and mobilize for an attack response. Most often, the foreign material is a small bacterial or viral microorganism.

Different types of antibodies have various means of fighting an infection and use a much more complex interaction than that seen in the cell-mediated response.

INFECTIONS

When bacteria or viruses are successful in penetrating the defense mechanisms in large numbers or are allowed to enter areas of the body where they are not usually found, the resulting disruption is known as an infection (Evans et al., 2000). Philip Smith, an infection control epidemiologist who has written extensively in this field, estimates that 1.5 million infections occur each year in United States nursing homes. This suggests an average of about one infection per resident per year and that, on average, 5% to 10% of residents will acquire an infection in any given year (Smith, 1989). Nursing home residents may be more prone to infections than other population groups because of

- age-related changes in their bodies
- the presence of multiple chronic diseases that weaken the defenses
- associated use of multiple medications with side effects that may compromise the body
- increased incidence of immobility and incontinence
- frequent use of invasive devices such as indwelling urinary catheters

These factors all increase nursing home resident/patients' susceptibility to infections and also serve to weaken the body's own natural defense mechanisms. Three researchers, Beck-Sague, Banerjee, and Jarvis (1993) estimate that risk of infection from residing in a nursing home ranges from 3.3% to more than 15%. Kane et al. (1989) remain unconvinced, however, that alterations in defense mechanisms predispose older persons to certain infections. They speculate that environmental factors, specific diseases, and physiological changes other than the immune system may account for the increased frequency of certain infections in older individuals (see also, Goldrick & Larson, 1992).

New infectious processes are being identified in nursing homes. More recently documented infections include bacteremia (bacteria in the bloodstream occurring with intravascular catheters), conjunctivitis, AIDS, streptococcal infection, Legionnaires' disease, and methicillin-resistant staphylococcus aureus (MRSA) (Evans et al., 2000). More and more nursing facilities are being asked to care for and are accepting MRSA residents/patients who have special care requirements relative to universal precautions. Of particular concern is whether the MRSA is colonized or noncolonized upon admission. A colonized MRSA means the infectious agents are encapsulated and much less likely to spread infection. Noncolonized MRSA can spread infection via airborne particles and contact with objects in the patient's physical vicinity.

Additional infection risk factors are emerging as nursing facilities accept transfer from hospitals of patients who are quite ill, some of whom have tracheostomies, central IV catheters, hyperalimentation, or AIDS. The emergence of vancomycin-resistance in *Staphylococcus* is of increasing concern for the nursing facility that receives such patients from the hospital (Evans et al., 2000).

Nosocomial Infections

Infections that are associated with institutionalization or acquired while in a health care facility are called nosocomial infections. Nursing home residents are considered to be at a particular risk of developing these infections because of the levels of group interaction and activities among residents (Garibaldi, Brodine, & Matsumiya, 1981).

Farber, Brennen, Punteri, and Brody (1982) found that half of all infections in the chronic-care facility they studied may be due to nosocomially acquired pneumonia or urinary tract infections and that these two infections are commonly responsible for morbidity (illness) in the older population (p. 502). Pneumonia immunization is recommended for persons over 65 (Evans et al., 2000,, 85). Some of the other types of nosocomial infections often seen in the nursing home include infections of the skin, soft tissues, and gastrointestinal tract (Farber et al., 1982; Nicolle, McIntyre, Zacharias & MacDonald, 1961). Because of more frequent and longer hospitalizations, nursing facility residents are at increased risk for *Staphylococcus* and gram-negative infections (Kane et al., 1989). Infection control has generally improved in recent years according to research by Raymond Otero who focused on methicillin-resistant *S. aureus* (MRSA) (Otero, 1993).

The Inflammation Response

Inflammation occurs in the physical responses by other body systems when fighting off infection of some external threat. The blood vessels dilate (expand) bringing more cells to combat the unwanted component. This if often the cause of redness surrounding areas of skin that may become infected. The debris from the antigen often become pus, which may drain from the infection as well (Groenwald, 1980).

SPECIAL DIFFICULTIES IN IDENTIFYING INFECTIONS

Infections in older persons may be more difficult to diagnose because it is possible to confuse the symptoms with those of other chronic diseases. Also, even when symptoms are present, the older resident/patient may be reluctant to complain about these disruptions, so they are less likely to be reported (Beck & Smith, 1983).

Most infections are not considered chronic diseases because they respond to treatment, and their damage to the body can often be reversed.

POSSIBLE EFFECTS OF AGING

The skin contains fibers that change as people age. These changes may make the skin and other connective tissue drier and less resilient (Balin & Lin, 1995; Kenney, 1982; Tonna, 1995b).

Skin, nail, and hair cells, which are among the fastest to grow during younger years, often do not replace themselves as quickly when people age (Carter & Belin, 1983). Together, these changes help explain why many older people have some degree of tough, dry, wrinkled skin (Kenney, 1982). Kligman (1979) also suggests that these types of changes work to diminish the barrier function of the skin as a person ages.

A study by Tindall and Smith (1963) of 163 persons 64 years of age and older showed that 94% of them had "lax" skin, secondary to changes in connective tissue, which contributed to wrinkling and other related manifestations.

The greatest alteration in the internal immune system is the involution (decrease in size) of the thymus gland (Felser & Raff, 1983; W. Smith, 1982; Weksler, 1981). This change is suspected to influence the function of the immune system, but it is still to early to determine the full range of implications this may have on the health of older individuals. However, in contrast to Kane et al. (1989) Weksler notes that some impairment of the immune response makes older individuals more susceptible to infection.

DISEASE PROCESSES

Some of the more prevalent diseases or disruptions that affect either of the body's defense mechanisms will be discussed here. (Tuberculosis and pneumonia have already been dealt with in greater detail in previous sections).

Facility Responses to the Presence of Infections: The Infection Control Program

The federal requirements in the Medicare program call for nursing facilities to establish infection control programs to monitor facility performance in this area. The Department of Labor has issued universal precautions required of all facilities.

Depending on the nature of the infection, various isolation precautions need to be taken to protect other residents/patients, staff, and visitors from acquiring the infection as well. The administrator must also make sure that residents with certain communicable diseases are reported to the state health department. Each state, in cooperation with the United States Public Health Service, specifies diseases that must be reported to the state health department.

Infections complicate the older residents' disease status and may even increase their chance of death (mortality). Besides this risk, infections may increase the likelihood that a resident will need to be transferred to a hospital for more intensive care (Irvine, Van Buren, & Crossley, 1984).

Risk Control, Infection Control, and the Infection Control Practitioner (ICP)

The risk of an epidemic is always present in the nursing facility. An epidemic is a cluster of infections involving multiple individuals. Nursing home epidemics include influenza, staph skin infections, antibiotic-resistant bacteria, infectious diarrhea, scabies, and tuberculosis (Smith, 1989). A survey of Nebraska nursing homes found more than 50% of the facilities experienced an epidemic in the previous year involving an average of 35 residents and 14 employees. Influenza was the most common cause (Smith, 1989). Carefully following of the Department of Labor's universal precautions bloodborne pathogens will do much to reduce epidemics. Along with federal and state requirements, each facility is expected to individualize and enforce its own infection control policies coordinated by a trained part-time or full-time infection control practitioner (ICP) (Bryant & Tuttle, 1989; Satterfield, 1989).

Skin Disease

One of the diseases that primarily affects older individuals is herpes zoster, more commonly known as shingles (Evans et al., 2000). This infection is caused by the herpes varicella virus (not to be confused with herpes simplex) which travels along nerve pathways to infect skin cells (Becker, 1979). The skin covering the chest region and areas surrounding the eye are among the areas more commonly infected by this disease. Residents who suffer from a debilitating disease such as cancer are also at greater risk of developing this infection.

Signs and symptoms include itching (usually preceding a rash) reddened areas of the skin (usually along a nerve pathway), vesicles (fluid-filled pimples) often erupting over reddened areas, and burning accompanied by stabbing pain.

At present there is no cure for this form of herpes infection, so **treatment** consists of attempts to alleviate the associated symptoms rather than effect a cure. Steroids are often used to reduce inflammation, which may shorten the length of the infection and provide comfort. Antibiotics are sometimes prescribed to prevent secondary infections, and analgesics to relieve pain (Beacham, 1989).

Decubitus Ulcers

Pressure sores is the federal government's preferred term for these infections known also as bedsores, decubitus ulcers, and stasis ulcers (ulcers resulting from tissue death due to reduced blood flow), all terms for the same process—tissue breakdown (Bergstrom, 1995). Stasis ulcers are the sores that result from extremely poor peripheral circulation or peripheral vascular disease (Evans et al., 2000; Garagusi, 1989).

Tissue breakdown often occurs over a bony prominence (buttocks, elbow, heel, hip, shoulder). These ulcers do not develop from an infection, but rather from some form of constant unrelieved pressure on one area of the body.

With all of these ulcers, the end result is the same: Tissues do not receive an adequate amount of oxygen, so they break down and begin to die. This process is similar to what happens to the heart muscle in coronary artery disease.

Residents at most risk for developing these ulcers are those chronically immobile (paralyzed) because of a stroke or some other incapacitating illness and those experiencing poor nutritional status, constant pain, incontinence, or dementia (Husain, 1953). These ulcers often enlarge to form cavities of dead tissue prone to the development of infection and once enlarged, are more difficult to heal (Kart et al., 1978).

Decubitus Ulcer Formation. The formation of an ulcer usually occurs when the weight of the body exerts pressure on internal soft tissues by compressing them between skeletal bone and another hard surface (Evans et al., 2000). Residents/patients who are immobilized or unable to move by themselves are particularly at risk for developing pressure sores. Because these patients cannot change position frequently on their own, there is the danger of continuous pressure on one area of the body.

Many of these residents/patients spend much of their time lying on their backs, also knows as the decubitus (lying down) position. When this occurs, the areas most likely to develop sores are the buttocks, hips, heels, shoulders, ears, and elbows. Similarly, residents who spend long periods sitting up in a chair without moving are also at risk of developing these sores.

The signs and symptoms of decubitus ulcers include tingling, pale skin color, or other signs that there is a loss of circulation to an area; reddened area of skin over a bony prominence; a sore that will not heal; edema (swelling) of the lower legs; and shiny skin.

However, these signs are often difficult to recognize before tissue has already died and the ulcer itself has already developed (Evans et al., 2000; Rowe & Besdine, 1982).

Pressure sores are typically classed as Grade I, I, III, and IV.

Grade I: acute inflammatory response, often over a bony prominence; skin red, but unbroken
Grade II: extension of the acute inflammatory response through the dermis to subcutaneous fat
Grade III: extension though fat to deep fascia, base of ulcer infected
Grade IV: deep ulceration reaching the bone (Kane et al., 1989).

The following are some of the treatments the facility may use:

- Providing special equipment, such as an air mattress.
- Keeping the resident/patient clean and dry.
- Eliminating the source of pressure.
- Working to improve the resident/patient's circulation.
- Ensuring frequent position change (at least every 2 hours) for those who are unable or unlikely to do so themselves.
- Padding feet, elbows, and other areas at high risk of tissue breakdown (e.g., using "bunny boots" on the feet).
- Frequently assessing the integrity of a resident/patient's skin.
- Changing diet to include foods higher in protein, vitamin C, and calorie content to promote healing.
- Preventing infection by applying dressings and dispensing antibiotic medications as prescribed.
- Using elastic stockings or Ace wrap bandages, which are often prescribed for the person with peripheral vascular insufficiency (poor blood circulation in their arms and legs)..
- Other: A number of experimental treatments are constantly being offered to nursing facilities, such as the use of a hypobaric chamber which facilitates the flow of oxygen to injured areas.

Both pressure sores and stasis ulcers are significant disruptions of the skin's protective barrier defense. A study by Garibaldi et al. (1981) concluded that 32% of infections originated from this source. One of the most severe types of infections that may result is called sepsis, a condition in which the circulating bloodstream carries infectious organisms throughout the body.

Residents Most at Risk

Residents who are bedfast or chair-bound for long periods of time are at high risk of developing pressure sores.

Figure 5-9 reveals that from the years 1993 to 1999, nearly half of all residents were chair-bound. This includes residents who were in a bed or recliner for 22 or more hours per day in the week before the federal survey. The percentage of bedfast residents increased from 5% of residents in 1993 to 7% of residents in 1999. The average percent of bedfast residents ranged from 2% in North Dakota to 16% in Hawaii in 1999. Even a slight increase in the number of such residents increases the nursing load carried by a facility.

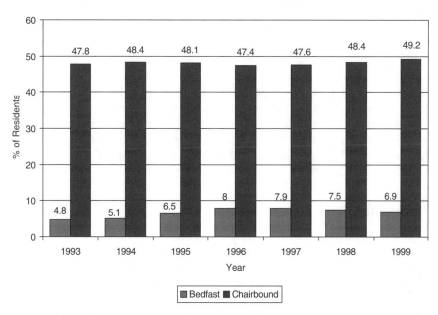

FIGURE 5-9. Percentage of residents in U.S. nursing homes who are bedfast or chairbound, 1993–1999.
Nursing Facilities, Staffing, Residents and Facility Deficiencies, 1993–1999, Department of Social & Behavioral Sciences, University of California San Francisco.

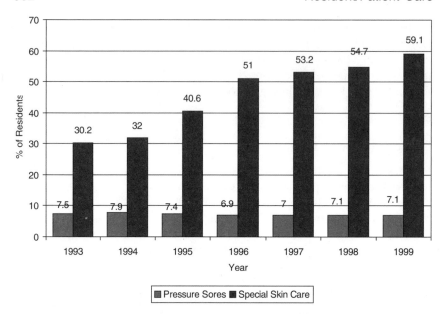

FIGURE 5-10. Percentage of residents with pressure sores and receiving special skin care in U.S. nursing homes, 1993–1999.
Nursing Facilities, Staffing, Residents and Facility Deficiencies, 1993–1999, Department of Social & Behavioral Sciences, University of California San Francisco.

A number of residents depend on a chair for mobility or are unable to walk without extensive or constant support from others. Figure 5-10 shows that the percentage of total residents who were chairbound was nearly 50% in the years 1993 to 1999. The percent who were chairbound ranged from 35% in Rhode Island to 52% in Washington in 1999 (Harrington et al., 2000).

Nonroutine Skin Care

Figure 5-10 reveals some headway in reducing the number of residents with pressure sores, dropping from 7.5% of residents in 1991 to 7.1% in 1999. This reduction in pressure sores may be due to the consistent increase of residents receiving special skin care from 30% in 1993 to 60% in 1999. Special skin care is nonroutine care according to a resident care plan or physician's order, usually designed to prevent or reduce pressure ulcers of the skin.

Facilities must ensure that residents without pressure sores do not develop them if avoidable. In both 1993 and 1999, about 18% of facilities received deficiencies for failing to meet this nursing care challenge.

The deficiency rate dropped during 1994 to 1996, but began rising in 1997 (Harrington et al., 2000).

Attention of the Administrator. The *in-house acquired preventable decubitus ulcer rate* is one of the three or four yardsticks by which the quality of the care given in the facility is judged. Good nursing care is the best form of overall treatment. One of the administrator's roles is to ensure that evaluation and screening is routinely done for residents at high risk for developing these ulcers. Approximately two thirds of these ulcers develop within the first weeks that a patient is institutionalized.

The Department of Health and Human Services' Agency for Health Care Policy and Research has developed clinical practice guidelines for the management of pressure sores (Agency for health Care Policy and Research [AHCPR], 1995).

Hypothermia

Hypothermia (low body temperature) is an issue of special concern to nursing home staff. Usually, the body temperature is maintained between 97° and 99° F. Patients in a nursing home facility may be endangered by subtle changes in temperature (Collins et al., 1977). The older resident often may have less insulation from body fat, increasing the risk of hypothermia.

Hypothermia is the sudden appearance of a low body temperature (less than 95°). Often it is difficult to diagnose hypothermia because symptoms may be similar to those of a minor stroke.

When the body temperature drops below 95°, residents are no longer able to feel cold and may be suffering from confusion, so they are often unable to complain of other symptoms, such as skin that is pale, dry, and cool with low pulse or blood pressure.

Many complications may result from hypothermia, including dehydration, renal failure (Evans et al., 2000), pneumonia, or cardiac arrhythmias (Evans et al., 2000). Treatment is aimed at slowly rewarming the patient back to a normal body temperature, usually with blankets. Residents with multiple chronic diseases may not survive an episode of hypothermia.

Because of the threat of hypothermia, loss of heat in the nursing facility can be a life-threatening situation for the resident/patients.

Cancer

Cancer is actually a group of chronic diseases that affect different areas of the body (Birchenall & Streight, 1982). Approximately 5% of nursing home residents suffer from some form of cancer. Cancer is discussed here as a disorder of the immune system because cancer cells act as antigens and are known to attack many organs or cells throughout the body.

The growth of cancer cells is markedly different from that of normal cells. They grow much more rapidly and are often released or break out from their initial area of growth (tumor) and travel into the bloodstream or lymphatic channels and then throughout the body. Damage may result either from this rapid cell growth, depletion of normal cell food supply, or from actual expansion and crushing of the organ affected.

Another mode for cancer growth occurs when cancerous cells travel from the initial growth to new sites, forming metastases or other cancer sites throughout the body. Metastasis is the transfer of disease from one organ or part of the body to another not directly connected with it, due either to transfer of pathogenic microorganisms or transfer of cells.

The cause of cancer is still unknown, but among the different factors believed to play possible roles in this disease are environmental exposure to harmful substances, chronic chemical or biologic irritation (drugs, alcohol, smoking, viral infections, radiation), inherited genetic predisposition to the disease, dietary (Beattie & Louie, 1989) and even behavioral factors.

It has been suggested that some combination of these factors probably best explains the cause of cancer (Fraumeni, 1979). Often these factors may expose the body to a substance known as a carcinogen, which alters the body's immune response capabilities and allows these substances to enter the body and promote the growth of cancerous cells.

According to Birchenall & Streight (1982), the leading types of cancer seen in nursing facility residents, listed in order of prevalence by gender, are as follows:

Males—lung, colon, rectum, and prostate
Females—breast, colon, rectum, and lung

Variations in Cancer Treatments. Physicians may choose to manage cancer patients with different forms of treatments, depending on the specifics of the disease. Surgery, radiation, and the use of chemical therapy are the three most common forms of cancer treatment. There are more than 250 different kinds of cancer; forms of treatment will vary for individual patients according to the severity of their illness.

Problems Associated with Cancer Treatments. There are many problems associated with cancer treatment. The patient with colon cancer may have undergone surgery to remove the diseased portion of the bowel. If a large enough area has been removed, then the patient will usually also have a colostomy, which is an opening on the abdomen where the end of the bowel is brought to the surface and digestive waste materials are collected in a bag attached to an appliance surrounding the site. Depending on the level of independence, residents with colostomies may require additional assistance with this special type of elimination process.

The two other types of cancer treatment (radiation and chemotherapy) may be quite painful for residents because of their associated side effects. One of these is anorexia (continual lack of appetite). When this persists, physicians may prescribe special high-calorie food supplements to maintain the patient's strength and energy, as well as treatments for pain and nausea.

5.3.7 Musculoskeletal System

The muscles and skeleton working together provide two important functions: (a) a supporting framework for all of the other body structures, and (b) mobility, which is closely related to the nursing facility resident's degree of independence and autonomy (Hofland, 1995; Maddox, 2001).

COMPONENTS OF THE SYSTEM

The Skeleton and Muscles

One of the basic elements of the supporting framework of the body is the skeleton, which is composed of the many bones that meet to form joints. The muscles are attached to the skeleton. The skeleton also protects soft tissues and organs inside the body. This framework dictates an individual's posture, directly affecting personal appearance.

Joints

In the body there are 68 joints, which are the points where the ends of two bones meet. These joint bones are covered by cartilage and surrounded by a capsule containing fluid that lubricates the area to enhance movement. The joint is held in place by ligaments.

MOVEMENT

In order for movement to occur, the muscles must first receive a nerve impulse from the brain directing them to contract, then relax. Because the muscles are attached to the bones, when they move, the bone moves also. The joints respond like mechanical levers to assist in completing this movement. Thus, mobility requires coordination between both the nervous and musculoskeletal systems.

POSSIBLE EFFECTS OF AGING

The individual bones contain an inner component—bone marrow—that produces the red blood cells. The remainder of bone consists of a network of fibrous tissue containing salts, which are primarily minerals, such as calcium, that serve to harden and strengthen the bone (Hayflick, 1995).

There is some consensus that during the aging process the total amount of bone in the body is decreased. However, to determine the loss one needs to have measured the amount of bone the individual had at age 35 (Heaney, 1982).

Higher Risk for Women

Women are at a high risk of experiencing some degree of bone loss following menopause (Evans et al., 2000). It has been established that this loss results from the depletion of estrogen, which apparently helps promote the body's use of dietary calcium for the purpose of bone growth (Evans et al., 2000; Heaney, 1982).

When bone loss occurs, some of the observable changes are shortened stature and a slumped posture due to a compression of the vertebrae (bones in the spine) and the cartilage discs between them (Grob, 1983).

Often, because of these changes, older individuals become stooped and appear to have a hump back. They are also more likely to fracture one of their bones (Glowacki, 1989).

Although a certain amount of bone loss is associated with aging, much of it in older individuals is a result of osteoporosis (Evans et al., 2000). There is considerable controversy over the extent to which these changes in the bone can be attributed to normal aging rather than to osteoporosis, which will be described further on.

Both muscles and bones are made up of connective tissue and collagen (Maddox, 2001). Similar to the collagen-related changes associated with age, muscles also become less elastic as a result of this same process. The most significant age-related muscle change for older persons is a decrease in the amount of muscle throughout the body. In addition, degenerative changes in the nervous system may disturb impulses, decreasing muscle skills. However, it is unclear to what extent, if any, these changes in bone and muscle size and strength are related to age, rather than to the possible effects of decreased activity (Weg, 1983).

DISEASE PROCESSES

The discussion of age-related changes in the musculoskeletal system reflects the considerable uncertainty as to whether the changes in bones are a manifestation of the aging process or a distinct disease process (V. Barzel, 1983).

The term *rheumatism* has often been used by older persons to describe any painful disorder of the muscles, joints, and their surrounding areas (Agate, 1975). Following is a discussion of some of the common disruptions of musculoskeletal functioning as experienced in the nursing home population.

Osteoporosis

Osteoporosis has already been described as a condition of decreased skeletal mass without alteration of any chemical components of bone (Rossman, 1979). Thus, while there may be less total amount of bone, the components of bone are still present in necessary proportions.

The cause of osteoporosis remains unclear, but the mechanism of bone loss apparently is through increased reabsorption of bone tissue by the body. Osteoporosis may result from prolonged use of medication, immobility, or some other underlying disease (Spencer, 1979).

Symptoms of osteoporosis include bone pain, often in the lower back, recurrent bone fractures, and frequent falls and related injuries.

Treatment can include managing the symptoms of pain, treating complications such as fractures, rehabilitation to correct physical inactivity, and increasing protein and vitamin intake. Medications often used are calcium supplements and hormones, usually estrogen, to improve the body's ability to absorb calcium.

Simply taking extra calcium without estrogen replacement appears to be dramatically less effective, according to Glowacki, who also believes that reports of estrogen replacement therapy causing endometrial (inner lining of the uterine wall) cancer are exaggerated. There is no evidence, he asserts, that estrogen replacement therapy causes breast cancer (Glowacki, 1989).

Arthritis

Arthritis is an inflammation of a joint (Evans; Evans et al., 2000; Maddox, 2001). Nearly 25% of nursing home residents suffer from some form of this disease. There are many different types of arthritis, and two that commonly afflict nursing home residents are listed below.

Osteoarthritis. This is the most prevalent form, also called degenerative joint disease. As the disease progresses, the cartilage and other components of the joint begin to wear away or degenerate (Evans et al., 2000). The joints that bear most of the weight on a continual basis are most commonly affected, including the knee, hips, and ankles.

Symptoms include aching pain in the affected joint, most often a backache, and decreased mobility because the pain becomes worse following exercise.

Treatment consists of relieving symptoms. Use of an anti-inflammatory agent such as enteric-coated aspirin is usually recommended (Kane et al., 1989). Continual degeneration of the hip joint may require a surgical replacement if the patient still has good walking skills.

Rheumatoid Arthritis. This is a much more serious form of arthritis. It can affect any age group. This is considered an autoimmune disease (Heidrick, 1995) because it is thought the body begins to attack its own cells in the joint, causing an inflammatory reaction.

Signs and symptoms include

- symmetric inflammation of joints on both sides of the body
- frequent flare-ups and remissions of pain
- stiffness and joint swelling, usually in the hands
- pain, often occurring in the morning hours and decreasing with exercise

Treatments include

- a balance of rest and exercise
- physical therapy
- heat and cold applications
- whirlpool baths
- medications, including aspirin, to decrease the inflammation and analgesics, to relieve the pain

FALLS

More than 70% of deaths that result from all falls occur among persons over 65 years of age. Falling is a major cause of disability and death in older individuals and may be due to factors such as chronic illness or orthostatic hypotension (decreased blood pressure upon standing) (Evans et al., 2000; Kennie & Warshaw, 1989; Kippenbrock & Soja, 1993; "Putting an End," 1994; Tideiksaar, 1995). This phenomenon is sometimes associated with reduced blood pressure among residents after eating, known as postprandial hypotension (Evans et al., 2000, 119).

Patients in the facility dining room who have just finished a large meal are especially vulnerable. It appears that the blood supply is being routed to the digestive system (H. J. Cohen, 1995), causing even lower blood pressure when the resident stands up from the meal.

Osteoporosis, gait disorders (Evans et al., 2000,p. 825), and decreased blood supply to the brain (Rodstein, 1983) may also be found in the typical nursing home resident, leaving them more prone to falls than the noninstitutionalized older population (Evans et al., 2000, 93).

It is estimated that due to privacy in rooms, only 25% of falls in institutions are witnessed and that 25% to 50% of residents fall each year. Eighty percent of all individuals falling are 75 or older.

The facility environment can often be unsafe (Kane et al., 1989). An emphasized and smoothly running risk management program focusing on incident reports can identify changes needed in the facility environment to reduce falls.

FRACTURES

Frequently, when facility residents fall, they fracture one of their bones. Often this is in either the spine or the hip. When a nursing home resident fractures the hip, two treatment approaches are used.

One is to place the resident on bed rest. Lyon and Nevins (1984) suggest that this conservative form of treatment is safer and less likely to lead to further mental decline or other complications. The other approach is for the resident to have surgery to repair the hip. Often the patient is provided with an artificial prosthesis. Gordon (1989) argues for definitive treatment within the first 24 to 72 hours, early ambulation with physical therapy.

The danger of hip fracture increases dramatically with age: In women ages 75 to 79 the incidence of hip fracture is 6 of 1,000 falls; for those 85 to 89 the incidence of hip fracture rises to 48.6 per 1,000 falls (Maddox, 2001; Pousada, 1995).

AMPUTEES

Amputees are another group of nursing facility residents who need special assistance when walking.

Three fourths of all amputations are performed on patients 65 years of age and older (Vallarino & Sherman, 1981). The most common type of amputation is the removal of the leg either above or below the knee (abbreviated as AKA or BKA). An amputation is the treatment of last resort for residents with a severe infection, peripheral vascular disease, or injury that is often related to diabetes. Many devices are available to restore lost function. In the absence of suitable prosthetic devices, the environment can be changed to accommodate to the resident's skills (Redford, 1989).

CONTRACTURES

Often patients with chronic rheumatoid arthritis develop contractures in their hands. Contractures are a deformity that result when the muscle has shortened and pulls the adjacent joint into a flexed position. After a period of time the joint becomes fixed in this position and results in a permanent deformity in which the joint cannot be straightened. Contractures are another disruption likely to occur in the immobilized resident.

Other joints that are likely to develop contractures, besides those in the hand and wrist, include the foot, hips, and legs.

The best form of treatment for contractures is to help prevent them by exercising the joints of those who are unable to do so for themselves. These are called passive range-of-motion exercises and can be taught to the resident's family. Proper positioning in bed helps prevent the development of these contractures. Special devices and splints are available for that purpose.

REHABILITATION SERVICES

Rehabilitation services are provided under the direction of a rehabilitation professional (usually a physical therapist, occupational therapist, or speech therapist) to improve functioning. The rate at which residents received these services declined slightly from 19% in 1993 to 16% in 1999. These services varied from 7% of residents in South Dakota facilities to 38% in Alaska (Harrington et al., 2000).

Limited Range of Motion Services

Residents with limited range of motion must receive appropriate treatment and services to increase their range and to prevent declines in range of motion. Through the years 1993—1999 between 8% and 9% of facilities received deficiencies for failure to provide sufficient range of motion therapies.

5.3.8 Genitourinary (Renal) System

The renal system consists of the two kidneys, which filter wastes from the blood, and two ureters, which transmit the filtered materials (urine) from the kidneys to the bladder, where the urine is stored until discharged through the urethra (Malone-Lee, 1995).

In addition to removing waste materials from the bloodstream, the kidneys also help regulate the amount of fluids in the body. At the same time, the kidneys also monitor the level of important electrolytes including sodium (Na), potassium (K+) and calcium (Ca+++).

Channels within the kidney filter the blood and collect a concentration of waste products and excess fluids. The newly filtered blood supply is returned to the general circulation by the renal vein and the concentration of waste materials or urine travels from within the kidney to the bladder by connecting tubes (ureters).

The bladder is a balloonlike muscular structure that serves as a holding tank for the continuous stream of urine produced by the kidneys. When a sufficient amount of urine has collected in the bladder, signals are sent to the brain identifying the need to urinate.

Individuals have voluntary control over the bladder in responding to this need to urinate. A nerve impulse sent back to the bladder signals it to contract and expel urine through the urethra, at which point it leaves the body. See Figure 5-11 for an illustration of the location of the renal system for both men and women.

EFFECTS OF AGING ON THE RENAL SYSTEM

According to some studies, the average 80-year-old adult has approximately one half of the renal function of a normal 30-year-old (Evans et al., 2000; Lindeman, 1989).

Because the kidneys are so closely associated with the circulatory system, age-associated atherosclerotic (hardening) changes in blood vessels can also affect the kidney. Because of the location of the renal organs, age-related changes in the reproductive organs also influence their ability to function. A diagram of the urinary system is presented in Figure 5-11.

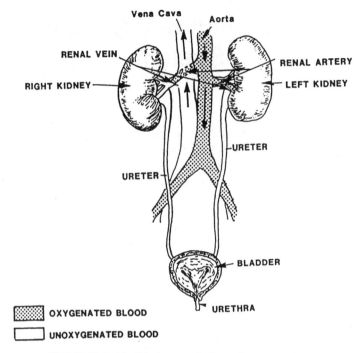

FIGURE 5-11. Diagram of the urinary system.

Studies have shown that the ability of the kidneys to concentrate urine probably decreases with age (McLachlan, 1978). A progressive loss of renal mass (size) is also believed to occur (Rowe, 1982). However, these changes have not been associated with an overall decline of kidney function. Because the bladder is a muscle, its capacity to hold large amounts of urine also seems to decrease with age.

Alterations in Renal Function

Disruptions in renal function may be caused by problems in an associated system or systems, such as arteriosclerotic changes in blood vessels and changes in body nutrients, as in diabetes, leading to renal failure.

A disruption may also be due to a malfunction of the kidney itself or to some type of internal blockage within the kidney and ureters, as with kidney stones or tumors. Approximately 10% of nursing home residents are estimated to have kidney problems.

Chronic Renal Failure

Renal failure is the inability of the kidney to filter out body waste products. This can be either an acute (short-term) or more likely, a chronic (long-term) process.

Chronic renal failure may be caused by cardiovascular changes leading to a decreasing amount of blood being filtered through the kidneys. This decrease in blood flow can result in permanent damage to some of the kidney's internal filtering mechanisms (nephrons) that require continual use for optimal functioning. The most obvious physical sign of renal failure is uremia (a decrease in urine output), which may progressively lead to oliguria (no urine output).

The **symptoms** of chronic renal failure, much like the disease itself, develop gradually. Some of the initial symptoms include dehydration, electrolyte imbalance, osteoporosis, nocturia (producing much urine at night), and anemia.

When little or no urine is produced by the body, toxic waste materials may build up, which could damage other organs and cause painful symptoms, including itching and dry skin, mental confusion, weakness, muscle cramps, nausea, vomiting, and diarrhea. Older individuals are particularly prone to developing end-stage renal disease and are the largest group entering kidney dialysis programs (Faubert, Shapiro, Porush, & Kahn, 1989).

End-Stage Renal Disease

Chronic renal failure that has progressed to the stage where little or no urine is being produced is called end-stage renal disease (ESRD). The two most common forms of treatment are kidney transplantation and dialysis (Maddox, 2001).

Kidney dialysis (hemodialysis, i.e., filtering the blood) requires special equipment that performs much like the kidney in filtering unwanted waste materials and fluids from the blood. The process is usually performed in special clinics and takes several hours. The patient's blood is circulated externally through a small machine that filters the blood in much the same fashion as the kidney itself. Feinstein and Friedman (1979) report that since its inception hemodialysis has been successful when used for older patients.

Renal Calculi

Kidney stones, or renal calculi, are formed in the kidney as a result of an imbalance in body chemistry. These stones are hard, crystalline, stone-

like substances that become a problem when they block urine flow out
of the kidney or block any other area of the renal system.

The group of residents most at risk for developing kidney stones are
those unable to move or who are on chronic bed rest. (In the previous
section we discussed how these residents are likely to suffer from increased osteoporosis.) The extra calcium that the body absorbs may also
form kidney stones when enough of this mineral is filtered.

Symptoms are blood in urine, decrease in urine outflow, and pain in
the back or side. **Treatment** consists of relieving pain symptoms and
medications to relax ureters, allowing the stones to pass. If retrieved, the
stones are analyzed to determine their composition and the necessity for
any further treatment. In recent years, the need for surgical removal of
kidney stones has been greatly reduced by the use of a machine called a
lithotripter that bombards and breaks the kidney stones into small fragments
by directing electrical shock waves that pass harmlessly through body tissue.

Urinary Incontinence

Urinary incontinence is the inability to control the timing of urination.
Bladder or urinary incontinence more often than one time a week is a
common problem in nursing facility residents (Harrington et al., 2000).
There are many reasons why a resident may become incontinent, including neurologic damage, chronic constipation, and impactions. A defect
in the nervous system (stroke patients who lose nervous control of the
bladder), urinary tract infections, constant pressure on the bladder from
other disorders such as constipation all may cause incontinence (Evans
et al., 2000; Kane et al., 1989).

Figure 5-12 indicate that a persistent half of all residents have bladder
incontinence. The percentage ranged from 38% in West Virginia to 67%
in Washington, D.C. (Harrington et al., 2000).

Problems in mobility that prevent the resident from reaching the toilet
in time may also lead to incontinence (Keegan & McNichols, 1982;
Williams & Fitzhugh, 1982). The nursing staff must be prompt in assisting the resident to the bathroom on a regular schedule. The resident is
more able to empty the bladder if placed on the commode.

Bladder retraining is used to assist the resident in using the bathroom
at appropriate times. There are several types of bladder retraining programs (Kane et al., 1989). Once assurance has been obtained that there
is no impaction, the nurses monitor the amount of fluid consumed by the
resident and assist the patient in using the toilet about 2 hours after-
wards. A persistent 5 to 6% of all residents were in a bladder training
program during the years 1993—1999 (Harrington et al., 2000).

Residents who are unable to void are catheterized. Urine is released
intermittently about every 2 hours following fluid intake. Special devices

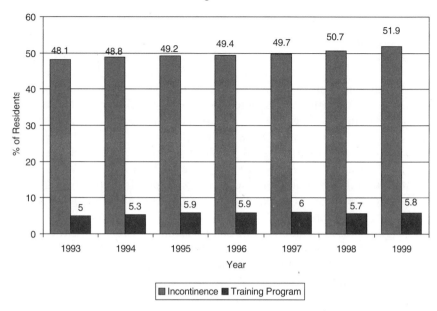

FIGURE 5-12. Percentage of residents in U.S. nursing homes with bladder incontinence and in training program, 1993–1999.
Nursing Facilities, Staffing, Residents and Facility Deficiencies, 1993–1999, Department of Social & Behavioral Sciences, University of California San Francisco.

are also used to assist the resident in voiding (urinating). These include bedpans, urinals for men, and bedside commodes for the resident who can get up out of bed.

If none of these treatments is successful, some type of drainage system can be ordered for the resident. Men may use either a condomlike or an indwelling type of catheter. Women may use only the indwelling catheter, which is inserted into the urethra and threaded up into the bladder. Urine flows out of the bladder and through the catheter. It is then collected in a clear plastic drainage bag. This is a closed system used to attempt to control the introduction of bacteria or other harmful microorganisms into the urinary tract, but it is a last choice because urinary tract infections are associated with this approach (Kane et al., 1989; Maddox, 2001).

Urinary Tract Infections

According to Kurtz (1982), of all age groups older persons most frequently have urinary tract infections (UTI) and associated illnesses. Together, urinary tract infections and pneumonia were found to be responsible for more than half of all infections in a chronic-care facility studied (Evans et al., 2000; Farber et al., 1982). Sterile catheter insertions tend to become infected within 3 weeks regardless of preventive efforts (Evans et al., 2000).

Infection from urinary catheters is, therefore, usually impossible to prevent. The bladder is usually sterile. Urinary tract infections are the most common form of catheter-related infections and account for 30% of all nosocomial infections. The female rate of urinary tract infections is higher than the male rate because pathogenic organisms traveling up the outside of the catheter have a shorter distance to travel in women (2") compared to men (6" to 8"). When urinary catheters are used for extended periods of time, the risk for acute UTI complicated by pyelonephritis (inflammation of the kidney) occurs. Sepsis from pyelonephritis is a major cause of death in patients with long indwelling catheters.

The most commonly associated causes of UTI, as identified by Bjork and Tight (1983), include lack of hand washing between patient contacts (an example of poor infection control practices by staff), close proximity of residents with catheters, and the prevalence of residents who have indwelling urinary catheters. Other causes, such as poor insertion techniques and poor positioning of drainage bags, have been identified as causes of infection.

Indwelling Catheter Rates

Indwelling catheters are tubes used to drain the bladder. In 1993, about 8% of facility residents were catherized, declining to 7% in 1999 (Harrington et al., 2000). There has been a constant push to reduce the number of residents with indwelling catheters.

Residents with urinary catheters often show no symptoms associated with the initial stages of this infection. Residents who do not have indwelling catheters may complain of **symptoms**, including burning and painful urination, cloudy and foul-smelling urine, fever, and chills (Garagusi, 1989). The indwelling catheter should be cleaned daily with soap and water where it enters the urethra and the catheter itself changed aseptically every month (Garagusi, 1989).

An initial form of **treatment** is to obtain a sample of urine that may be studied to determine the organisms present. Antibiotic therapy is usually held off for as long as possible. There is only a limited number of antibiotics available to treat UTI, and residents with chronic indwelling catheters are likely to become resistant to these antibiotics quickly, at which point there is little alternative treatment available. As many as 50% of urinary tract infections are recurrent.

A frequently encountered nursing facility problem is that many older women have asymptomatic bacteriuria (Evans et al., 2000). Treatment protocols may indicate a constant need for treatment in these cases. However, chronic suppressive antibiotic administration to these residents can be counterproductive because it can lead to development of antibiotic-resistant organisms, which results in a superinfection (Garagusi, 1989).

In an effort to avoid overuse of antibiotics, a new trend among geriatric physicians is to treat UTI only if it is symptomatic (that is, burning discomfort or pain), not treating when the culture is positive but the patient is asympotomatic.

UTI is an ongoing treatment challenge in the nursing facility, and new approaches are constantly being sought. Practical experience suggests that no matter how careful or sterile the procedures, infection often spreads, not on the inside but along the outside of the inserted tube. Despite every staff effort, an incontinent female patient may be at risk of infection within minutes after incontinence occurs.

Facilities have been cited at about the rate of 11% of facilities for the years 1993 to 1999 for improper bladder care (Harrington et al., 2000).

Bowel Incontinence Rates

Bowel incontinence more often than one time a week is also a common problem among nursing facility residents. Over the years 1993 through 1999, a persistent 42% of all residents were affected by bowel incontinence (Harrington et al., 2000). About 4% of residents were in a bowel-training program.

Ostomy Care Rate

Ostomy care includes special care for a skin opening to the intestine and/or urinary tract such as a colostomy (opening to the colon). Ostomy care was provided to between 2% and 3% of residents during the years 1993 to 1999 (Harrington, 2000).

5.3.9 Reproductive System

The reproductive system in the younger adult has the potential to promote the creation of new life and facilitate the expression of intimacy through human contact. Some of the most notable changes in older persons include the woman's loss of reproductive capabilities following menopause (cessation of menses), whereas a man retains his reproductive capabilities. However, both have a continuing need to express their sexuality throughout the life span (Wallace, 1992).

The first part of this section is a description of the reproductive organs and age-associated changes for each sex; the second is a discussion of sexuality and the nursing home resident.

WOMEN

The reproductive organs in women include the ovaries, which produce eggs that travel down the fallopian tubes to the uterus about once every month. Hormones act to control these reproductive cycles. Estrogen is the female sex hormone that directs most of these processes.

The organs of the lower reproductive tract are the cervix, the uterus, and the vagina. The cervix is the opening of the uterus leading into the vagina. The vagina is a barrel-shaped organ that leads to the external genitals in the female reproductive tract, the labia and the clitoris. During midlife most women go through menopause (cessation of egg production and therefore of menstruation) and are no longer fertile.

Diseases of the uterus tend to decrease with age (Rossman, 1979). Changes in the reproductive system are closely related to decreases in secretions of the hormone estrogen.

Some of the physical changes that may be experienced by older women include a loss of tone and elasticity in the breast, uterus, cervix, and vagina; a thinning and drying of the vaginal walls, which may cause uncomfortable irritations; infections and bleeding; decrease in size of the uterus, fallopian tubes, and vagina (U.S. Barzel, 1989); loss of pubic hair; and decrease in the number of ducts or milk glands of the breasts (Butler & Lewis, 1977; Goldfarb, 1979; Kart et al., 1978; Kay & Neeley; Kenney & Kenny, 1982; Stilwell & O'Conner, 1989).

Older women do not tend to suffer from diseases of the uterus or reproductive tract per se (Rossman, 1979). However, the incidence of breast cancer does continue to rise with age, and it remains the most common type of cancer affecting older women. The **signs and symptoms** of breast cancer are a hardened lump or thickening in the breast or change in size of the breast and the nipples. **Treatment** depends of the extent of the disease and may include surgery, radiation, or chemotherapy, as well as the relief of associated symptoms.

Another age-related change is genital prolapse. This occurs when the tone of the genital organs becomes so weakened that they begin to drop and may seem to fall out of the vagina. Women with weak muscles are at risk. Some of the **signs and symptoms** associated with genital prolapse include constant pressure on the bladder, incontinence of urine, and a sense of weight in the pelvis. Usually this disorder can be repaired surgically.

A decrease in the production of the female sex hormone estrogen may also lead to osteoporosis (discussed in the section on the musculoskeletal system). With the exception of arthritis, the rate of chronic disease among women is about equal to the rates of men (Evans et al., 2000).

MEN

The primary organs of the male reproductive tract are the testes, scrotum, prostate, and penis.

The testes are encased within the scrotum and produce the male hormone testosterone and sperm cells. These cells mature as they travel through the surrounding epididymis until released into the vas deferens. The sperm travel through the vas deferens until they are released from the ejaculatory ducts into the urethra. Nearby ducts secrete seminal fluid from the prostate gland, which provides food for the sperm as well as enhancing their motility. When the male ejaculates, the sperm travel down the urethra through the penis and are emitted from the body (Maddox, 2001).

Some of the age-related changes in the male reproductive tract are an enlargement of the prostate gland, decreased production of testosterone, which may result in slight decreases in sexual desire, and a reduction in muscle bulk and strength. Sperm production, and therefore the ability to procreate, continues into advanced old age (Barzel, 1982; Kay & Neeley, 1982).

Problems with the prostate gland are a major concern for many older men (Kart et al., 1978). Enlargement of the prostate is a common age-related change in men (Kart et al., 1978; Reichel, 1983; Rossman, 1979). For some men, this enlargement may interfere with the ability to urinate or may cause incontinence (Maddox, 2001). Prostatitis is an inflammation of this gland that often develops following the initial enlargement of the prostate gland and can be very painful. Other **symptoms** include painful urination and blood in the urine.

This enlargement may develop into cancer of the prostate, which is the second most common form of cancer in older men. Cancer of the prostate is considered a "geriatric disease," with 95% of all cases seen in older men (Breschi, 1983; Rowe, 1982). The initial **symptoms** for this disease are the same as those experienced with prostatitis, including a decrease in urination and discomfort. A combination of surgery and radiation is often used to treat the cancerous or extremely large prostate. Chemotherapy or hormone treatments may also be used.

COPING WITH SEXUALITY

Sexual needs persist into old age, with continued activity considered healthy and health-preserving (Griggs, 1978; Snowden, 1983). The older nursing home resident, like those in the community, continues to have needs for a positive self-image and self-esteem (Maddox, 2001), which are closely associated with the needs for intimacy and sexuality (Butler, 1975; Griggs, 1978). Too often, society and individuals discourage sexual activity in the nursing home because of existing stereotypes and misunderstandings about sex and old age (Huntley, 1979; Wasow & Loeb, 1979).

Sexuality is not achieved exclusively by sexual intercourse, but may also incorporate a variety of activities related to touch and displays of affection. Older people may be more likely to express their sexuality in these more diffuse and varied terms (Boyer & Boyer, 1982; Huntley, 1989).

The sexual partners of those who have confirmed HIV antibody tests are themselves at risk for developing AIDS. Education to prevent disease transmission in the facility may become important (O'Conner & Stilwell, 1989).

Impotence, or the inability to perform sexually, is more often attributed to the male. The extent of this disorder in old age is not known, but an early American Medical Association report revealed that, rather than organic problems, anxiety and internalization of societal pressures account for most of the problems related to impotence (Breschi, 1983; Evans et al., 2000; Kay & Neeley, 1982). Nursing homes are often perceived as disapproving and actively discouraging of displays of love or affection among residents. A frequent suggestion in the literature is that nursing home staff be educated concerning sexuality in old age and that more efforts be made to deal with problems of morality that may arise.

Stillwell and O'Conner (1989) attempt to dispel some of the myths concerning sexuality with the observation that

1. older people do remain interested in sex
2. older people find each other physically attractive
3. sexuality contributes to overall well-being

Contrary to public perceptions, the incidence of a heart attack or stroke during sexual intercourse is actually very low, and sexual activity is sometimes recommended for patients with diseases such as arthritis because of the therapeutic effects of exercise and intimacy (Huntley, 1989).

One research study suggests allowing for privacy of some residents to develop closer relationships (Kay & Neeley, 1982). Another encourages the development of programs to deal with quality-of-life issues such as loneliness and isolation that are important to residents. Sexual expression would be only one component of this effort (Huntley, 1989; B. Kahana, 1995).

5.3.10 Emotional and Mental Well-Being

A number of the physical system disruptions already discussed can have profound effects on the mental well-being of the nursing home resident.

EFFECTS OF AGING

There are differences of opinion about whether intelligence declines with age. One difficulty is the use of tests that may not be appropriate measures for older individuals (Botwinick, 1978).

Aging is associated with special problems that may not be as disruptive for younger individuals. Burnside (1981) identifies two of these as behavioral problems and mental illness. The range of behaviors residents employ to cope with these problems will vary, but studies often show that many of the recurrent problems in a nursing home are related to behavioral problems (Stotsky, 1973).

As discussed next, when residents are admitted to the facility, they may display initial symptoms of anxiety and apprehension regarding their new surroundings (Trella, 1994) (discussed below). Chronic illness and the process of dying are anxiety-provoking and necessarily are an aspect of life with which nursing home residents must constantly cope.

Anxiety may be experienced by most individuals, and each deals with it in a particular way. Some manifestations of anxiety include fantasizing, hostile or dependent behavior, avoidance of eye contact, fidgeting, insomnia, and isolation from other.

INSOMNIA

Insomnia, or sleep disorder, is common among older individuals. Studies of human sleep patterns have shown that older persons spend more time in bed, have more difficulty getting to sleep, or tend to awaken during sleep periods (Busse & Pfeiffer, 1973; Dement, Miles, & Bliwise, 1982).

Sleep problems may result from the use of multiple medications as well as from anxiety. To assist the residents in coping, sleeping medications may be prescribed, along with increases in daily activities and attempts to alleviate the source of anxiety.

LONELINESS

Behaviors associated with loneliness are similar to those of a mild depressive mood and include isolation, constipation, weight loss, insomnia, fatigue, and loss of appetite. Depression is often associated with losses, some of which are depicted in Figure 5-13.

Treatment for these residents is to discern the cause of depression and try to help them cope effectively with those feelings (Aller & Van Ess Coeling 1995; Moore & Gilbert, 1995, p 7). If these behaviors persist and worsen, the resident may be progressing toward mental illness. Antidepressive medications may also be prescribed in these cases (see Ade-Ridder & Kaplan, 1993; Engle & Graney, 1993).

LOSSES	→ ADJUSTMENTS →	GAINS
Familiar Surroundings—"home" whatever it was.	Adapt to new room, roommate(s)	An environment adapted to their needs
Loss of family contacts or caregiver contact pattern	Accept new caregivers as new "family"	Personnel available 24 hours, who try to care
Loss of contact pattern with friends	Reduced contact, especially if frail	New friends one's own age and condition
Loss of control over one's life, including		Expert caregivers who take over this function
meal timing choice of snacks	Accept the facility food choices	Predictable meals, snacks, 24 hours.

Range of decision making losses
   Independence,
   e.g., eat or not,
   take medicines or not
	Accept physician's nearly total control over diet, activities	An array of concerned staff, assisting decision making

Personalization
   Losses in clothing,
   life style, timing,
   activities or daily
   living
	Conformity to time schedule, food choices, daily schedule	Not much—An intense struggle to repersonalize oneself in a potentially depersonalizing institutional environment

FIGURE 5-13. Losses, adjustments, and gains of patient admitted to long-term care.

MENTAL ILLNESS

Some studies have revealed that about 10% of older citizens have severe mental illness (Palmore, 1973), and the incidence of mental illness tends to increase as people age (Butler & Lewis, 1977). It is estimated that the rate of mental illness in nursing homes is somewhere between one fourth and one half of all residents. This high prevalence of mental illness may be a result of preexisting problems (Birren, 1964).

The term *senile* often is used to describe a variety of behaviors in mental illness, ranging from slight forgetfulness to a generalized decline in mental functioning of older persons. Butler and Lewis (1977) describe two different groups of older persons suffering from mental illness as (a) those with a history of mental illness and (b) those who develop mental illness for the first time later in life.

Those with a history of mental illness often have been transferred to the nursing home from a psychiatric facility, a phenomenon brought about by the development of psychotropic drugs in the 1950s and 1960s. This population may also be suffering from mental retardation (E. Kahana, 1995a).

Psychotrophic drugs are those that exert an effect on the mind. They are usually used to calm and control patient behavior. Equipped with these new medications and a belief that persons with mental illness are better cared for in the community setting, most states dramatically reduced the number of persons held in state psychiatric hospitals. It is believed that a significant portion of persons who were deinstitutionalized during this movement have entered the nursing home as a substitute for the psychiatric hospital. As time passes, and the states continue to lower the number of hospital beds available for those with mental illness, this phenomenon is likely to continue (Mosher-Ashley & Henrikson, 1993).

PSYCHOACTIVE DRUG RATES

The percentage of residents receiving psychoactive drugs is rising (see Figure 5-14). By 1999 half of all residents were on psychoactive medications. Such drugs include antidepressants, antianxiety drugs, sedatives and hypnotics, and antipsychotics. There has been pressure from the federal government for facilities to use fewer psychoactive drugs while at the same time encouraging facilities to diagnose and get prescriptions for more antidepressant drugs.

The second group of patients with mental illness often become emotionally disturbed because they are no longer able to cope with the physical and social changes associated with the aging process (Miller, 1994).

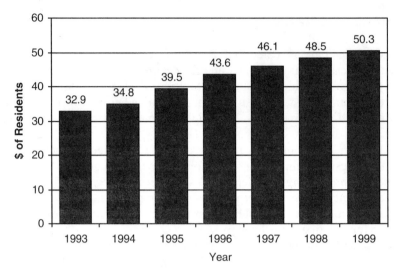

FIGURE 5-14. Residents in U.S. nursing facilities receiving psychoactive medications, 1993–1999.

Who is mentally ill? What is mental illness? These are difficult questions in the setting of the nursing facility (Haight, 1995; Scott, Bramble, & Goodyear, 1991). The changes brought about by chronic physical illnesses and by the "normal" social changes faced by older persons are sometimes powerful enough to overwhelm even a well-adjusted person. The line between disabling mental illnesses and the day-to-day effects of attempting to cope with aging, especially in the institutionalized setting of the nursing facility, is often blurred.

ORGANIC BRAIN SYNDROME

Organic brain syndrome, brain failure, and *senility* are all different words describing the same disorder (Burnside, 1981; Golden & Cohen, 1995; Gwyther, 1995). (Dementia and Alzheimer's disease have already been discussed as problems of the nervous system.)

The two most common causes of organic brain syndrome are Alzheimer's disease and cerebrovascular insufficiency, or reduced blood flow to the brain. The brain tissue responds to any impairments resulting from these disorders with a variety of **symptoms** that initially can involve memory loss, leading to levels of disorientation and confusion and to difficulty following even simple directions. These symptoms of confusion progress until the resident is no longer aware of reality (Blustein, 1993; Emanuel & Emanuel, 1992).

Affected residents may engage in such problematic behaviors as suicidal threats or attempts, destructiveness, hostility, nosiness, and wandering off (Busse & Pfeiffer, 1973; Rantz & McShane, 1995, p 23). These behaviors can become especially troublesome in the group setting of a nursing home. Psychiatric consultation is usually desirable in these instances.

Treatment can include

- reality orientation (continually reminding residents of the date, time and place to keep the oriented to their environment) (Maddox, 2001)
- choosing compatible roommates and company for these residents
- avoiding sudden changes or surprises
- increasing the amount of assistance available to these residents to perform the activities of daily living (Fillenbaum, 1995)
- providing a supportive environment

The most disoriented patients are typically those with advanced dementia (Baldwin, 1995). Results of a study of Rhode Island facilities showed that about 26% of nursing home residents studied were disruptive at least once in two weeks, for example, physical abuse, screaming, wandering (Maddox, 2001; National Center for Health Services, 1989).

RESTRAINTS

The restraint issue is one of the most debated in the nursing home industry (Strumpf & Evans, 1995). Restraints are variously defined. In essence, a restraint is anything that restricts a resident/patient beyond their will (Maddox, 2001). Restraints may be physical, like a vest or a gerichair that keeps the resident/patient from getting out of the chair; or mental such as the use of psychotropic drugs to control anxiety or agitation. Some nursing chains have achieved a restraint-free environment in groups of facilities after consciously mounting a program (Technical Assistance Series, 1995).

The use of restraints, particularly physical restraints, is one of the thorniest issues in long-term care. Cogent arguments for and against them can be marshaled (Brooke, 1991–1992; Burger, 1994; Aller & Coeling, 1995; Johnson, 1995; Magee, Hyatt, Hardin, Stratmann, Vinson & Owen, 1993; Menscher, 1993; Moss & Puma, 1991; Scherer, Janelli, Kanski, Neary, & Morth, 1991; Stolley et al., 1993; Watzke & Wister, 1993; Werner, Cohen-Mansfield, Koroknay & Braun, 1994). Reducing chemical restraints has also been of concern (Burger, 1992) and is a source of contention.

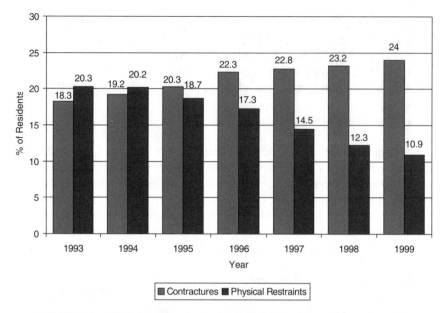

FIGURE 5-15. Percentage of U.S. residents in nursing homes with contractures and physical restraints, 1993–1999.
Nursing Facilities, Staffing, Residents and Facility Deficiencies, 1993–1999, Department of Social & Behavioral Sciences, University of California San Francisco.

Restraint use is now closely regulated, with monthly reviews and justifications mandated under nursing home reform requirements. Many facilities have moved toward a restraint-free environment, because in the their view restraints kill the human spirit.

Figure 5-15 reveals an increase in the number of contractures identified among residents during the years 1993 to 1999. Restraint use, however, has decreased 50% over these same years, from 20% in 1993 to 10% in 1999. In 1999, 11% of facilities were cited for improper use of restraints (Harrington et al., 2000). The pressure on facilities to become restraint free seems clear when one considers that in 1999, 11% of facilities were still restraining residents and 11% of facilities were receiving deficiencies for improper use of restraints (Harrington et al., 2000).

DEPRESSION

Depression is probably the most common mental illness in older persons (Blazer, 1995; M. Blumenthal, 1980; Tueth, 1995). Residents must be assessed to determine whether they are merely in a depressed mood or if the disease has progressed to a mental illness (Kane et al., 1989; Lazar

& Karasu, 1980). Often depression may be associated with another underlying chronic disease (e.g., arthritis or Parkinson's disease) or may be a result of a reaction to medications (M. Blumenthal, 1980; Lazar & Karasu, 1980). Busse and Pfeiffer (1973) also implicate depression as a symptom or precursor of other chronic diseases.

Additional **signs** of depression include loss of appetite resulting in weight loss, feelings of sadness, loss of interest in people, and a sense of needing great effort to perform daily activities (M. Blumenthal, 1980). Older individuals may also complain of symptoms that are actually attributable to depression. Often the real problem is loss of control over their daily lives and a lack of decision-making opportunities (Everard, Rowles, & High, 1994).

Treatment of depression can include the use of antidepressant medications, usually tricyclic antidepressant drugs or newer ones such as Prozac and Paxil ("Listening," 1995). These drugs themselves, however also have strong side effects (Kane et al., 1989).

Electrocortical shock treatment (ECT) is a powerful form of treatment used to stimulate a specified area of the brain. M. Blumenthal (1980) suggests that ECT may be safer than drug therapy. However, use of electroshock treatments for depression and other mental disorders has been a subject of intense controversy for decades (Kane et al., 1989).

Counseling, group activities and social functions appear to be productive therapeutic techniques available to the nursing home staff (Busse & Pfeiffer, 1973; Shore, 1978).

In essence, efforts by the staff to restore a sense of worth and importance to the resident may be among the most powerful tools available. Some of these include daily exercise, such as aerobics geared to the resident's level of physical capacity, dance therapy, recreation therapy, work therapy, and bibliotherapy (reading books) (Kane et al., 1989; Kennie & Warshaw, 1989; Maddox, 2001; Osgood, 1995; Waldo, Ide & Thomas, 1995).

Observations on a Career in Nursing Home Administration

FIX IT (THE FACILITY) ALL THE TIME

Nobel laureate Albert Szent-Gyorgyi observed that there is a tendency for all living things to keep growing, changing, evolving (Kriegel, 1991).

Everything around us is constantly changing: the health system, the economic system, the aging population itself, and its relationship to everything else. The relationships among hospitals, nursing homes, assisted living facilities, life-care communities, home health agencies, third-party payers, health maintenance organizations, managed care processes, and government regulations are always in flux. If the nursing facility does not change and grow, improve and evolve, it will face extinction. The nursing facility is a living organism. Treat it as alive, and you and it will survive.

Fix It (Your Own Career) All the Time

In the unlikely event that you feel yourself on a plateau at some point in your career in nursing home administration, having achieved all you had hoped in your facility, consider the following.

An aboriginal tribe made it a practice to move on whenever the food was plentiful because of lush harvests. When life was this easy they knew they were in danger of becoming fat, lazy, and unprepared for the inevitable seasons of scarcity when their survival skills would be necessary.

Finished Never Is

The Japanese concept of *kaizen* means continuous improvement, a commitment to the idea that "finished never is."

David Harrington, a violinist with the avant-garde Kronos Quartet, finds being an artist a source of perpetual renewal because it is a task that has no ending point (Kriegel, 1991).

The cellist Pablo Casals was asked why, at the age of 94, he continued to practice as hard each day as he had decades earlier, since he remained clearly the preeminent cellist in the world. He replied that he practiced because he hoped to improve.

REFERENCES: PART FIVE

Adams, G. (1981). *Essentials of geriatric medicine* (2nd ed.). Oxford, England: Oxford University Press.

Ade-Ridder, L., & Kaplan, L. (1993). Marriage, spousal care giving, and a husband's move to a nursing home. *Journal of Gerontological Nursing, 19*(10), 13–23.

Agate, J. (1979). *Geriatrics for nurses and social workers* (2nd ed.). London: Heinemann.

Agency for Health Care Policy and Research. (1995, March-April). Guidelines on pressure sores released. *Research Activities p. 15.* (Agency for Health Care Policy and Research, No. 183, AHCPR Pub. No. 95–0051).

Albanese, A. A. (1980). *Nutrition for the elderly.* New York: Liss.

Albert, M. (1995). Alzheimer's disease: Clinical. In G. L. Maddox (Ed.), *The encyclopedia of aging* (2nd. ed., pp. 56–57). New York: Springer.

Allen, J. E. (2000). Federal requirements and guidelines to surveyors (4th ed., Appendix A). New York: Springer.

Aller, L. J., & Van Ess Coeling, H. (1995). Quality of life: Its meaning to the long-term care resident. *Journal of Gerontological Nursing, 21*(2), 20–25.

American Medical Association. (1967). *The extended care facility: A handbook for the medical society.* Chicago: Author.

Anderson, W. F. (1976). *Practical management of the elderly* (3rd ed.). Oxford, England: Blackwell.

Andres, R. (1989). Relation of physiologic changing in aging to medical changes of disease in the aged. In W. Reichel (Ed.), *Clinical aspects of aging* (3rd ed.). Baltimore: Williams & Wilkins.

Baldwin, B. A. (1995). Disruptive behaviors. In G. L. Maddox (Ed.), *The encyclopedia of aging* (2nd ed., pp. 284–286). New York: Springer.

Balin, A. K., & Lin, A. N. (1995). Connective tissues. In G. L. Maddox (Ed.), *The encyclopedia of aging* (2nd ed., pp. 220–222). New York: Springer.

Barzel, U. S. (1989). Endocrinology and aging. In W. Reichel (Ed.), *Clinical aspects of aging* (3rd ed.). Baltimore: Williams & Wilkins.

Barzel, U. S. (1995). Osteoporosis. In G. L. Maddox (Ed.), *The encyclopedia of aging* (2nd ed., pp. 722–723). New York: Springer.

Barzel, V. (1983). Common metabolic disorders of the skeleton. In W. Reichel (Ed.), *Clinical aspects of aging* (2nd ed., pp.). Baltimore: Williams & Wilkins.

Basen, M. (1977). The elderly and drugs: Problem overview and program strategy. *Public Health Reports, 92*(1),43–48.

Bazzare, T. (1983). Nutritional requirements of the elderly. In McCue (Ed.), *Medical care of the elderly: A practical approach.* Lexington, MA: Callamore.

Beacham, B. E. (1989). Geriatric dermatology. In W. Reichel (Ed.), *Clinical aspects of aging* (3rd ed., pp.). Baltimore: Williams & Wilkins.

Beattie, B. L., & Louie, V. Y. (1989). Nutrition and health in the elderly. In W. Reichel (Ed.), *Clinical aspects of aging* (3rd ed., pp. 207–228). Baltimore: Williams & Wilkins.

Beck, S., & Smith, J. (1983). Infectious diseases in the elderly. *Medical Clinics of North America, 67,* 273–289.

Beck-Sague, C., Banerjee, S., & Jarvis, W. R. (1993). Infectious diseases and mortality among U.S. nursing home residents. *American Journal of Public Health, 83,* 1739–1742.

Becker, L. (1979). Herpes zoster: A geriatric disease. *Geriatrics, 34*(9), 41–47.

Bennett, D. A., & Knopman, D. S. (1994). Alzheimer's disease: A comprehensive approach to patient management. *Geriatrics, 49*(8), 20–26.

Bergstrom, N. (1995). Pressure ulcers. In G. L. Maddox (Ed.), *The encyclopedia of aging* (2nd ed., pp. 751–752). New York: Springer.

Best drugs for hypertension. (1995). *Johns Hopkins Medical Letter, 7*(4), 1.

Birchenall, J. M., & Streight, M. E. (1982). *Care of the older adults* (2nd ed.). Philadelphia: Lippincott.

Birren, J. (1964). *The psychology of aging.* Englewood Cliffs, NJ: Prentice-Hall.

Bjork, D., & Tight, R. (1983). Nursing home hazard of chronic indwelling urinary catheters. *Archives of Internal Medicine, 143,* 1675–1676.

Blazer, D. G. (1995). Depression. In G. L. Maddox (Ed.), *The encyclopedia of aging* (2nd ed., pp. 265–266). New York: Springer.

Blumenthal, H. T. (1968). Some biomedical aspects of aging. *Gerontologist, 8,* 34.

Blumenthal, M. (1980). Depressive illness in old age: Getting behind the mark. *Geriatrics, 35*(4), 34–43.

Blustein, J. (1993). The family in medical decision making. *Hastings Center Report, 23*(3), 6–13.

Botwinick, C. (1978). *Aging and behavior: A comprehensive integration of research findings.* New York: Springer.

Boyer, G., & Boyer, J. (1982). Sexuality and the elderly. *Nursing Clinics of North America, 17,* 421–427.

Breschi, L. (1989). Common lower urinary tract problems in the elderly. In W. Reichel (Ed.), *Clinical aspects of aging* (3rd ed., pp. 264–278). Baltimore: Williams & Wilkins.

Brody, H. (1995a). Central nervous system (brain and spinal cord). In G. L. Maddox (Ed.), *The encyclopedia of aging* (2nd ed., pp. 166–171). New York: Springer.

Brody, H. (1995b). Nerves. In G. L. Maddox (Ed.), *The encyclopedia of aging* (2nd ed., pp. 674–675). New York: Springer.

Brooke, V. (1991–1992, Winter). Meeting the challenge: Involuntary restraints in the nursing home. *Journal of Long Term Care Administration,* pp. 9–14.

Bruns, H. J. (1995). Gastrointestinal system. In G. L. Maddox (Ed.), *The encyclopedia of aging* (2nd ed., pp. 390–392). New York: Springer.

Bryant, J., & Tuttle, K. (1989). Setting up top facility policies and procedures. *Provider, 15*(12), 13–14.

Burger, S. G. (1992, Summer). Eliminating inappropriate use of chemical restraints. *Journal of Long Term Care Administration,* pp. 31–35.

Burger, S. G. (1994). Avoiding physical restraint use: New standards in care. In *Long Term Care Advances, 5*(2), 1–9. (Duke University Center for the Study of Aging and Human Development).

Burnside, I. (Ed.). (1981). *Nursing and the aged.* New York: McGraw-Hill.

Busse, E., & Pfeiffer, E. (1973). *Mental illness in later life.* Washington, DC: American Psychological Association.

Butler, R., & Lewis, M. (1977). *Aging and mental health.* St. Louis, MO: Mosby.

Butler, W. (1975). Psychology and the elderly: An overview. *American Journal of Psychiatry, 132,* 893–900.

Carter, D., & Balin, A. (1983). Dermatological aspects of aging. *Medical Clinics of North America, 67,* 531–534.

Chui, H. (1995a). Cerebrovascular disease. In G. L. Maddox (Ed.), *The encyclopedia of aging* (2nd ed., pp. 171–172). New York: Springer.

Chui, H. (1995b). Vascular dementia. In G. L. Maddox (Ed.), *The encyclopedia of aging* (2nd ed., pp. 173–174). New York: Springer.

Cohan, S. L. (1989). Neurologic diseases in the elderly. In W. Reichel (Ed.), *Clinical aspects of aging* (3rd ed., pp. 163–174). Baltimore: Williams & Wilkins.

Cohen, F. L. (1995a). Survival. In G. L. Maddox (Ed.), *The encyclopedia of aging* (2nd ed., p. 50). New York: Springer.

Cohen, F. L. (1995b). Tuberculosis. In G. L. Maddox (Ed.), *The encyclopedia of aging* (2nd ed., pp. 945–947). New York: Springer.

Cohen, H. J. (1995). Blood. In G. L. Maddox (Ed.), *The encyclopedia of aging* (2nd ed., pp. 121–123). New York: Springer.

Cooper, J. (1978). Drug therapy in the elderly: Is it all it could be? *American Pharmacist, 18*(7), 25–33.

Corso, J. (1981). *Aging: Sensory systems and perception.* New York: Praeger.

Crow. (1984). *Pharmacology for the elderly.* New York: Teachers College Press.

Delague, J., Guay, D., Straub, K., & Luxemberg, M. G. (1995). Effectiveness of oral antibiotic treatment in nursing home-acquired pneumonia. *Journal of the American Geriatrics Society, 43,* 245–251.

Dement, W., Miles, L., & Bliwise, D. (1982, April). Physiological markers of aging: Human sleep patterns. In Reff and Schneider (Eds.), *Biological markers of aging* (pp. 177–187). Washington, DC: U.S. Department of Health and Human Services, National Institutes of Health, Public Health Service.

deVries, H. A. (1989a). Physiological effects of an exercise training regimen upon men aged 52 to 88. In W. Reichel (Ed.), *Clinical aspects of aging* (3rd ed., p. 89). Baltimore: Williams & Wilkins.

deVries, H. A. (1989b). Physiology of physical conditioning for the elderly. In W. Reichel (Ed.), *Clinical aspects of aging* (3rd ed., p. 90). Baltimore: Williams & Wilkins.

deVries, H. A. (1989c). Vigor regained. In W. Reichel (Ed.), *Clinical aspects of aging* (3rd ed., p. 90). Baltimore: Williams & Wilkins.

Emanuel, E. J., & Emanuel, L. L. (1992). Proxy decision making for incompetent patients. *Journal of the American Medical Association, 267,* 2067–2071.

Engel, B. T. (1995). Incontinence. In G. L. Maddox (Ed.), *The encyclopedia of aging* (2nd ed., pp. 501–502). New York: Springer.

Engel, V. F., & Graney, M. J. (1993). Stability and improvement of health after nursing home admission. *Journal of Gerontology, 48*(1), (Social Sciences section, pp. S17–S23).

Everad, K., Rowles, G. D., & High, D. (1994). Nursing home room changes: Toward a decision-making model. *Gerontologist, 34,* 520–527.

Evans, J. G., Williams, T. F., Beattie, B. L., Michel, J.-P., & Wilcock, G. K. (2000). *Oxford textbook of geriatric medicine* (2nd ed.). New York: Oxford University Press.

Farber, B., Brennen, C., Punteri, A., & Brody, J. (1982). Nosocomial infections in a chronic care facility. *Journal of the American Geriatric Society, 32,* 513–519.

Faubert, P. F., Shapiro, W. B., Porush, J. G., & Kahn, A. I. (1989). Medical renal disease in the aged. In W. Reichel (Ed.), *Clinical aspects of aging* (3rd ed., pp. 228–247). Baltimore: Williams & Wilkins.

Feinstein, E., & Friedman, E. (1979). Renal disease in the elderly. In I. Rossman (Ed.), *Clinical geriatrics* (2nd ed.). Philadelphia: Lippincott.

Felser, J., & Raff, M. (1983). Infectious diseases and aging. *Journal of the American Geriatrics Society, 13,* 802–806.

Fillenbaum, G. G. (1995). Activities of daily living. In G. L. Maddox (Ed.), *The encyclopedia of aging* (2nd ed., pp. 7–9). New York: Springer.

Finch, C., & Hayflick, L. (1977). *Handbook of the biology of aging.* New York: Van Nostrand Reinhold.

Foley, C. (1981). Nutrition and the elderly. In L. Libow (Ed.), *The core of geriatric medicine: A guide for students and practitioners.* St. Louis, MO: Mosby.

Franz, M. (1981, Summer). Nutritional requirements of the elderly. *Journal of Nutrition for the Elderly, 1.*

Franz, R. A., & Gardner, S. (1994, September). Clinical concerns: Management of dry skin. *Journal of Gerontological Nursing,* pp. 15–18.

Fraumeni, J. (1979). Epidemiological studies of cancer. In Griffen and Shaw (Eds.), *Carcinogens: Identification and mechanism of action* (p. 61). New York: Raven.

Freedman, M. (1982). Anemias in the elderly: Physiological or pathological? *Hospital Practice, 17*(5), 121–136.

Gambert, S. R. (1983). A clinician's guide to the physiology of aging. *Wisconsin Medical Journal, 82*(8), 13–15.

Garagusi, V. F. (1989). Infectious disease problems in the elderly. In W. Reichel (Ed.), *Clinical aspects of aging* (3rd ed., p. 204). Baltimore: Williams & Wilkins.

Garibaldi, R., Brodine, S., & Matsumiya, S. (1981). Infections among patients in nursing homes. *New England Journal of Medicine, 305,* 731–735.

Gibbons, J. C., & Levy, S. M. (1989). Gastrointestinal diseases in the aged. In W. Reichel (Ed.), *Clinical aspects of aging* (3rd ed., p. 197). Baltimore: Williams & Wilkins.

Glowacki, G. A. (1989). Geriatric gynecology. In W. Reichel (Ed.), *Clinical aspects of aging* (3rd ed.). Baltimore: Williams & Wilkins.

Golden, C. J. (1995). Atherosclerosis. In G. L. Maddox (Ed.), *The encyclopedia of aging* (2nd ed., pp. 90–91). New York: Springer.

Golden, C. J., & Cohen, D. I. (1995). Organic brain syndrome. In G. L. Maddox (Ed.), *The encyclopedia of aging* (2nd ed., pp. 686–687). New York: Springer.

Goldfarb, A. (1979). Geriatric gynecology. In I. Rossman (Ed.), *Clinical geriatrics* (2nd ed., p. 336). Philadelphia: Lippincott.

Goldrick, B. A., & Larson, E. (1992). Assessing the need for infection control programs: A diagnostic approach. *Journal of Long Term Care Administration, 20*(1), 20–23.

Gordon, J. C. (1989). Musculoskeletal injuries in the elderly. In W. Reichel (Ed.), *Clinical aspects of aging* (3rd ed.). Baltimore: Williams & Wilkins.

Gotz, B., & Gotz, V. (1978). Drugs and the elderly. *American Journal of Nursing, 78,* 1347–1350.

Griggs, W. (1978). Sex and the elderly. *American Journal of Nursing, 78,* 1352–1354.

Grob, D. (1989). Common disorders of muscles in the aged. In W. Reichel (Ed.), *Clinical aspects of aging* (3rd ed., pp. 314–330). Baltimore: Williams & Wilkins.

Groenwald, S. (1980). Physiology of the immune system. *Journal of the Heart and Lung, 9,* 645–650.

Gwyther, L. (1983). Alzheimer's disease. *North Carolina Medical Journal, 44,* 435–436.

Gwyther, L. P. (1995). Alzheimer's disease: Special care units. In G. L. Maddox (Ed.), *The encyclopedia of aging* (2nd ed., pp. 60–62). New York: Springer.

Gwyther, L., & Matteson, M. A. (1983). Care for the caregivers. *Journal of Gerontological Nursing, 9*(2), 93.

Haight, B. K. (1995). Suicide risk in frail elderly people relocated to nursing homes. *Geriatric Nursing, 16,* 104–107.

Halter, J. B. (1995). Carbohydrates. In G. L. Maddox (Ed.), *The encyclopedia of aging* (2nd ed., pp. 131–133). New York: Springer.

Harrington, C. H., Carrillo, M. S., Thollaug, S. C., Summers, P. R., & Wellin, V. (2000). *Nursing facilities, staffing, residents, and facility deficiencies, 1993 through 1999.* University of California at San Francisco, Department of Social & Behavioral Sciences.

Harris, R. (1989). Exercise and physical fitness for the elderly. In W. Reichel (Ed.), *Clinical aspects of aging* (3rd ed., pp. 90–91). Baltimore: Williams & Wilkins.

Hayflick, L. (1965). The limited in vitro lifetime of human diploid cell strains. *Experimental Cell Research, 37,* 614–636.

Hayflick, L. (1995). Biological aging theories. In G. L. Maddox (Ed.), *The encyclopedia of aging* (2nd ed., pp. 113–118). New York: Springer.

Heaney, R. (April, 1982). Age-related bone loss. In Reff and Schneider (Eds.), *Biological markers of aging.* Washington, DC: U.S. Department of Health and Human Services, National Institutes of Health, Public Health Service.

Hefti, F. (1995). Neurotrophic factors and aging. In G. L. Maddox (Ed.), *The encyclopedia of aging* (2nd ed., pp. 686–687). New York: Springer.

Heidrick, M. L. (1995). Autoimmunity. In G. L. Maddox (Ed.), *The encyclopedia of aging* (2nd ed., pp. 99–100). New York: Springer.

Hing, E. (1977). *Characteristics of nursing home residents' health status and care received* (NCHS Series 13, No. 51). Washington, DC: U.S. Public Health Service.

Hofland, B. F. (1995). Autonomy and aging. In G. L. Maddox (Ed.), *The encyclopedia of aging* (2nd ed., pp. 100–101). New York: Springer.

Huntley, R. R. (1989). Common complaints of the elderly. In W. Reichel (Ed.), *Clinical aspects of aging* (3rd ed., pp. 61–64). Baltimore: Williams & Wilkins.

Husain, T. (1953). An experimental study of some pressure effects on tissues with reference to the bed sore problem. *Journal of Pathology and Bacteriology, 66,* 347.

Irvine, P., Van Buren, N., & Crossley, K. (1984). Causes for hospitalization of nursing home residents: The role of infection. *Journal of the American Geriatrics Society, 32,* 103–107.

Janelli, L. M., Kanski, G. W., & Neary, M. A. (19__, June). Physical restraints: Has OBRA made a difference? *Journal of Gerontological Nursing,* pp. 17–21.

Johnson, S. H. (1995, Fall). Law and quality in long-term care. *Journal of Long Term Care Administration,* pp. 75–77.

Jokl, E. (1989). Abstract, XII International Congress of Gerontology, Hamburg, July 12–17. In W. Reichel (Ed.), *Clinical aspects of aging* (3rd ed., pp. 41–43). Baltimore: Williams & Wilkins.

Jones, J. K. (1989). Drugs and the elderly. In W. Reichel (Ed.), *Clinical aspects of aging* (3rd ed., pp. 50–60). Baltimore: Williams & Wilkins.

Kahana, B. (1995). Isolation. In G. L. Maddox (Ed.), *The encyclopedia of aging* (2nd ed., pp. 526–527). New York: Springer.

Kahana, E. (1995a). Deinstitutionalization. In G. L. Maddox (Ed.), *The encyclopedia of aging* (2nd ed., p. 254–256). New York: Springer.

Kahana, E. (1995b). Institutionalization. In G. L. Maddox (Ed.), *The encyclopedia of aging* (2nd ed., pp. 510–513). New York: Springer.

Kane, R. L., Ouslander, J. G., & Abrass, I. B. (1989). *Essentials of clinical geriatrics* (2nd ed.). New York: McGraw-Hill.

Karcher, K. A. (1993, March). Is your risk management program designed to deal with Alzheimer's disease? *Nursing Homes,* pp. 34–36.

Kart, C., Metress, E., & Metress, J. (1978). *Aging and health: Biological and social perspectives.* Menlo Park, CA: Addison Wesley.

Kasper, R. L. (1989). Eye problems of the aged. In W. Reichel (Ed.), *Clinical aspects of aging* (3rd ed., p. 448). Baltimore: Williams & Wilkins.

Kaszniak, A. W. (1995). Parkinson's disease. In G. L. Maddox (Ed.), *The encyclopedia of aging* (2nd ed., pp. 727–729). New York: Springer.

Kay, B., & Neeley, J. (1982). Sexuality and aging: A review of current literature. *Sexuality and Disability, 5*(1), 38–46.

Keegan, G., & McNichols, D. (1982). The evaluation and treatment of urinary incontinence in the elderly. *Surgical Clinics of North America, 62,* 261–269.

Keeping active with oxygen therapy. (1994, December). *The Johns Hopkins Medical Letter, 6*(10), 52.

Kenney, R. (1982). *Physiology of aging: A synopsis.* Chicago: Year Book Medical.

Kennie, D. S., & Warshaw, G. (1989). Health maintenance and health screening in the elderly. In W. Reichel (Ed.), *Clinical aspects of aging* (3rd ed., p. 24).

Baltimore: Williams & Wilkins.

Kippenbrock, T., & Soja, M. E. (1993). Preventing falls in the elderly: Interviewing patients who have fallen. *Geriatric Nursing, 14,* 205–209.

Kleiger, R. (1976). Cardiovascular disorders. In Steinberg (Ed.), *Cowdry's: The care of the geriatric patient* (5th ed.). St. Louis, MO: Mosby.

Kligman, A. (1979). Perspectives and problems in cutaneous gerontology. *Journal of Investigative Dermatology, 73*(1), 39–46.

Kraus, H. (1977). Preservation of physical fitness. In R. Harris & L. J. Frankel (Eds.), *Guide to fitness after 50* (p. 35). New York: Plenum.

Kravitz, S. C. (1989). Anemia in the elderly. In W. Reichel (Ed.), *Clinical aspects of aging* (3rd ed., pp. 412–421). Baltimore: Williams & Wilkins.

Kriegel, R. J. (1991). *If it ain't broke, break it.* New York: Warner Brothers Books.

Kurtz, S. (1982). Urinary tract infection in older persons. *Comprehensive Therapy, 8*(2), 54–58.

Landfield, P. W. (1995). Stress theory of aging. In G. L. Maddox (Ed.), *The encyclopedia of aging* (2nd ed., pp. 903–905). New York: Springer.

Lazar, I., & Karasu, T. (1980). Evaluation and management of depression in the elderly. *Geriatrics, 35*(12), 49.

Leaf, A. (1973). Getting old. *Scientific American, 229*(3).

Lehman, K. Administrator's role in prevention and care of decubitus ulcers. *Journal of Long Term Care Administration, 11*(2), 22.

Leone & Siegenthaler. (1994). In *Alzheimer's disease and associated disorders* (AHCPR Vol. 8, Suppl. 1 (AHCPR Pub. No. 94–0106), pp. S58–S71).

Libow, L. (1981). *The core of geriatric medicine: A guide for students and practitioners.* St. Louis, MO: Mosby.

Lindeman, R. D. (1989). Application of fluid and electrolyte balance principles to the older patient. In W. Reichel (Ed.), *Clinical aspects of aging* (3rd ed., p. 286). Baltimore: Williams & Wilkins.

Listening to depression: The new medicine. (1995). *Johns Hopkins Medical Letter, 6*(11), 4.

Lo, B., & Dornbrand, L. (1986). The case of Claire Conroy: Will administrative review safeguard incompetent patients? *Annals of Internal Medicine, 104,* 869–873.

Logemann, J. A. (1995). Dysphagia. In G. L. Maddox (Ed.), *The encyclopedia of aging* (2nd ed., pp. 297–298). New York: Springer.

Lung cancer is always treatable. (1995). *Johns Hopkins Medical Letter, 7*(6), 1–2.

Lyon, L., & Nevins, M. (1984). Management of hip fracture in nursing home patients: To treat or not to treat? *Journal of the American Geriatrics Society, 32,* 391–395.

MacHudis, M. (1983). In W. Reichel (Ed.), *Clinical aspects of aging: A comprehensive text* (2nd ed.). Baltimore: Williams & Wilkins.

Maddox, G. L. (2001). *The encyclopedia of aging* (3rd. ed.). New York: Springer.

Magee, R. (1993, April). Institutional policy use of restraints in extended care and nursing homes. *Journal of Gerontological Nursing,* pp. 31–39.

Malone-Lee, J. (1995). Genitourinary system. In G. L. Maddox (Ed.), *The encyclopedia of aging* (2nd ed., pp. 400–402). New York: Springer.

McCaddon, A., & Kelly, C. L. (1994). Familial Alzheimer's disease and vitamin B12 deficiency. *Age and Aging, 23,* 334–337.

McLachlan, M. (1978). The aging kidney. *Lancet, 2,* 43.

Medvedev, Z. A. (1995). Wear-and-tear theories. In G. L. Maddox (Ed.), *The encyclopedia of aging* (2nd ed., pp. 964–965). New York: Springer.

Meites, J., & Quadri, S. K. (1995). Neuroendocrine theory of aging. In G. L. Maddox (Ed.), *The encyclopedia of aging* (2nd ed., pp. 677–681). New York: Springer.

Menscher, D. (1993). Let the people go: Caring for the demented elderly without using restraints. *North Carolina Medical Journal, 54,* 145–150.

Meza, J., Peggs, J., & O'Brien, J. (1984). Constipation in the elderly patient. *Journal of Family Practice, 18,* 695–703.

Miller, R. I. (1994). Managing disruptive responses to bathing by elderly residents. *Journal of Gerontological Nursing, 20*(11), 35–39.

Moore, J. R., & Gilbert, D. A. (1995). Elderly residents: Perceptions of nurses' comforting touch. *Journal of Gerontological Nursing, 21*(1), 6–13.

Mosher-Ashley, P. E., & Henrikson, N. M. (1993, July-August). Long term care alternatives for the mentally ill. *Nursing Homes,* pp. 34–36.

Moss, A. J. (1989). Diagnosis and management of heart disease in the elderly. In W. Reichel (Ed.), *Clinical aspects of aging* (3rd ed., p. 65). Baltimore: Williams & Wilkins.

Moss, R. J., & La Puma, J. (1991, January-February). The ethics of mechanical restraints. *Hastings Center Report,* pp. 22–24.

National Center for Health Services research and health care technology assessment. (1989, March). *Research activities* no. 115. Rockville, MD: National Center for Health Services.

National Center for Health Services research and health care technology assessment. (September, 1989). *Research activities* no. 121. Rockville, MD: National Center for Health Services.

Nicolle, L., McIntyre, M., Zacharias, H., & MacDonald, J. (1961). Twelve months of surveillance of infections in institutionalized elderly men. *Journal of the American Geriatrics Society, 9,* 654–680.

O'Brien, A. A. J., & Bulpitt, C. J. (1995). Hypertension in the elderly. In G. L. Maddox (Ed.), *The encyclopedia of aging* (2nd ed., pp. 489–491). New York: Springer.

O'Connor, C. E., & Stilwell, E. M. (1989). Sexuality, intimacy and touch in older adults. In W. Reichel (Ed.), *Clinical aspects of aging* (3rd ed., p. 542). Baltimore: Williams & Wilkins.

Office of Long Term Care. (1976, June). *Physician prescribing patterns in skilled nursing facilities* (Long Term Care Facility Improvement Campaign Monograph no. 2). Washington, DC: Author.

Orentreich, D. S. (1995). Skin. In G. L. Maddox (Ed.), *The encyclopedia of aging* (2nd ed., pp. 860–861). New York: Springer.

Osgood, N. J. (1995). Leisure programs. In G. L. Maddox (Ed.), *The encyclopedia of aging* (2nd ed., pp. 546–548). New York: Springer.

Ostfeld, A., & Gibson, D. (Eds.). (1972). *Epidemiology of aging* (NIH Pub. No. 75–7111). Washington, DC: Public Health Service.

Otero, R. B. (1993, May). Current approaches to infection control. *Nursing Homes,* pp. 48–49.

Ouslander, J. G., Schapira, Schnelle, Uman, Fingold, Tuico, & Nigam. (1995). Does eradicating bacteriuria affect the severity of chronic urinary incontinence in nursing home residents? *Annals of Internal Medicine, 122,* 749–754.

Paffenbarger, R. S., Wing, A. L., & Hsieh, C. (1986). Physical activity, all-cause mortality and longevity of college alumni. *New England Journal of Medicine, 314,* 605.

Palmer, M. H., Bennett, Marks, McCormick, & Engel. (1994). Urinary incontinence: A program that works. *Journal of Long Term Care Administration,* pp. 19–25. Palmore, J. (1973). In Busse & Lewis (Eds.), *Mental illness in later life,* pp. . Washington, DC: American Psychological Association.

Pierce, R. I. (1995). Pulmonary system. In G. L. Maddox (Ed.), *The encyclopedia of aging* (2nd ed., pp. 783–786). New York: Springer.

Poe, W., & Holloway, D. (1980). *Drugs and the aged.* New York: McGraw-Hill.

Pousada, L. (1995). Hip fracture. In G. L. Maddox (Ed.), *The encyclopedia of aging* (2nd ed., pp. 456–457). New York: Springer.

Putting an end to dizziness. (1994). *Johns Hopkins Medical Letter, 6*(9), 4–5.

Rantz, M. J., & McShane, R. E. (1995). Nursing interventions for chronically confused nursing home residents. *Geriatric Nursing, 16*(1), 22–27.

Ray, W. A. (1993). Reducing antipsychotic drug use in nursing homes. *Archives of Internal Medicine, 153,* 713–720.

Redford, J. B. (1989). Rehabilitation and the aged. In W. Reichel (Ed.), *Clinical aspects of aging* (3rd ed., pp. 177–186). Baltimore: Williams & Wilkins.

Reichel, W. (Ed.). (1983). *Clinical aspects of aging: A comprehensive text* (2nd ed.). Baltimore: Williams & Wilkins.

Reichel, W., & Rabins, E. V. (1989). Evaluation and management of the confused, disoriented or demented elderly patient. In W. Reichel (Ed.), *Clinical aspects of aging* (3rd ed., pp. 137–153). Baltimore: Williams & Wilkins.

Reisberg, B. (1995). Senile dementia. In G. L. Maddox (Ed.), *The encyclopedia of aging* (2nd ed., pp. 837–847). New York: Springer.

Rimer, B. K. (1995). Cancer control and aging. In G. L. Maddox (Ed.), *The encyclopedia of aging* (2nd ed., pp. 130–131). New York: Springer.

Ripich, D. N., Wykle, M., & Niles, S. (1995). Alzheimer's disease caregivers: The focused program. *Geriatric Nursing, 16*(1), 15–19.

Roberts, J., & Snyder, D. L. (1995). Drug interactions. In G. L. Maddox (Ed.), *The encyclopedia of aging* (2nd ed., pp. 289–291). New York: Springer.

Rodman, M., & Smith, D. (1977). *Clinical pharmacology in nursing.* Philadelphia: Lippincott.

Rodstein, E. (1983). Falls by the aged. In I. Rossman (Ed.), *Fundamentals of geriatric medicine.* New York: Raven.

Rosendorff, C. (1983). *Clinical cardiovascular and pulmonary physiology.* New York: Raven.

Rossman, I. (Ed.). (1979). *Clinical geriatrics* (2nd ed.). Philadelphia: Lippincott.

Rowe, J. (1982). Renal function and aging. In Reff and Schneiderb (Eds.), *Biological markers of aging.* Washington, DC: U.S. Department of Health and Human Services, National Institutes of Health, Public Health Service.

Rowe, J., & Besdine, R. (1982). *Health and disease in old age.* Boston: Little, Brown.

Rubin, P. (1981). Management of hypertension in the elderly. In F. Ebaugh (Ed.), *Management of common problems in geriatric medicine,* p. 309. Menlo Park, CA: Addison Wesley.

Satterfield, N. (1989). New regulations bring changes to facilities. *Provider, 15*(12), 10–11.

Scherer, Y. K. (1991). The nursing dilemma of restraints. *Journal of Gerontological Nursing, 17*(2), 14–17.

Schneck, M. (1982). An overview of current concepts of Alzheimer's disease. *Psychiatry, 139*(2).

Schnelle, J. F., Ouslander, J. G., Simmons, Alessi, & Gravel. (1993). The nighttime environment, incontinence care and sleep disruption in nursing homes. *Journal of the American Geriatrics Society, 41,* 910–914.

Scott, R. R., Bramble, K. J., & Goodyear, N. (1991). How knowledge and labeling of dementia affect nurses' expectations. *Journal of Gerontological Nursing, 17*(1), 21–24.

Segal, J., Thompson, J., & Floyd, R. (1979). Drug utilization and prescribing patterns in a skilled nursing facility: The need for a rational approach to therapeutics. *Journal of the American Geriatric Society, 27,* 117–122.

Selma, T. P., Palla, K., Padding, B., & Brauner, D. J. (1994). Effect of OBRA 1987 on antipsychotic prescribing in nursing home residents. *Journal of the American Geriatrics Society, 42,* 648–652.

Sengstaken, E. A., & King, S. A. (1993). The problems of pain and its detection among geriatric nursing home residents. *Journal of the American Geriatrics Society, 41,* 541–544.

Shashaty, G. G. (1989). Thromboembolism in the elderly. In W. Reichel (Ed.), *Clinical aspects of aging* (3rd ed., p. 101). Baltimore: Williams & Wilkins.

Shore, H. (1978). Group programs in long-term care facilities. In Burnside (Ed.), *Working with the elderly: Group process and techniques.* North Scituate, MA: Duxbury.

Sinclair, A. J. (1995). Diabetes mellitus. In G. L. Maddox (Ed.), *The encyclopedia of aging* (2nd ed., pp. 274–276). New York: Springer.

Sinex, M. F. (1977). The molecular genetics of aging. In C. Finch & L. Hayflick (Eds.), *Handbook of the biology of aging*. New York: Van Nostrand Reinhold.

Sklar. (1983). Gastrointestinal diseases in the aged. In W. Reichel (Ed.), *Clinical aspects of aging: A comprehensive text* (2nd ed., p. 206). Baltimore: Williams & Wilkins.

Smith, P. W. (1989). Making infection control an art. *Provider, 15*(12), 7–9.

Smith, W. (1982). Infections in the elderly. *Hospital Practice, 17,* 69–85.

Snowden, J. (1983). Sex in nursing homes. *The Australian Nurse's Journal, 12*(8), 55–56.

Spencer, H. (1979). The skeletal system. In I. Rossman (Ed.), *Clinical geriatrics* (2nd ed., p. 296). Philadelphia: Lippincott.

Starr, I. (1964). An essay on the strength of the heart. *American Journal of Cardiology, 14,* 771–783.

Steffl, B. (Ed.). (1984). *Handbook of gerontological nursing*. New York: Van Nostrand Reinhold.

Sterritt, P. F., & Pokorny, M. E. (1994). Art activities for patients with Alzheimer's and related disorders. *Geriatric Nursing, 15,* 155–159.

Stillwell, E., & O'Conner, C. (1989). Sexuality, intimacy, and touch. In W. Reichel (Ed.), *Clinical aspects of aging* (2nd ed., p. 542). Baltimore: Williams & Wilkins.

Stolley, J. M. (1993). Developing a restraint use policy for acute care. *Journal of Nursing, 23*(12), 49–54.

Stopgap benefits of tacrine for Alzheimer's. (1995). *Johns Hopkins Medical Letter, 7*(3), 3.

Stotsky, B. (1973). In E. Busse & E. Pfeiffer (Eds.), *Mental illness in later life* (p. 172). Washington, DC: American Psychological Association.

Strehler, B. (1962). *Time, cells, and aging*. New York: Academic Press.

Sullivan, R. J. (1995). Cardiovascular system. In G. L. Maddox (Ed.), *The encyclopedia of aging* (2nd ed., pp. 133–138). New York: Springer.

Swanson, E. A., Maas, M. S., & Buckwalter, K. C. (1993). Catastrophic reactions and other behaviors of Alzheimer's residents: Special unit compared with traditional units. *Archives of Psychiatric Nursing, 7,* 292–299.

Talbott, J. (1985). Clinical and policy issues. *Bulletin of the New York Academy of Medicine, 61,* 445.

Technical Assistance Services. (1995, March, April). Washington, DC: National Citizens Coalition for Nursing Home Reform.

Teuth, M. J. (1995). How to manage depression and psychosis in Alzheimer's disease. *Geriatrics, 50*(1), 43–49.

Tideiksaar, R. (1995). Falls. In G. L. Maddox (Ed.), *The encyclopedia of aging* (2nd ed., pp. 359–361). New York: Springer.

Tindall, J., & Smith, J. (1963). Skin lesions of the aged. *Journal of the American Medical Association, 186,* 1037–1040.

Tonna, E. A. (1995). Collagen. In G. L. Maddox (Ed.), *The encyclopedia of aging* (2nd ed., pp. 146–147). New York: Springer.

Trella, R. (1994). From hospital to nursing home: Bridging the gaps in care. *Geriatric Nursing, 15*(6), 313–316.

Tuberculosis. (1995). *Johns Hopkins Medical Letter, 7*(9), 8.

Vallarino & Sherman. (1981). Stroke, hip fractures, amputations, pressure sores, and incontinence. In L. Libow (Ed.), *The core of geriatric medicine: A guide for students and practitioners.* St. Louis, MO: Mosby.

Van Vliet, L. (1995a). Aphasia. In G. L. Maddox (Ed.), *The encyclopedia of aging* (2nd ed., pp. 75–76). New York: Springer.

Van Vliet, L. (1995b). Communication disorders. In G. L. Maddox (Ed.), *The encyclopedia of aging* (2nd ed., pp. 198–200). New York: Springer.

Waldo, M. J., Ide, B. A., & Thomas, D. P. (1995, February). Postcardiac-event elderly: Effect of exercise on cardiopulmonary function. *Journal of Gerontological Nursing,* pp. 12–19.

Wallace, M. (1992). Management of sexual relationships among elderly residents of long-term care facilities. *Geriatric Nursing,* 308–322.

Wasow, M., & Loeb, M. (1979). Sexuality in nursing homes. *Journal of the American Geriatrics Society, 27,* 73–79.

Watzke, J. R., & Wister, A. V. (1993, November). Staff attitudes: Monitoring technology in long-term care. *Journal of Gerontological Nursing,* pp. 23–29.

Weg, P. (1983). Changing physiology of aging. In D. Woodruff & J. Biren (Eds.), *Aging: Scientific perspectives and social issues* (2nd ed., p. 270). Monterey, CA: Brooks-Cole.

Weindruch, R. (1995). Diet restriction. In G. L. Maddox (Ed.), *The encyclopedia of aging* (2nd ed., pp. 276–279). New York: Springer.

Weksler, E. (1981). The senescence of the immune system. *Hospital Practice, 16,* 53–58.

Williams, M., & Fitzhugh, C. (1982). Urinary incontinence in the elderly. *Annals of Internal Medicine, 97,* 895–907.

Woodruff, D., & Birren, J. (1975). *Aging—scientific perspectives and social issues.* New York: Van Nostrand.

Yoder, M. G. (1989). Geriatric ear nose and throat problems. In W. Reichel (Ed.), *Clinical aspects of aging* (3rd ed., p. 457). Baltimore: Williams & Wilkins.

Zinn, J. S., & Mor, V. (1994). Nursing home special care units: Distribution by type, state, and facility characteristics. *Geriatrics, 34,* 371–376.

Index